Blockchain for Healthcare 4.0

Blockchain is a type of distributed ledger technology that consists of a growing list of records that are securely linked together using cryptography and numerous applications in every field, including healthcare. *Blockchain for Healthcare 4.0: Technology, Challenges, and Applications* presents an overview of the recent advances in blockchain technology which have led to new breakthroughs in the healthcare industry, the application of artificial intelligence (AI) with blockchain, challenges, and prospects.

Key Features

- Highlights blockchain applications in the biomedical and pharmaceutical industries and remote healthcare.
- Discusses applications and advancement in blockchain framework to track diseases and outbreaks.
- Elaborates the role of blockchain in managing health records, tracing, and securing medical supplies.
- Focuses on efficient and secure medical data sharing through blockchain and secure cloud-based electronic health record (EHR), a system using an attribute-based cryptosystem.
- Presents techniques and methods to utilize blockchain technology for clinical studies and facilitates the transition to patient-driven interoperability.

The text is primarily written for graduate students and academic researchers in the fields of computer science and engineering, biomedical engineering, electrical engineering, and information technology.

Blockchain for Healthcare 4.0
Technology, Challenges, and Applications

Edited by Rishabha Malviya and Sonali Sundram

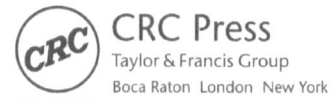

CRC Press is an imprint of the
Taylor & Francis Group, an **informa** business

A CHAPMAN & HALL BOOK

Designed cover image: Shutterstock

First edition published 2024
by CRC Press
2385 NW Executive Center Drive, Suite 320, Boca Raton FL 33431

and by CRC Press
4 Park Square, Milton Park, Abingdon, Oxon, OX14 4RN

CRC Press is an imprint of Taylor & Francis Group, LLC

© 2024 selection and editorial matter, Rishabha Malviya and Sonali Sundram; individual chapters, the contributors

Reasonable efforts have been made to publish reliable data and information, but the author and publisher cannot assume responsibility for the validity of all materials or the consequences of their use. The authors and publishers have attempted to trace the copyright holders of all material reproduced in this publication and apologize to copyright holders if permission to publish in this form has not been obtained. If any copyright material has not been acknowledged please write and let us know so we may rectify in any future reprint.

Except as permitted under U.S. Copyright Law, no part of this book may be reprinted, reproduced, transmitted, or utilized in any form by any electronic, mechanical, or other means, now known or hereafter invented, including photocopying, microfilming, and recording, or in any information storage or retrieval system, without written permission from the publishers.

For permission to photocopy or use material electronically from this work, access www.copyright.com or contact the Copyright Clearance Center, Inc. (CCC), 222 Rosewood Drive, Danvers, MA 01923, 978–750–8400. For works that are not available on CCC please contact mpkbookspermissions@tandf.co.uk

Trademark notice: Product or corporate names may be trademarks or registered trademarks and are used only for identification and explanation without intent to infringe.

ISBN: 978-1-032-52486-3 (hbk)
ISBN: 978-1-032-52758-1 (pbk)
ISBN: 978-1-003-40824-6 (ebk)

DOI: 10.1201/9781003408246

Typeset in Palatino
by Apex CoVantage, LLC

Dear healthcare professionals,

We are dedicating this book to you. Our love for profession shall live forever.

This book is also dedicated to friendship of editors. We work together and edited a fruitful book.

Contents

Foreword xix
Preface xxi
Editors xxiii
List of Contributors xxv

1 **Blockchain: A Digital Breakthrough in Healthcare** 1
  Anu Sayal, Janhvi Jha, and Chaithra N
  1.1 Introduction 1
  1.2 Applications 2
       1.2.1 Medical Records Management 2
       1.2.2 Supply Chain Management and Drug Traceability 4
       1.2.3 Telemedicine and Remote Patient Monitoring 6
       1.2.4 Clinical Trials and Research 7
       1.2.5 Medical Device Management 8
       1.2.6 Billing and Insurance 10
       1.2.7 Genomics 11
       1.2.8 Dental Industry 12
       1.2.9 Organ Transplant Management 14
  1.3 Advantages 14
  1.4 Challenges and Solutions 16
       1.4.1 Data Sharing and Interoperability 17
       1.4.2 Applying Blockchain Technology to Pre-Existing Hospital Infrastructure 18
       1.4.3 Scalability and Speed 18
       1.4.4 Security and Disclosure of Confidentiality 19
       1.4.5 Lack of Proficiency among Medical Professionals 19
       1.4.6 Lack of Legislation 20
  1.5 User Response and Acceptance 20
  1.6 Conclusion 21

2 **Application of Blockchain in Medical Industry** 26
  Naru Venkata Pavan Saish, Vijayashree J., and Jayashree J.
  2.1 Introduction 26
  2.2 Use of Blockchain in Medical and Pharmaceuticals 28
  2.3 Diseases and Outbreaks 30
  2.4 Analyzing Records 35
       2.4.1 Secure Data Sharing 36
       2.4.2 Real-Time Data Analysis 37
       2.4.3 Improved Patient Privacy and Security 37
       2.4.4 Reduced Costs 38
       2.4.5 Algorithm to Store Data in a Blockchain Way 38
  2.5 Building a Blockchain Network 39

	2.6	Scaling Blockchain Network	42
		2.6.1 Data Integrity and Usage	43
	2.7	Conclusion	44

3 Blockchain: A Decentralized, Persistent, Immutable, Consensus, and Irrevocable System in Healthcare 48
Dipa K. Israni and Mansi K. Shah

3.1	Introduction		48
3.2	Type of Blockchains		49
	3.2.1	Un-Permissioned or Public Blockchains	49
	3.2.2	Permissioned or Private Blockchains	49
	3.2.3	Hybrid Blockchain	50
	3.2.4	Consortium or Federated Blockchain	50
3.3	Advantages of Utilizing Blockchain Technology in Healthcare		50
	3.3.1	Immutability and Data Integrity	50
	3.3.2	Decentralized Technology	51
	3.3.3	Enhanced Speed and Efficiency	51
	3.3.4	Transparency	51
	3.3.5	Scalable and Dispersed	51
	3.3.6	Security and Privacy	51
	3.3.7	Distributed Ledgers	51
	3.3.8	Consensus	51
	3.3.9	Open Source	51
	3.3.10	Anonymity	51
	3.3.11	Uniqueness and Ownership	52
	3.3.12	Provenance	52
	3.3.13	Smart Contracting	52
3.4	Blockchain Technologies		52
	3.4.1	Ethereum	52
	3.4.2	Smart Contract	52
	3.4.3	Solidity	52
	3.4.4	Express.js	53
	3.4.5	Ganache	53
	3.4.6	React	53
	3.4.7	MetaMask	53
3.5	Blockchain Technology Components		53
	3.5.1	Data Block	53
	3.5.2	Distributed Ledger	53
	3.5.3	Consensus Algorithm	53
3.6	Working of Blockchain		54
3.7	Blockchain Structure		55
	3.7.1	Module for Data Source	55
	3.7.2	Transaction Module	55
	3.7.3	Module for Block Creation	55
	3.7.4	Consensus Module	56
	3.7.5	Module for Connection and Interface	56
3.8	Applications of Blockchain in Healthcare		56
	3.8.1	Patient Consent Management	56
	3.8.2	Remote Treatment Traceability	57
	3.8.3	Remote Monitoring IOT Security	57

	3.8.4	Managing and Maintaining Patients' Health Records 58
	3.8.5	Managing the Supply Chain 59
	3.8.6	In-Home Medical Gadgets and Kits for Patient Monitoring 59
	3.8.7	Access to Private Health Data in a Secure Manner 59
	3.8.8	Payments on Automatic Basis 59
	3.8.9	Dependable Supervision of Elderly Patients 60
	3.8.10	Traceability of Medication Distribution and Pharmacy Fill-Ups 60
	3.8.11	Trustworthy Health Insurance Services 61
	3.8.12	Reputation-Aware Specialist Referral Services 61
	3.8.13	Automated Patient Follow-Up Service 61
	3.8.14	Pharmaceutical Research and Development 62
	3.8.15	Medical Staff Credential Verification 62
	3.8.16	Supply Chain Transparency 62
	3.8.17	Tracking Clinical Trials and Pharmaceuticals 62
	3.8.18	Disease Surveillance at the Community Level 63
	3.8.19	Treatment Optimization 64
	3.8.20	Doctor Management 64
3.9	Barriers in Leveraging Blockchain Technology in Healthcare 65
	3.9.1	Regulation, Both Internal and External 65
	3.9.2	Challenges in Medical Care Information Transfer and Lack of Interoperability 65
	3.9.3	Interoperability Assistance for Cross-Platform Transactions 66
	3.9.4	Challenges to Blockchain Adoption in Institutions 66
	3.9.5	Difficulties in Ensuring Data Confidentiality and Privacy 66
	3.9.6	Safety Susceptibilities of Smart Contracts 66
	3.9.7	Data Ownership 67
	3.9.8	Patient Data Overload 67
3.10	Conclusion 67

4 Application of Blockchain in Tracking Diseases and Outbreaks 72
Phool Chandra, Zeeshan Ali, Neetu Sachan, Vaibhav Rastogi, Mayur Porwal, and Anurag Verma

4.1	Introduction 72
4.2	Healthcare 74
4.3	Blockchain Technology's Capabilities in Healthcare 75
4.4	Functions for Storing and Tracking Information about Infectious Diseases 77
	4.4.1 At Hospital Level 81
	4.4.2 Resource Management in Health Systems 81
	4.4.3 Patient-Level Applications 82
	4.4.4 Disease Surveillance at the Community Level 82
	4.4.5 In the Early Detection and Surveillance of Infectious Diseases 84
	4.4.6 Utilizing Blockchain Technology to Streamline the Reporting, Establishing a Distributed Procedure for Infectious Diseases 84
4.5	Blockchain Technology in the Pharmaceutical Industry 85
	4.5.1 Counterfeit Prevention 86
	4.5.2 Product Distribution 86
	4.5.3 Tracking and Tracing 87
	4.5.4 Safety and Security 87
4.6	Conclusion 87

5 Building Efficient Smart Contract for Healthcare 4.0 94
Kanika Agrawal and Mayank Aggarwal
- 5.1 Introduction 94
  - 5.1.1 Blockchain Overview 95
  - 5.1.2 Blockchain 95
  - 5.1.3 Blockchain Architecture 96
  - 5.1.4 Blockchain Characteristics 96
  - 5.1.5 Blockchain Consensus Mechanisms 96
- 5.2 Applications of Blockchain System in the Healthcare Domain 97
  - 5.2.1 Biomedical 97
  - 5.2.2 Prediction of Diseases 98
  - 5.2.3 Electronic Health Record (EHR) 100
  - 5.2.4 Genomics 103
  - 5.2.5 Pharmaceuticals 103
- 5.3 Tools for Blockchain Systems 105
  - 5.3.1 Hyperledger Fabric 105
  - 5.3.2 Hyperledger Sawtooth 105
  - 5.3.3 Ethereum 107
  - 5.3.4 InterPlanetary File System (IPFS) 107
  - 5.3.5 Postman 107
  - 5.3.6 Ganache 107
  - 5.3.7 Blockchain Testnet 107
  - 5.3.8 Iroha 107
  - 5.3.9 Geth 108
  - 5.3.10 Hyperledger Composer 108
  - 5.3.11 MATLAB 108
  - 5.3.12 Truffle 108
  - 5.3.13 Wireshark 108
  - 5.3.14 Spyder IDE 109
  - 5.3.15 SPSS 109
- 5.4 Analysis Tools for Blockchain Ethereum Smart Contracts 109
  - 5.4.1 Echidna 109
  - 5.4.2 Eth2Vec 109
  - 5.4.3 Gastap 110
  - 5.4.4 Remix IDE 110
  - 5.4.5 Slither 110
  - 5.4.6 SmartAnvil 110
  - 5.4.7 SmartBugs 110
  - 5.4.8 SmartCheck 110
  - 5.4.9 DefectChecker 111
  - 5.4.10 GasChecker 111
  - 5.4.11 Gasper 111
  - 5.4.12 HoneyBadger 111
  - 5.4.13 MadMax 111
  - 5.4.14 Mythril 111
  - 5.4.15 Oyente 111
  - 5.4.16 Securify 112
  - 5.4.17 Vandal 112
  - 5.4.18 Manticore 112

5.5	Building Smart Contracts		112
	5.5.1	Speed and Accuracy	112
	5.5.2	Transparency and Trust	112
	5.5.3	Security	113
	5.5.4	Savings	113
5.6	Solidity Static Analysis		113
5.7	Research Challenges in Healthcare		116
	5.7.1	Patient Data Management	116
	5.7.2	Clinical Trials	116
	5.7.3	Drug Traceability	116
	5.7.4	Latency	116
	5.7.5	Scalability	117
	5.7.6	Interoperability	117
	5.7.7	Security and Privacy	117
5.8	Conclusion		117

6 Blockchain Technology: Reinventing the Management of Information Infrastructure 124
Shashimala Tiwari

6.1	Introduction		124
6.2	Background		125
	6.2.1	Blockchain Technology	125
	6.2.2	Literature Survey	126
6.3	Medical Data Supervision on Blockchain		127
	6.3.1	Invoking the Transaction	128
	6.3.2	Creation of New Records	129
	6.3.3	Record Validation	129
6.4	Why Is Blockchain Technology Needed in the Healthcare Industry?		129
6.5	Top 10 Blockchain Use Cases in the Healthcare Area		129
	6.5.1	Increasing Access to Medical Records	130
	6.5.2	Preventing Counterfeit Drug	130
	6.5.3	Tracking Medical Staff Credentials	130
	6.5.4	Patient-Centric Electronic Health Record	131
	6.5.5	Smart Contracts for Insurance	131
	6.5.6	Remote Monitoring by IoT Security	131
	6.5.7	Reducing Costs	131
	6.5.8	Tracking Clinical Trials	132
	6.5.9	Enhancing Data Security and Management	132
	6.5.10	Providing Supply Chain Transparency	133
6.6	Blockchain Prevents Medical Errors		133
6.7	Challenges Faced by Blockchain Technology		133
6.8	Associated Work		134
	6.8.1	Theoretical/Analytical Blockchain-Based Research	135
	6.8.2	Prototype/Implementation Blockchain-Based Research	136
6.9	System Implementation		136
6.10	Advanced Contracts		137
6.11	Convention Scenario for Algorithm 1		137
6.12	Conclusion and Future Work		138

7 Potential of Blockchain in Disease Surveillance 141
Mohamed Yousuff, Jayashree J., Vijayashree J., and Anusha R.
- 7.1 Introduction 141
  - 7.1.1 The Three Fundamental Tenants of Blockchain Technology 142
- 7.2 Cryptographically Secure Blockchain-Based Disease Surveillance 143
  - 7.2.1 Contact-Tracking Infrastructure Using Blockchain 144
  - 7.2.2 Blockchain-Based Geosocial Data Sharing and Artificial Intelligence-Based Epidemic Control 145
  - 7.2.3 WeChat GeoAI Blockchain-Based System 146
- 7.3 Safety Measures Monitoring Using IoT 146
  - 7.3.1 Enterprise Network Infrastructure 147
  - 7.3.2 Cloud Computing and Service Provision 148
  - 7.3.3 Superlative Network 148
- 7.4 Disease Surveillance and Control Using AI and Blockchain 149
  - 7.4.1 Data Sharing in Secure Mode Using Blockchain 149
- 7.5 Blockchain-Based Contact Tracing 149
  - 7.5.1 Blockchain with IoMT (Internet of Medical Things) 150
  - 7.5.2 Blockchain in Communicable Diseases Tracking 152
- 7.6 Blockchain in Patient Tracking System 153
  - 7.6.1 Healthcare Blockchain Applications 154
- 7.7 Use of Blockchain and AI 155
- 7.8 Blockchain in Diseases Health Surveillance 155
- 7.9 Disease Management Infrastructure Based on IoT and Blockchain 156
- 7.10 Mobile Health Infrastructure on Blockchain (mHealth) 156
- 7.11 Benefits of Blockchain 157
  - 7.11.1 Challenges on Blockchain 157
- 7.12 Conclusion 158

8 Postmortem Concentrations: Distributed Privacy-Preserving Blockchain Authentication Framework in Cloud Forensics 161
Rohit Kaushik and Eva Kaushik
- 8.1 Introduction 161
- 8.2 Problem Statement 163
- 8.3 Literature Review 163
- 8.4 Background of Related Work 164
- 8.5 Methodology 165
  - 8.5.1 Modules 166
- 8.6 Key Terminologies 167
- 8.7 Cloud Forensics Challenges 168
  - 8.7.1 Technical 168
  - 8.7.2 Procedural 169
  - 8.7.3 Custody Forensic 170
- 8.8 Concepts in Cloud Forensics 171
  - 8.8.1 Kind of Crime 171
  - 8.8.2 Conducting Investigations 171
  - 8.8.3 Performing Investigation on Cloud 172
- 8.9 Cloud Security 172
  - 8.9.1 Cloud Architecture 172
  - 8.9.2 Cloud Security Attacks 173

8.10		The Necessity of Digital Forensics	174
8.11		Case Studies	175
	8.11.1	Traditional Forensics vs. Cloud Forensics	177
8.12		Way Forward/Solutions	178
	8.12.1	Traditional	178
	8.12.2	Blockchain-Based	179
8.13		Future Scope	180
8.14		Conclusion	180
8.15		Discussion	181

9 Blockchain in Tracing and Securing Medical Supplies ... 185
Tamanna Rai, Rishabha Malviya, Niranjan Kaushik, and Pramod Kumar Sharma

9.1	Introduction	185
9.2	Background	186
	9.2.1 Blockchain Technology in Brief	186
9.3	The Blockchain Technology	186
9.4	Blockchain's Benefits: Blockchain Technology's Advantages Make It Suited for Medical Record Management	187
9.5	Blockchain Networks	187
	9.5.1 Public Blockchain	187
	9.5.2 Permissioned Blockchain	187
	9.5.3 Consortium Blockchain	188
9.6	Blockchain's Verification Procedure	188
	9.6.1 Practical Byzantine Fault Tolerance (PBFT)	188
	9.6.2 Proof-of-Stake (PoS)	188
	9.6.3 Proof-of-Work (PoW)	188
9.7	Insights into Blockchain-Based Tracking Methods	189
	9.7.1 The Aims of Drug Traceability	189
9.8	The Need for Blockchain in Medication Traceability Is Described by the Issues That Follow Conventional Techniques of Tracking Drugs	189
	9.8.1 Consenting to Regulations	189
	9.8.2 Cold Chain Shipping	190
9.9	Using Blockchain Technology to Track Pharmaceuticals	190
	9.9.1 Hyperledger Besu Architecture	190
	9.9.2 Hyperledger Fabric Architecture	190
9.10	Steps Involved during the Transaction in Drug Safety	191
9.11	Proposed Method for Blockchain in Personal Health Records	191
9.12	Applying Blockchain to Healthcare Supply Chains	192
9.13	Blockchain and IoT for Supply Chain	194
9.14	Conclusion	195

10 Leveraging Blockchain in Sharing and Managing Health Record Credential ... 199
Atul B. Kathole, Sonali D. Patil, Vinod V. Kimbahune, and Avinash P. Jadhav

10.1	Introduction	199
10.2	Literature Review	200
	10.2.1 EHR Structures	200

		10.2.2	Blockchain	201
	10.3	Blockchain-Based EHR Systems		202
		10.3.1	Information Storage	203
		10.3.2	Information Sharing	205
		10.3.3	Information Audit	206
		10.3.4	Identity Manager	207
	10.4	Future Movements		207
		10.4.1	Big Information	207
		10.4.2	Machine Learning	208
		10.4.3	Internet of Things (IoT)	208
	10.5	Conclusion		209

11 Healthcare Record Management for Healthcare 4.0 via Blockchain: A Review of Current Applications, Opportunities, Challenges, and Future Potential 211

Shalom Akhai

	11.1	Introduction to Healthcare 4.0: Embracing Digital Transformation in Healthcare		211
		11.1.1	The Progression of Healthcare Delivery: From Industry 1.0 to Healthcare 4.0	211
		11.1.2	Healthcare 4.0: Definition, Characteristics, and Goals	212
		11.1.3	Key Drivers of Healthcare 4.0	213
	11.2	Blockchain Technology and Its Application in Health Record Management		214
		11.2.1	Decentralized Storage	214
		11.2.2	Improved Data Security	214
		11.2.3	Interoperability	215
		11.2.4	Patient Control	215
		11.2.5	Research and Analytics	215
	11.3	BcT Advantages and Challenges in Healthcare Delivery		215
		11.3.1	Benefits	215
		11.3.2	Challenges	216
	11.4	Healthcare Use Cases for Blockchain Technology		216
		11.4.1	Patient-Centered Health Data Management	216
		11.4.2	Clinical Trials and Research	217
		11.4.3	Supply Chain Management	217
		11.4.4	Claims and Payment Processing	217
		11.4.5	Telemedicine	217
	11.5	Legislative and Ethical Concerns Surrounding Blockchain in Healthcare		217
		11.5.1	Data Protection and Privacy	217
		11.5.2	Security and Ownership	218
		11.5.3	Interoperability and Standardization	218
		11.5.4	Regulatory Compliance	218
		11.5.5	Informed Consent	218
	11.6	Obstacles and Future Directions for Blockchain in Healthcare		218
		11.6.1	Interoperability and Standardization	218
		11.6.2	Adoption and Implementation	219
		11.6.3	Cost and Complexity	219
		11.6.4	Regulatory Compliance	219

Contents

	11.6.5 Trust and Security	219
11.7	Conclusions	219
11.8	Research Directions for Blockchain in Healthcare	220

12 Benefits and Roles of Blockchain in Genomics 224
Dablu Kumar

- 12.1 Introduction 224
- 12.2 What Is Genomics? 225
- 12.3 Blockchain Technology and Blockchain-Based System 225
- 12.4 Types of Blockchain 226
  - 12.4.1 Public Blockchain (Open-Access and Permissionless) 226
  - 12.4.2 Private Blockchain (Private and Permissioned) 226
  - 12.4.3 Consortium Blockchain (Public and Permission-Granted) ...226
- 12.5 Why Blockchain in Genomics 227
  - 12.5.1 Genetic Data Security 227
  - 12.5.2 Genomic Data Sharing 228
  - 12.5.3 Electronic Health Record–Sharing System 231
- 12.6 Commercial Scenario of Blockchain 234
- 12.7 Non-Commercial Blockchain Genomic Marketplaces 235
- 12.8 Advantages 237
- 12.9 Future Direction 238
- 12.10 Limitations of Blockchain 239
- 12.11 Conclusions 240

13 Blockchain for Transaction of Large-Scale Clinical Information 245
Anusha R., Jayashree J., Vijayashree J., and Mohamed Yousuff

- 13.1 Introduction 245
  - 13.1.1 How Does Blockchain Work? 246
  - 13.1.2 Consensus 246
- 13.2 Generations of Blockchain 247
  - 13.2.1 Blockchain 1.0 247
  - 13.2.2 Blockchain 2.0 247
  - 13.2.3 Blockchain 3.0 247
  - 13.2.4 Hyperledger Fabric 247
  - 13.2.5 Blockchain X.0 248
- 13.3 A Smart Contracts–Based Blockchain-Based Electronic Medical Health Record 249
  - 13.3.1 Smart Contracts for Phases of Clinical Trials 249
  - 13.3.2 EHR Characteristics 250
  - 13.3.3 FHIRChain: Using Blockchain to Share Clinical Data in a Secure and Scalable Way 250
  - 13.3.4 Clinical Data Sharing Based on Blockchain Requirements ...251
- 13.4 How Blockchain and AI Are Revolutionizing Healthcare Solutions 252
  - 13.4.1 Blockchain Applications in Medical Care 252
  - 13.4.2 AI Applications in Medical Services 252
  - 13.4.3 Drawbacks 252
  - 13.4.4 Clinical Trials 253
  - 13.4.5 Gartner Hype Cycle 253
  - 13.4.6 Evolutions in Technology 254

- 13.5 A Blockchain Future for Secure Clinical Data Sharing 254
  - 13.5.1 Blockchain to Improve the Quality of Clinical Research 255
  - 13.5.2 Sharing Data in Community-Driven Medicine 255
  - 13.5.3 Sharing Key Information on a Blockchain 255
  - 13.5.4 Cloud-Based Methodologies...255
- 13.6 Solutions with Blockchain Technology....................................256
- 13.7 Blockchain to Establish IoT-Based Healthcare..............................256
  - 13.7.1 Useful Features of Blockchain That Can Be Used in e-Health 256
- 13.8 IoT Blockchain-Based e-Healthcare..257
  - 13.8.1 Blockchain to Enable Secure Medical Record Access 257
  - 13.8.2 Assessing Claims and Billings 257
  - 13.8.3 Medicinal Drug Supply Chain Management 257
- 13.9 Challenges and Solutions of Integrating Blockchain in Healthcare................258
  - 13.9.1 Privacy Concerns Over Healthcare Data 258
  - 13.9.2 Blockchain Applied to Secure Clinical Big Data 258
  - 13.9.3 Challenges of Blockchain 259
- 13.10 Conclusion..259

14 Sharing and Interpretation of Genomic Datasets Using Blockchain 262
Mohamed Yousuff, Jayashree J., Vijayashree J., and Anusha R.
- 14.1 Introduction 262
- 14.2 Genomics..263
  - 14.2.1 Challenges in Genomics 264
  - 14.2.2 Applications of Genomics 265
- 14.3 Blockchain 266
- 14.4 Blockchain in Genomics..267
- 14.5 The Genesy Model for a Blockchain-Based Fair Ecosystem of Genomic Data 269
  - 14.5.1 Features, Benefits, and Potential Impact of the Genesy Model...269
- 14.6 Blockchain in Genomics Applications 271
  - 14.6.1 Commercial Genomics Marketplace 271
  - 14.6.2 Non-Commercial Applications 271
- 14.7 Motives for Blockchain Application in Genomics..........................273
- 14.8 Current Problems, Difficulties, and Future Scope 274
- 14.9 Conclusion..275

15 Improved Data Transmission Technique for Healthcare Emergency Vehicle Using Blockchain in VANET..278
R. M. Rajeshwari and S. Rajesh
- 15.1 Introduction 278
- 15.2 Motivation..279
- 15.3 Objectives of the Proposed Work..279
  - 15.3.1 Related Works 280
  - 15.3.2 Proposed Work 281
  - 15.3.3 Algorithms Used 283
- 15.4 Results and Discussion 285
  - 15.4.1 Data Collected per User...285
  - 15.4.2 Message Delivery Ratio 286

		15.4.3	Total Amount of Data Collected	286
		15.4.4	End-to-End Delay	287
		15.4.5	Energy Consumption	287
	15.5	Conclusion		287

16 Blockchain-Based Digital Twin to Predict Heart Attacks 291
Venkatesh Upadrista, Sajid Nazir, and Huaglory Tianfield

	16.1	Introduction		291
	16.2	Literature Review		292
		16.2.1	Abdominal Aortic Aneurysm (AAA)	292
		16.2.2	Occlusive (Ischemic) Heart Disease and Hypertension	293
		16.2.3	Arrhythmia	294
		16.2.4	Heart Failure	295
	16.3	Blockchain-Based Digital Twin Architecture		295
	16.4	Experimental Evaluation		298
		16.4.1	Systems Setup	298
		16.4.2	Prediction Accuracy	299
		16.4.3	Data Analysis and Notifications	299
		16.4.4	Data Visualization	300
	16.5	Discussion		302
	16.6	Conclusion		303

Index 307

Foreword

Blockchain is growing immensely in the field of healthcare. This book states and covers the aspects of blockchain in healthcare and wellness. This book aims to explain and present the ideology and beliefs around blockchain technology and its connection to health preservation, management, and protection. Blockchain has a bright future ahead and many upcoming opportunities, about which the readers will come to know through this book. This book will guide the students and prove to be helpful for those working and studying blockchain in healthcare. The secure supply and tracking of exported medical devices, biomedical applications, use in genomics, and effectively raising smart contracts for healthcare are applications of blockchain in medicine that are thoroughly detailed here.

The book's chapters highlight each component of blockchain applications in healthcare. Along with the benefits and opportunities, the authors have mentioned the challenges so that readers learn about them and try to overcome them in the future.

I am pleased to write a foreword for the book ***Blockchain for Healthcare 4.0: Technology, Challenges, and Applications***, edited by Dr. Rishabha Malviya.

The pattern and manner of sequence and flow in this book are systematic, and information has been given to the point that the content does not become much more complex for the readers to understand and correctly interpret the information.

I appreciate the authors and editors for making great efforts to write and edit this book.

I congratulate Dr. Rishabha Malviya and the authors for their journey and wish them all success.

Best wishes!

Dr. (Prof.) Seifedine Kadry
Professor Noroff University College, Norway FIET, SMIEEE, ACM

Preface

The blockchain is an effectual and high-powered topic procuring a lot of heed latterly. Blockchain is a technology growing ineffably in every sector, including healthcare. It is being used in clinical trials, display of information, and maintenance of health records. The basic rationale behind the involvement of blockchain in healthcare is transparent sharing of information that are linked together. Applications of blockchain are growing wider gradually with time. The recent advances of blockchain in healthcare include its applications in precision medicines, which will revolutionize the strategy and planning of personal treatment. The motive of this book is to lay out and portray the practice, ideology, and beliefs concerning blockchain technology and its link with protection, maintenance, and management of health. Other applications of blockchain in healthcare, such as secure supply and tracking of exported medical device, biomedical applications, use in genomics, and efficiently raising smart contract for healthcare, are well explained here. The chapters in this book foreground each aspect of blockchain application in healthcare separately. It is also being applied to the pharmaceutical industrial scale for the distribution of database, recording of transactions, and providing easy access as well as security to the data. The primary theme of this book is to furnish and enlighten statistics about blockchain technologies, along with further opportunities of the same, although there are still some challenges associated with blockchain technology and its actual implementations in healthcare, which are also addressed here. The readers of this book will get a comprehensive and complete idea about how, when, and where blockchain can have relevance in wellness and healthcare, and as well, they will get a brief idea about futuristic opportunities with regards to blockchain. The suitable and accurate arrangement of chapters, sequencing of headings, and flow pattern of the content make it easy for the readers to interpret information provided inside the book. Considerable endeavor has been made by us to reduce the complexity of the topics so that the information could be served in an uncomplicated manner. Illustrations of figures and given tables make it better to explicate data in a concise manner. The ongoing aspects of developments relating to blockchain in healthcare are included here. This information will be useful to students and researchers as well. We are thankful to the authors for appreciably writing chapters for our book. We are also very thankful to CRC Press, Taylor & Francis Group, for supporting us during the publication process.

Editors

Editors

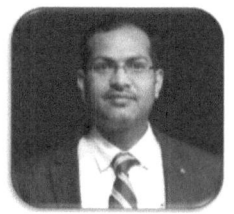

Dr. Rishabha Malviya completed bachelor of pharmacy from Uttar Pradesh Technical University and master of pharmacy (pharmaceutics) from Gautam Buddha Technical University, Lucknow, Uttar Pradesh. His PhD (pharmacy) work was in the area of novel formulation development techniques. He has 12 years of research experience and is presently working as an associate professor in the Department of Pharmacy, School of Medical and Allied Sciences, Galgotias University, doing so for the past 8 years. His area of interest includes formulation optimization, nanoformulation, targeted drug delivery, localized drug delivery, and characterization of natural polymers as pharmaceutical excipients. He has authored more than 200 research/review papers for national/international journals of repute. He has 58 patents (19 grants, 38 published, 1 filed) and publications in reputed national and international journals, with total of 191 cumulative impact factor. He has also received an Outstanding Reviewer award from Elsevier. He has authored/has edited/is editing 50 books (Wiley, CRC Press/Taylor & Francis, Springer, River Publisher, IOP Publishing, and OMICS Publication) and authored 31 book chapters. His name has been included in the world's top 2% scientist list for the years 2020 and 2021 by Elsevier BV and Stanford University. He is a reviewer/editor/editorial board member of more than 50 national and international journals of repute. He has been invited as an author for *Atlas of Science* and *Pharma* magazine, dealing with industry (B2B) *Ingredients South Asia* magazine.

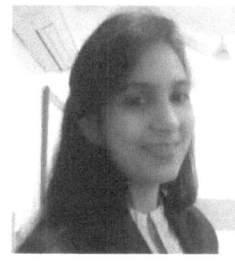

Prof. Sonali Sundram completed bachelor of pharmacy and master of pharmacy (pharmacology) from AKTU, Lucknow. She has worked as a research scientist in a project of ICMR in King George's Medical University, Lucknow. After that, she has joined BBDNIIT. Currently, she is working in Galgotias University, Greater Noida. Her PhD (pharmacy) work was in the area of neurodegeneration and nanoformulation. Her areas of interest are neurodegeneration, clinical research, and artificial intelligence. She has authored/has edited/is editing more than 15 books (Wiley, CRC Press/Taylor & Francis, IOP Publishing, Apple Academic Press/Taylor & Francis, Springer Nature, and River Publisher). She has attended as well as organized more than 15 national and international seminars/conferences/workshops. She has more than eight patents, national and international, in her credit. She has published six SCI indexed manuscripts (cumulative impact factor: 20.71) with reputed international publishers. She has delivered oral presentations in international conferences organized in different European countries.

Contributors

Anu Sayal
School of Accounting and Finance
Taylor's Business School
Taylor's University
Malaysia.

Anurag Verma
Teerthanker Mahaveer University
Moradabad, Uttar Pradesh, India

Anusha R.
School of Computer Science and Engineering
VIT, Vellore Campus
Tamil Nadu, India

Atul B. Kathole
Computer Engineering
Dr. D. Y. Patil Institute of Technology
Pune, India

Avinash P. Jadhav
Computer Science and Engineering
DRGIT and R Amravati, India

Chaithra N
Department of CSE (AI and ML)
JAIN (Deemed-to-be University)
Bangalore, Karnataka, India

Dablu Kumar
Shakuni Choudhary College of Health and Sciences
Tarapur Munger, Bihar, India

Dipa K. Israni
Department of Pharmacology
L. J. Institute of Pharmacy
L. J. University
Ahmedabad, Gujarat, India

Eva Kaushik
Department of Engineering (Information Technology)
Dr. Akhilesh Das Gupta Institute of Technology and Management
Lucknow, Uttar Pradesh, India

Huaglory Tianfield
Department of Computing
Glasgow Caledonian University
Glasgow, Scotland

Janhvi Jha
Department of CSE (AI and ML)
JAIN (Deemed-to-Be University)
Bangalore, Karnataka, India

Jayashree J.
School of Computer Science and Engineering (SCOPE)
Vellore Institute of Technology
Vellore, India

Jayashree J.
School of Computer Science and Engineering
VIT, Vellore Campus
Tamil Nadu, India

Kanika Agrawal
Department of Computer Science and Engineering
Faculty of Engineering and Technology
Gurukula Kangri (Deemed-to-Be University)
Haridwar, India

Mansi K. Shah
Department of Pharmacology
L. J. Institute of Pharmacy
L. J. University
Ahmedabad, Gujarat, India

Mayank Aggarwal
Department of Computer Science and Engineering
Faculty of Engineering and Technology
Gurukula Kangri (Deemed-to-Be University)
Haridwar, India

Mayur Porwal
Teerthanker Mahaveer University
Moradabad, Uttar Pradesh, India

Mohamed Yousuff
Madanapalle Institute of Technology and Science
Andhra Pradesh, India

Naru Venkata Pavan Saish
Computer Science Department Specialized in Data Science
Vellore Institute of Technology
Chennai, Tamil Nadu, India

Neetu Sachan
Maharana Pratap College of Pharmacy, Mandhana
Kanpur, Uttar Pradesh, India

Niranjan Kaushik
Department of Pharmacy
School of Medical and Allied Sciences
Galgotias University, Greater Noida
Gautam Budh Nagar, Uttar Pradesh, India

Phool Chandra
Teerthanker Mahaveer University
Moradabad, Uttar Pradesh, India

Pramod Kumar Sharma
Department of Pharmacy, School of Medical and Allied Sciences
Galgotias University, Greater Noida
Gautam Budh Nagar, Uttar Pradesh, India

R. M. Rajeshwari
Sri Vidya College of Engineering and Technology
Virudhunagar, Tamil Nadu, India

Rishabha Malviya
Department of Pharmacy, School of Medical and Allied Sciences
Galgotias University, Greater Noida
Gautam Budh Nagar, Uttar Pradesh, India

Rohit Kaushik
Department of CS and Mathematics (Data Analytics)
University of Illinois, Springfield

S. Rajesh
Mepco Schlenk Engineering College
Virudhunagar, Tamil Nadu, India

Sajid Nazir
Department of Computing, Glasgow Caledonian University
Glasgow, Scotland

Shalom Akhai
Department of Mechanical Engineering
Chandigarh Engineering College
Jhanjeri, Mohali, India

Shashimala Tiwari
India Health Action Trust
Uttar Pradesh Technical Support Unit
Lucknow, Uttar Pradesh, India

Sonali D. Patil
Information Technology Department
Pimpri Chinchwad College of Engineering
Pune, India

Tamanna Rai
Department of Pharmacy
School of Medical and Allied Sciences
Galgotias University, Greater Noida
Gautam Budh Nagar, Uttar Pradesh, India

Vaibhav Rastogi
Teerthanker Mahaveer University
Moradabad, Uttar Pradesh, India

Venkatesh Upadrista
Department of Computing
Glasgow Caledonian University
Glasgow, Scotland

Vijayashree J.
School of Computer Science and Engineering (SCOPE)
Vellore Institute of Technology
Vellore, India

Vijayashree J.
School of Computer Science and Engineering
VIT, Vellore Campus
Tiruvalam Rd, Katpadi
Vellore, Tamil Nadu, India

Vinod V. Kimbahune
Artificial Intelligence and Data Science
Dr. D. Y. Patil Institute of Technology
Pune, India

Zeeshan Ali
Teerthanker Mahaveer University
Moradabad, Uttar Pradesh, India

1
Blockchain: A Digital Breakthrough in Healthcare

Anu Sayal, Janhvi Jha, and Chaithra N

1.1 Introduction

Blockchain, a 2009-developed distributed ledger system, is a novel form of the decentralized ledger. A blockchain is a decentralized database that logs and verifies transactions conducted over a peer-to-peer network, in which both consumers and criminals participate. All network miners contribute to the maintenance of the distributed ledger by computing encrypted hashes at random locations. As a result of its use of consensus procedures, cryptographic signature, and hash networks in its design, the blockchain database provides highly secure data storage. Blockchain's sophisticated design enables it to store data in a public, decentralized manner while preserving users' anonymity and enabling a vast array of services, including audibility, privacy, and security [1]. Through the use of blockchain technology, consumers can engage in secure, third-party-free interactions. The distributed agreement is utilized to verify transactions in the absence of a central authority. Validators, also known as miners, are employed to accomplish this objective. Consequently, the issue of a digital token being spent twice without independent verification is resolved. The term "blockchain" refers to a distributed ledger that consists of time-stamped, encrypted blocks. Each shareholder, or node, in a peer-to-peer network, has its own pair of public and private keys for encrypting and decrypting communications. This procedure lends blockchains their credibility as immutable and unalterable transaction ledgers.

There are three broad categories for blockchains: consortium (public permission), public permissionless, and private. Public permissionless blockchains, such as Bitcoin and Ethereum, are accessible to anyone and open to the public. Consortium blockchains enable the participation of a finite number of nodes in the distributed agreement process, whether within a single industry or across multiple industries. Private blockchains are managed and maintained by a singular entity, and only a limited number of servers are permitted to join the network. It is also possible to classify blockchains based on whether they are used to track digital assets or to execute smart contracts. Despite its promise, one of the impediments preventing the widespread adoption of blockchain technology in the healthcare industry is its incorporation with existing systems. This requires significant adjustments to the extant infrastructure, including time, money, and personnel. It is possible that blockchain and healthcare systems will never be compatible, necessitating the purchase of potentially expensive new systems [2].

DOI: 10.1201/9781003408246-1

For the healthcare industry to provide quality care to patients, data and personnel are indispensable. Diverse teams with the necessary expertise utilizing cutting-edge technology to achieve the desired outcomes for patients are successful in healthcare operations. Collaboration with educational institutions and research and manufacturing firms is highly advantageous for both the education of personnel and the improvement of knowledge and instruments. Access control, data security, and compatibility are also essential for the successful exchange of information while maintaining the confidentiality of the involved parties. The distributed ledger and immutability of its data are two of blockchain's thrilling features that have the potential to boost confidence in the system and its participants. Increased demand for real-world data, unlawful data sharing, and healthcare system abuses all pose challenges for healthcare organizations, necessitating the exploration of new data administration techniques [3]. Electronic health records, supply chain management, telehealth, clinical studies, medical device management, billing and payments, etc. are just some of the areas on which this chapter provides a summary of the challenges and prospective benefits of implementing this technology. We also discuss the advantages and disadvantages of blockchain technology, including its potential advantages in areas such as security, data veracity, process simplification, and enhancement of healthcare quality. Then, we draw a conclusion regarding blockchain's potential effects on the healthcare industry by analyzing user reaction and acceptance, environmental concerns, and future reach.

1.2 Applications

Multiple applications are utilized in the healthcare industry to improve patient care, streamline administrative tasks, and reduce costs. Examples of such software include electronic health records (EHRs), supply chain management, telemedicine, clinical trials, research, medical device management, and insurance and claims processing. Each of these programs is indispensable to the delivery of professional medical care.

1.2.1 Medical Records Management

Blockchain integration is best for managing health data access, but methods vary. The system could link the scattered systems by storing an index of health records and metadata connected to private data. Boston's MedRec system allows statistical researchers and many healthcare practitioners to obtain data with the patient's consent. The blockchain tracks patient–provider interactions by linking cloud-based medical records with viewing rights and data access guidance. Before being added to a smart contract, a medical record is checked for veracity, and the patient chooses its recipients. The document will never be changed if most network sites oppose it. (Inconvenient and probabilistically unlikely.) Third parties like healthcare providers and insurance companies can use user-generated codes to briefly restrict access [4]. Electronic health record (EHR) systems were initially designed to resolve the inefficiencies of paper-based healthcare data and to provide a more efficient system that would revolutionize the healthcare industry. Electronic health record (EHR) systems have been adopted by numerous medical facilities around the world due to their numerous benefits, most notably increased security and reduced operating costs. They are considered indispensable to the healthcare system because they serve so many

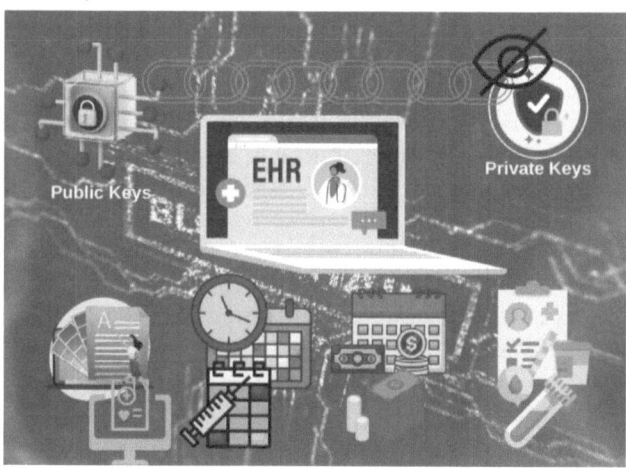

FIGURE 1.1
EHR characteristics and traits.

functions. Functionalities include electronic medical document storage, scheduling of appointments, billing and payment processing, and laboratory analysis. They are present in the vast majority of electronic health record systems currently in use in the medical field. The primary objective is to ensure that patient's medical records are secure, unalterable, and readily transferable between systems. In hospitals and other healthcare facilities, electronic health record (EHR) systems were implemented with the intention of improving patient care, but they ultimately fell short of their objectives. The results of a survey of nursing staff in Finland regarding their experiences with electronic health records (EHR) revealed that the systems had reliability issues and were not user-friendly [5]. Figure 1.1 shows EHR functionality.

Government directives and policies in the United Kingdom and elsewhere have started to be influenced by the possibilities offered by a mainly digitalized healthcare sector, stimulating the creation of new health applications and certification requirements, and leading to improvements in consumer hardware. In spite of this, ambitious plans for the industry's overall transformation have had little impact. The sharing of data between various applications, data sources, and systems, or interoperability, is a significant barrier to the digitalization of healthcare [6]. Patients' health data can be stored on the blockchain network using their public keys, along with their unique identifiers and public keys, and transactions involving these records can also be stored. Healthcare providers can only use smart contracts to obtain de-identified data if the two IDs match. Patients can, if necessary, provide health groups with the public key, but without the private key, the information can never be attributed to a specific individual. Smart contracts are necessary to ensure user consent for the sharing and retrieval of data [7].

Azaria A. et al. detailed the development of a blockchain-based health records system [8]. The register contract (RC), the patient–provider relationship contract (PPR), and the summary contract (SC) are the three legal documents that make up this system. The RC is responsible for translating user-supplied identifiers into Ethereum addresses. This paves the way for the use of pre-existing identification methods, while predefined contract policies can govern the registration of new IDs and the modification of existing mappings. When one network node functions as a medical data repository and manager for another,

PPR is granted between those nodes. The medical professional's records are defined by a set of data references and the rights associated with those references. The SC serves as a "breadcrumb trail" for users to locate their personal health records. It contains a collection of PPR references that reflect the participant's historical and ongoing interactions with other system nodes. The system component was designed to be compatible with existing EMR (electronic medical record) systems. Backend library, Ethereum client, database gatekeeper, and EMR manager are the diverse components of the system. These operations can be performed on remote computers as part of a larger, distributed, unified system. The prototype for these features is a web-based user interface that communicates with an SQLite database. The HealthBank, a global digital health company headquartered in Switzerland, is implementing an innovative, new method for managing data transmissions and the exchange of sensitive medical information. This new business venture offers its consumers a secure location to store their medical records. The user has full control over the dataset. Using blockchain-enabled health applications or smart clothing, patients will soon be able to securely document their own health data (blood pressure, medications consumed, heart rate, sleep patterns, dietary habits, etc.) in the cloud [9].

1.2.2 Supply Chain Management and Drug Traceability

The healthcare supply chain is a complex system that spans organizational and geographical boundaries to provide support for life's most fundamental needs. Due to their inherent complexity and unreliable information sources, impurities, such as erroneous information or a lack of transparency, can be introduced into such systems. The proliferation of counterfeit medications, which has detrimental effects on human health and costs the healthcare system billions of dollars annually, is one consequence of the current supply network constraints. Therefore, prior research has emphasized the importance of a comprehensive tracking and tracing system for the medication supply chain. It is crucial, therefore, to implement a comprehensive method for monitoring pharmaceutical products from the point of manufacture throughout the entire supply chain. Concerns regarding data privacy, accessibility, and legitimacy in healthcare supply networks are exacerbated by the centralization of the majority of current surveillance and tracking systems [10]. These applications take advantage of the blockchain's decentralized database of transaction records and its built-in cryptographic validation of transactions between peers. It is shown by Nakamoto S. that it is exceedingly difficult to alter the records once they have been established as a chain of blocks connected by cryptographic structures (hashes), since the rebuild from the genesis to the most current block transfer would be highly costly [11]. Mohana M. et al. represent one of the earliest initiatives to use blockchain technology to trace the origin of pharmaceuticals [12]. Drug tracking and supply chain management issues and their potential remedies are illustrated in Figure 1.2.

Scientists have done a plethora of in-depth analyses and investigations into the potential of distributed ledgers in the drug supply chain. There are three main steps: learning what makes blockchain technology useful, designing a system to support its use, and launching the system for the first time. Preliminary studies have already shown the advantages, possibilities, and success factors of using blockchain solutions in the pharmaceutical sector. Implementing a system to track the distribution of drugs is challenging yet necessary. Many problems, including data tampering and knowledge obscurity, have been exposed by integrated surveillance systems. The unique properties of blockchain, such as immutability, openness, and security, imply that it may be able to help us address these issues. Potential benefits, process design, and experimental modelling are a few of the aspects of

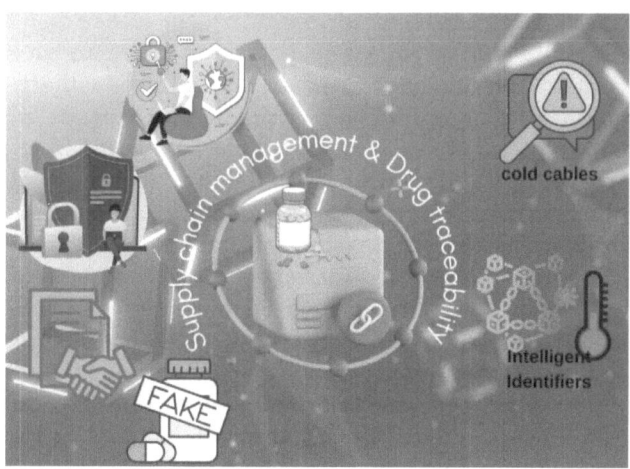

FIGURE 1.2
Issues and potential answers.

blockchain application and development that have been studied. In addition, there are few real-world implementations of blockchain technology for drug trafficking [13].

First, when a novel medical treatment or treatment method is created, an obstruction consisting of copyright protection and a protracted clinical trial procedure is erected. The digital register keeps track of this data as a record of the transaction. After the clinical study is complete, stage 2 will have the idea sent to the manufacturer for prototype testing and, if successful, mass manufacturing. With its digital fingerprint, each item may be linked to a specific record in the decentralized ledger. When pharmaceuticals have been manufactured in large quantities and packaged, they are kept in a warehouse until they are ready to be sent. The time, batch number, identifier, and expiry date are all recorded on the blockchain. Fourth, the blockchain documents the logistics of moving goods from one distribution center (IN) to another, including the time it takes, the means of transportation used, the authorized agent, and any other relevant details. Fifth, the delivery of medicines and medical supplies to pharmacies and shops is often handled by a third-party distribution grid. All delivery nodes are linked to a central storage (referred to as an "OUT") that functions as the gateway for all external parties. Additionally, the database contains a second exchange. Sixth, healthcare services, such as hospitals and clinics, must provide batch numbers, lot numbers, product proprietor, and expiration dates in order to verify and prevent counterfeiting. This information is also contained in the database. In step 7, a store operates similarly to how it was described in step 6. Eighth, the blockchain distribution network provides patients with open, verifiable information that they can use to determine the validity of the entire process [14].

In the pharmaceutical industry, cold cables are prevalent. A "cold chain" is an example of a supply chain in which products must always be maintained within a limited temperature range. There are numerous vulnerable points in the conventional refrigeration chain that can be exploited at any time. Until they are delivered, finalized medications must be stored at the appropriate temperature and relative humidity. During transport, the refrigerated transport lorry must be outfitted to the medication standard. When the product is transferred to a secondary storage location, temperature and humidity regulation are once again required. Traditional refrigerated chains fall short in their monitoring of these crucial areas, making it difficult to determine who was responsible for a deviation. Unbeknownst to consumers, they are compelled to purchase medications regardless of their quality. Integration of blockchain-based smart contracts with the Internet of Things could be the solution. The sections that follow will go into greater detail regarding the cold chain situation that was considered, the proposed blockchain-IoT framework, the development of the proof-of-concept, and a summary of the smart contract [15].

Intelligent identifiers or barcodes may be scanned at each supply chain process node. After this information is entered into a system, a complete audit trace of the drug's distribution network is created and recorded (based on blockchain). These components allow for the tracing of an item to its original source. People may succumb if they do not know the optimal temperature, pressure, and other parameters for storing medications. Perhaps sensors are the solution to this problem. They can be incorporated into the network, with information on pressure, temperature, and other parameters recorded in a distributed database. Together with these instruments, Gangwar, Bali, and Kumar's long short-term memory (LSTM) and support vector machines (SVM) deep learning algorithms are used to create accurate wind speed predictions. This is especially essential for insulin and other medications that must be stored at a calm temperature, as well as for custom-made medications that adhere to general preservation guidelines. If a medication fails to satisfy the established requirements at any point in the supply chain, the pharmacist and patient will be able to trace it back to the location where the parameters were not met. With their knowledge, they can determine whether the medications are from a legitimate manufacturer or whether they were smuggled in. By scanning the barcode or entering the hash code on that portion of the packaging, the user will gain access to additional essential medication instructions [16].

1.2.3 Telemedicine and Remote Patient Monitoring

In light of the present difficulties and global spread of the coronavirus (COVID-19), there is an immediate need for dependable, resilient, and robust patient treatment and medical facilities. Telehealth and telemedicine have benefited from the COVID-19 pandemic because they enable patients to communicate securely with physicians and specialists via digital platforms, thereby reducing the risk of further infection. Utilizing telehealth and online consultations, which facilitate simpler access to medical care, can result in improved care coordination and therapeutic outcomes. Existing telehealth and system dependencies on a central center increase the likelihood of a calamitous failure. Moreover, there are several external and internal data breaches that threaten the data in present videoconferencing and telemedicine systems, which in turn reduce system reliability and accessibility. Blockchain technology's implementation may help with such vital problems. The healthcare industry faces many challenges, many of which can be mitigated with the help of blockchain technology. This includes, but is not limited to, keeping track of the locations that infected patients have visited, protecting remote patient–doctor consultations, tracking medical supplies, validating the source of faulty medical test kits, and validating the credentials of medical professionals. Telemedicine is a low-cost alternative to in-person medical treatment that allows doctors to monitor, diagnose, and treat patients from afar, thereby improving access, expanding healthcare providers' skill sets, and decreasing patients' chances of contracting the influenza A virus subtype 19 (COVID-19). Moreover, telehealth makes use of digital communication technology to aid patients in managing their diseases by giving them access to resources for learning about and dealing with their conditions, as well as improving their ability to care for themselves [17].

Remote patient monitoring applications may benefit from blockchain technology because of its encryption capabilities for data flows between patients and tracking technologies like cloud, fog, and edge computing. To store RPM (remote patient monitoring) e-health records securely, Faruk MJ. et al. propose using Ethereum as a data repository [18]. Patients could rely on the security of their data throughout the upload, storage, analysis, recovery, and transmission processes of the data repository. The proposed distributed ledger technique is advantageous for both inpatients and outpatients. MedHypChain, proposed by Kumar M. et al., is a solution to the cloud computing compatibility issue [19]. Each data exchange in MedHypChain is encrypted using an identity-based broadcast group method to ensure patient privacy. According to Pighini C. et al., SynCare is an insightful, patient-centered private data collection and remote patient monitoring application [20]. Connecting patients, healthcare providers, and caregivers, constructing secure data-sharing networks, and providing patients with control over their own health information were the primary objectives of this study. The distributed ledger's immutability makes it an ideal platform for a system that records and verifies every transaction that occurs within the blockchain. High execution costs, complex integration, and high energy requirements are all disadvantages of the architecture [21].

1.2.4 Clinical Trials and Research

Clinical trials determine whether an experimental technique or new use of a substance is safer for preventing, diagnosing, and treating disease. Prior to using a novel substance in a clinical study, preclinical tests are necessary. All test-tube and animal trials fall under preclinical testing. Drug development study requires complex patient enrolment for clinical trials. According to a recent study, medication development costs $2.6 billion, the majority of which is spent recruiting patients and determining how to retain them in clinical trials; 80% of clinical trials are slowed by delays in patient enrolment, according to a study. Patients, funders, and leading scientists are unable to convene at the same time because these trials involve numerous complex concerns. Insufficient patient recruitment can lead to ineffective results and abrupt trial termination. During patient enrolment, blockchain technology safeguards patient data and privacy. Blockchain-distributed ledgers connect patients who are enrolled in secrecy to clinical study sites, thereby reducing the enrolment time for patients. Thus, the researcher is able to select participants based on the design of the study. The blockchain infrastructure, together with a slew of clinical trial contracts, has been made available for use in recruiting participants and coordinating research. The resistance of potential test subjects is a major roadblock in clinical research. Just 10% of these trials run into problems with patient assent, such as forged permission forms or failure to resubmit consent after protocol changes. By incorporating cryptographic verification into each step, the blockchain was able to track and verify each time-stamped patient assent to the streamlined clinical research design. Normal database characteristics (e.g., unread, shown, approved), indeed a component of the clinical trial beginning process, establish consent for the acquisition of sensitive data. Using blockchain to monitor clinical trials increases confidence in the results and encourages others to participate in clinical research. Transparency in novel drug research can reduce the number of trial sites that report favorable outcomes selectively. Thus, blockchain technology in clinical trials promotes data security, transparency, and collaboration between sponsors and sites [22]. Figure 1.3 depicts the blockchain's potential and proposed methodology for use in clinical trials and research.

There is a great deal of optimism that the pharmaceutical industry's research will be enhanced if they use this technique to manage clinical trial datasets. Blockchain

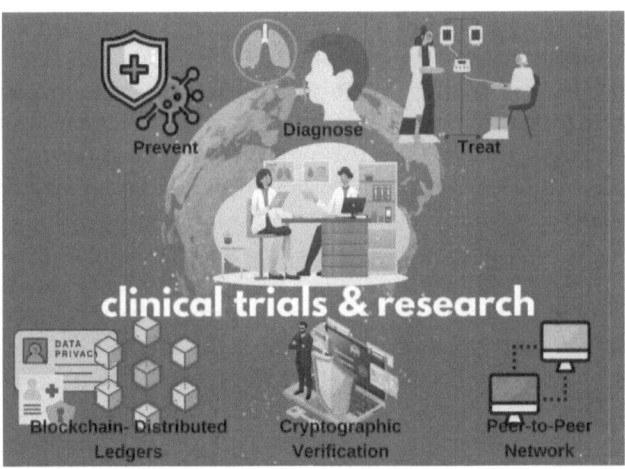

FIGURE 1.3
Goals and suggested methodology for using blockchain in clinical trials.

technology has the potential to improve the administration of clinical studies by regulatory agencies and research organizations, thereby resolving the current issues associated with clinical trials. In addition, it has the potential to improve the technology underlying clinical trial research, thereby enhancing the validity of such studies. Using blockchain technology, a P2P network can be created in clinical trials, enabling the recording of data exchanges, the facilitation of data exchange, and the transparency and irreversibility of trial data. Using the smart contract, which is an autonomous software maintained on the blockchain, these procedures can be automated. It could orchestrate the application's business logic without the need for a third party, guarantee the authenticity of data, generate immutable audit logs, and impose obligations on an action if certain conditions are met. Instantaneously communicate and share medical records with other institutes and institutions using blockchain-based tools. A belief in the immutability of blockchain-stored clinical trial data can result in safer medications and a higher level of confidence in scientific research [23].

1.2.5 Medical Device Management

The Internet of Medical Things (IoMT) is revolutionizing the medical industry by making remote and ubiquitous healthcare services available. Injectors, implantable cardiac, ECGs, and thermometer sensors are only few examples of IoMT devices that are often used to identify and treat a broad range of ailments via automated monitoring of patients' physiological parameters and so reduce the burden on healthcare professionals. It might be challenging to implement fine-grained permissions for diagnostic instruments and various types of users due to the fluid and complex nature of the healthcare ecosystem. It is important to implement fine-grained access control that takes into account factors like the moment during the day, the user's whereabouts, the kind of information being accessed, and the type of user using the device. It's not helped by the fact that there are so many people involved, each with their own agendas and obligations. Essential element authorization, position remote access, and potential access control are not enough to guarantee the security of IoMT devices. Smart contracts, a relatively new breakthrough of blockchain technology, may be utilized to resolve several permission difficulties in healthcare management by enabling detailed user access to clinical data and medical equipment. Metadata like information privacy, privileges, and data security may all be generated as sophisticated depictions of medical information via the use of contracts. Smart contract functions may handle registration and access control based on actors' responsibilities and locations, ensuring that only those with the appropriate permissions can obtain and edit health information. Future research and development into smart contracts is a fascinating field because of the many new healthcare management application scenarios they might enable [24].

In recent years, the quantity of data that must be evaluated within the context of a post-market monitoring (PMS) system for medical devices has skyrocketed. This is due to health authorities' increasingly stringent and complex requirements for evaluating the safety of medical devices. As authorities increase their oversight of device security, proactive PMS procedures are becoming increasingly vital. Some of the challenges caused by this altering regulatory landscape have prompted the exploration of innovative technological solutions. The widespread adoption of the unique device identifier may be facilitated by blockchain technology. Blockchain technology enables the real-time monitoring of manufacturing data as well as usage and maintenance records. The manufacturers of medical devices will benefit from the procedure's dependability and consistency, as it will enable comprehensiveness. As the need for monitoring and auditing increases, this technology is gaining ground [25]. In Table 1.1 a comprehensive view of some existing literature review has been provided.

TABLE 1.1

Comparison of Existing Literature Regarding Medical Equipment Management

Paper Title	Year	Approach	Advantages	Limitations	Citation
A Blockchain Framework for the Management of Medical Equipment in Healthcare	2020	Designed a blockchain-based solution for managing medical equipment that use smart contracts for monitoring equipment health and scheduling regular maintenance	Improved transparency, accountability, and efficiency in equipment management	No real-world implementation or validation was conducted	[26]
Blockchain-Based Asset Management System for Medical Equipment in Hospitals	2020	Presented a blockchain-based solution for hospital equipment management that leverages smart contracts to automate maintenance and calibration of medical devices	Improved equipment maintenance and calibration efficiency, reduced equipment downtime	No real-world implementation or validation was conducted	[27]
A Blockchain-Based Medical Equipment Management System for Enhancing Patient Safety in Healthcare	2021	Developed a blockchain-based system that uses smart contracts to track medical equipment maintenance and usage records, and to monitor equipment performance in real time	Improved patient safety, enhanced equipment maintenance efficiency	No real-world implementation or validation was conducted	[28]

(Continued)

TABLE 1.1 (*Continued*)
Comparison of Existing Literature Regarding Medical Equipment Management

Paper Title	Year	Approach	Advantages	Limitations	Citation
Blockchain Technology for Secure Medical Device Management	2020	The potential applications of blockchain in the medical device business were highlighted, including supply chain management, post-market monitoring, and device tracking	Improved traceability, security, and efficiency in medical device management	No specific framework or implementation was proposed	[29]
A forensics-by-design management framework for medical devices based on blockchain	2019	Provides a blockchain-based framework for the administration of forensics-by-design in medical equipment; framework contains many features to enhance the security and traceability of medical devices, such as encrypted data storage, immutable audit trails, and real-time device operation monitoring	Proposed framework provides security, transparency, traceability; data is tamper-proof and verifiable, audit-proof	No real-world implementation or practical use	[24]

Source: [24], [26], [27], [28], [29].

1.2.6 Billing and Insurance

There are numerous faults in this sector of healthcare funding, the majority of which are associated with a lack of confidence and transparency; however, the implementation of blockchain technology could ameliorate these issues. Integrated into the distributed ledger system, the blockchain is a system of implicit trust that facilitates direct connections between claimants and those responsible for processing those claims. The process of determining premiums is an ideal time to employ smart contracts. Insights into contemporary health, medication use, lifestyle routines, etc. are linked via blockchain to smart contract-based price adjustments. When multiple parties or intermediaries are engaged in the processing of a claim, the ultimate consumer may be subject to repetitive tasks and reviews. As a consequence of these systemic flaws, it has been proposed to implement blockchain technology in the areas of billing claims administration and the broader financial aspects of care delivery [30].

The health insurance claims procedure is one of the most aggravating problems in the healthcare industry. Falsified claims squander both patients' and physicians' time. The claims procedure begins when a consumer requires the services of a healthcare practitioner (such as a doctor or hospital). The supplier determines initial service costs after examining the patient's insurance policy. Before resolving a final service charge, the health insurer will compare the services received from the provider to their joint payment arrangement, taking a number of previously recorded variables into account (such as deductible, co-payment, and coinsurance amounts). The insurance company notifies the practitioner and client of the results. Attempting to calculate a patient's total cost without access to their complete medical history from all their physicians frequently wastes time.

Permissioned blockchain is an attractive solution for resolving the problems of monitoring and openness in a distributed health insurance claim system in which multiple parties exchange information and collaborate. Permissioned blockchains vet potential participants prior to permitting them to participate in the network or conduct transactions, as opposed to public blockchains, which anyone can join without restriction. Blockchain is based on a decentralized, shared database known as a ledger, which consists of a series of interconnected blocks that hold encrypted, time-stamped events. By storing all transactions in a centralized database, insurers will have ready access to aggregated data from multiple sources, allowing them to make policy adjustments on the run. Another essential component of the blockchain, the smart contract is a self-executing piece of software that can be used to execute business logic or legal agreements on the decentralized network. Using SCs, it is possible to automate both insurance policies and access control policies [31].

1.2.7 Genomics

DNA, or deoxyribose nucleic acid, is the foundation of genomics and is used globally for this objective. To examine genomic datasets, substantial and time-consuming computing and sequencing efforts are required [32]. Researchers are becoming more worried about the reliability of genetic data and the speed with which it is collected for use in medication development, virus prevention, disease prediction, better diagnostics, etc. With the platform of Nebula Genomics, data may be easily shared, saved, and accessible as buyers peruse the arrangement, so enhancing efficiency and ensuring data accuracy [33]. Nebula is built on the Ethereum blockchain and the Blockstack platform, enabling the construction of decentralized apps and smart transactions in an environment that is accessible and pleasant to developers. It helps maintain the privacy of genetic information while reducing the cost of sequencing. Genomic data may be received by data owners using Nebula sequencing facilities, which connect them to data buyers through a peer-to-peer network that is cryptographically protected, therefore easing the strain on third parties. The Nebula assessment tool based on smart contracts will assist data buyers in structuring surveys with complimentary questions and generating trustworthy responses. The Nebula token, the network's native currency, may be traded for commodities and information. Decentralized sequencing makes it easy to buy DNA sequencing machines and sequence one's own samples, allowing for the early discovery of privacy issues [34].

Genotyping, or a patient's DNA, holds the most intimate information about their existence at any given moment. Many DNA testing organizations now create money by selling client information to other parties without their knowledge or payment. This strategy exposes the consumer's most sensitive information. EncrypGen, the first blockchain-based genomic data market, puts users in command of their own genetic information through a decentralized blockchain-based ledger. Individuals who have registered with EncrypGen, such as researchers, institutions, etc., have the option of making their information available to the public, for a short time, to earn money, which will help them and the individual offering the information grow in their respective industries [36]. It also has the ability to reduce the expense of genetics and medical research. If data owners can communicate directly with data buyers without going via an intermediary firm, analysis expenses are reduced and data owners are compensated. These same considerations are applicable to digital healthcare applications. Blockchain technology enables the execution of transactions more rapidly and efficiently than conventional techniques. Data recorded in centralized systems may be changed, but the blockchain's immutable ledger is generated collectively by all users. Being a decentralized system, blockchain improves the

TABLE 1.2

Comparison between the Papers Reviewed for Studying the Application of Blockchain in Genomics

Paper Title	'Opportunities for solving real-world problems in healthcare and Biomedical Sciences' [32]	'Accelerating genomic data generation and facilitating genomic data access using decentralization, privacy-preserving technologies and equitable compensation' [33]	'Realizing the potential of blockchain technologies in Genomics' [34]
'Opportunities for solving real-world problems in healthcare and Biomedical Sciences' [32]	In this research, we explore numerous scenarios where distributed ledger technology might improve medical care delivery. It also includes clinical trials and the administration of the medication supply chain. We investigate how blockchain technology might improve supply chain efficiency, protect patient privacy, and facilitate data sharing.	Investigation of how distributed systems enhance the accessibility and exchange of genetic data without jeopardizing individual privacy. It proposes using blockchain technology to create a financially motivated, decentralized environment where genetic data may be exchanged and studied.	This study examines the benefits and drawbacks of applying blockchain technology in genomics, including data security, patient confidentiality, and researchers' fair compensation. This article discusses a number of blockchain applications, including data provenance, data sharing, and data privacy.
'Blockchain technology in healthcare: A comprehensive review and directions for future research' [35]	The administration of electronic health record (EHR) systems, the management of the medical supply chain, and clinical trials are a few of the areas where blockchain may be beneficial, according to this paper. Interoperability, scalability, and regulatory compliance are all discussed as obstacles to blockchain's use in the healthcare industry.	The article proposes a blockchain-based system for transferring genetic data using smart contracts to manage data access and compensation. There is speculation that blockchain technology might encourage data providers and facilitate data sharing, hence accelerating the development of genetic data.	In this work, the viability of using blockchain technology to promote the secure, transparent, and decentralized exchange of genomics data is investigated. It proposes using blockchain technology to create a platform for data interchange and analysis that offers granular data access control and privacy protection.

Source: [32], [33], [34], [35].

transparency and auditability of prior transactions. It is more effective than other systems in preventing dishonest transactions and unlawful acts. Any verification system must conform to stringent public accessibility and auditability criteria [37,38].

1.2.8 Dental Industry

Dental care has a great chance to influence the development of the standards and technology it will rely on in the future, as well as the ways in which these resources are going to be utilized. There are a number of words that have been used to represent the idea of a paperless medical file, and "electronic health record" as used in the EHR definition is only one of them. Yet the concept of an electronic health record makes no demands on the technology used or the form of the presentation itself, whether it is a layout chart or a display. Electronic versions of paper-based health records (EHRs) may include non-EHR data, such as comparators for diagnostic lab tests, to better meet the needs of providers, other authorized personnel, and in some cases, patients; these records are known as "electronic medical records" (EMRs) and "electronic dental records," respectively. Another way of looking at the ideas is via the provision of EHR samples with other crucial information in an EMR. In the healthcare system, we need the distinctive edition to be reliable for protracted usages, and it has to be accessible for swapping information or data to the shared system for distributing the data affiliated, like a photo or an image sharing, and the functionalities that need to collaborate to develop, maintain, and hold the EHR. A dental clinic equipped with an EDR system, on the other hand, would be able to import and export data from patients' electronic health records, as well as display and record the relevant data extract. A critical feature of such a system is the capacity to send health information quickly and securely to an authorized practitioner or the system across several companies, or maybe various healthcare venues [39].

Currently, everything within oral healthcare system is performed manually, from examination and X-rays through patient invoices and prescriptions. This pattern suggests that the person's information may be edited as the data thief sees fit. Patients have restricted applicability to and comprehension of their data, and the current infrastructure for conveying clinical records is grossly insufficient. The patient's end connects with the dental specialist, whose end stores the patient's dental embedded clinical data in the blockchain. It enhances inventiveness and commitment to therapeutic abilities. The patient is ultimately accountable for his or her own patient history, and they are most equipped for self-sufficiency if they have open access to their health information through system connection [40]. With the quantity of data in the dentistry sector and the extensive usage of Internet of Things (IoT) networks made of varied smart devices, it is evident that blockchain technology might have substantial beneficial impacts in this understudied but valuable industry. There is an immediate need to expand the technical understanding of blockchain in dentistry via future research partnerships, despite the fact that dental practitioners are currently inexperienced with this platform. There is a critical requirement to establish a more effective and trustworthy means of collecting, maintaining, manipulating, archiving, and transmitting patients' health data given by a wide range of equipment and platforms in dentistry, just as there is in healthcare, as it makes the move to digitization. Many blockchain features set it apart from conventional or cloud data storage, proving its viability and usefulness in the dental field. As blockchain transactions and data transfers may be recorded and authenticated by other network users, a trusted third party is unnecessary. Because all patient data are now stored in a resolute, highly confidential, and safe manner and there is a verifiable log of how and when healthcare professionals access these records, the implementation of blockchain in dentistry has the potential to overcome many established challenges and encourage additional future advancements for dentistry and the broader healthcare industry in terms of data ownership, confidentiality, and safety. Due to the time and effort necessary to prepare dental records and thoroughly examine and document each patient's unique oral, dental, etc. condition, dentists may suffer with inefficiency and treatment delays. When a patient is referred from one dentist to another, they may get an inaccurate diagnosis. Due to blockchain technology, patients and dentists can now schedule fewer dental visits, resulting in reduced stress for both parties [41].

1.2.9 Organ Transplant Management

When an organ fails or is injured because of a mishap or an illness, this is referred to as organ failure or organ damage. Living with this illness reduces your quality of life and may be deadly. The donation of organs to be transplanted is one of the highest forms of human kindness. The organs need to be in good-enough shape to be transplanted, the receiver must be a suitable match for the donor, and the donor's life must not be in risk if the organ is removed. Enrollment, recipient compatibility, organ extraction, organ distribution, and implantation each have unique requirements and hurdles in modern organ transplants and donation systems due to legislative, clinical, ethical, and technological restrictions. With a comprehensive organ donation and transplantation system, we can provide a fair and efficient procedure, improve the patient experience, and build trust [42]. Yet the key issue with organ donation is that the security and reliability of such data entirely depend on the ability of transplantation institutions to keep their systems secure and notice probable harm to donors and recipients. There can be no trust in the waiting list data without people having faith in the facilities' ability to keep their information secure from hackers and dishonest staff members. Therefore, transparency prevents organ donations. The current system's lack of transparency allows for illegal organ sales and acquisitions as well as unethical actions on the part of medical specialists. Also, there are hospitals that take advantage of the vulnerable character of organ donors by providing transfers to those who can pay more to the facility, while the sufferer at the pinnacle of the waiting list is neglected. The current transplant system's inefficiency is intolerable when time is of the essence [43].

Blockchain has the ability to revolutionize this system. Due to blockchain's openness and automated monitoring features, no one party will have control over the ranking of prospective beneficiaries. Every user has complete insight into every transaction. In addition to simplifying the communication of medical information between donors and receivers in a safe and secure manner, this technology has the potential to prevent criminal organ trafficking. It has the ability to drastically increase the efficiency of the transplantation network by eliminating many of the present intermediaries and allowing any organization to immediately access transaction information [44]. While comparing volunteer matching within and outside of the blockchain, Jain U. proposed OrganChain as a model [45]. They've decided to evaluate the success of their blockchain-based system using four criteria: maximum batch time out, maximum block size, endorsement policy, and transaction rate. The findings of this study suggest that, compared to using a conventional database, using blockchain to match donors and applicants produces more desirable outcomes. IPFS, or the Interplanetary Shared Folder, is a peer-to-peer network and encrypted distributed file system proposed in [46]. Focusing on lowering the cost of uploading donor and patient medical information was their main priority. Donor and patient information will be protected and kept private under their planned double-hashing system.

1.3 Advantages

While technological advancements have enabled the move from physical to electronic medical records (EMR), which substantially improves information sharing and archiving, more care must be taken to safeguard patient privacy [47]. The absence of privacy and security around patient health information raises further concerns. Visiting patients, for example, must undergo further screening if they transfer to a new hospital. Due to this practice, money and resources are being frittered away. Since sensitive patient information cannot be shared with research institutes, medical advancement is impeded. Many patient records are maintained in medical records, and this information is vital for both present treatment and research directions. To maintain the security of the information, it must be stored securely and shared with only authorized persons. The immutability and transparency of blockchain have made it a popular option for handling patient data [48]. Healthcare information is available in several formats, not only electronic health records. Data from pharmaceutical and medicine manufacturing, as well as information from clinical trials, are examples of what may be found in a patient's personal health record; health insurance data includes the patient's insurance policy information, payment information, and data on insurance-related services received; and data generated and used for research include information such as the patient's physiological health parameters and allergy information. As a consequence of this mountain of data, physicians may learn more about their patients and enhance their care. Despite this, several parties gain from healthcare data in various ways. Safeguarding this sensitive healthcare data from cyber risks, such as infiltration and manipulation, is a top priority. Due to the vast array of services offered in the healthcare industry, including medical diagnosis, medical testing, and administrative tasks, it is important to assign separate duties and rights to the participating nodes based on the service they provide. Hence, permissioned blockchains are favored for safeguarding sensitive medical data. Several initialization steps are required when the healthcare business adopts blockchain for data protection. The assignment of preset responsibilities and permissions to entities like doctors, nurses, and patients is one example of such a job. Further work remains once an application has been implemented, including the incorporation of user feedback and the management of new and updated health information. Blockchain technology empowers patients to take control of their health records by allowing them to define access permissions via smart contracts. Any changes to a patient's medical records, such as when new information was added or when older records were read, are recorded in an audit log. When hospitals employ blockchain for inter-organizational communication and data exchange, it benefits not only patients by providing a secure standard format for the speedy processing of healthcare-related services [49].

A blockchain-based "medichain" strategy was proposed in 2022. With this architecture, the blockchain acts as a database where all pertinent patient case information is stored. By hashing the transaction records and keeping the resultant hash values in a Merkle tree, disparities in clinical decision-making may be reduced. The proposed architecture maintains all information in a single hyperfield to address the problem of medical data originating from several locations and having diverse forms. The data is immediately saved on the blockchain [50]. Wu H. et al. have addressed the authentication process of sensitive information in healthcare systems by proposing a patient-centric confidentiality admittance control method [51]. In addition, a unique infrastructure for data storage is developed utilizing blockchain technology, and data transport is accomplished using industry-standard encryption. A file permission clause is used to safeguard critical patient information from unauthorized access. The model proposes a discriminating access control system that may discriminate between users on the basis of their species while maintaining their privacy. A third-party cloud service provider manages the database that stores electronic medical records. When data is saved to the Internet, a hash is formed. The subsequent step is to upload the hash to the distributed ledger. If modifications have been made, cloud-based data may be compared to the original using the hash value saved on the blockchain. Since the PoW technique requires the nodes to make several incorrect computations in order to establish consensus, this model cannot be regarded as totally practical. Many pieces of software medical equipment are included into the IOMT to concurrently monitor health status and record a variety of data. IOMT is of considerable value to patients, and early disease detection via the evaluation of physical signs is vital. Yet the market is flooded with IOMT systems that lack defined management standards, leaving them susceptible to data breaches. Blockchain technology offers a solution to the challenge of safeguarding IOMT for medical purposes. Smart contracts reduce the need for intermediaries by enabling the parties engaged in a transaction. Thanks to the unique addresses and accounts used by each smart contract, any IoT device may independently access the blockchain-stored directives of the smart contract [52].

The allure of immutable blockchain resides in its auditability and transparency, two characteristics that have the ability to entice customers. Only the patient in possession of the private key may decode the data, which is why the consensus mechanism and cryptographic keys of blockchain technology allow secure access under patient control. The patient has complete authority over who has access to his or her medical data and may modify this list at any moment (including healthcare professionals, insurance companies, and researchers) [53].

In today's high-tech society, mobile applications and remote monitoring devices play a significant role in patient care. Using blockchain technology might improve the safety and dependability of industrial equipment. Obtaining and exchanging patient medical information is another potential use of blockchain technology. Medical records for patients are often housed in many places, making them difficult to obtain. The use of blockchain technology might facilitate patients' access to their whole medical history in a secure and trustworthy way. Many blockchain-based solutions for the storage and retrieval of medical records have been proposed. MedBlock, a blockchain-based information management system, promotes quick EMR access and retrieval by using distributed blockchain technologies. The increased consensus mechanism of the program avoids the network from being overloaded. Adding software that grows over time, such as blockchain, might increase network congestion. In addition, encryption and access control make MedBlock an extremely secure environment [54].

1.4 Challenges and Solutions

Regulatory impediments, compatibility issues, the need for regulation, limited approval, and a lack of technological knowledge among healthcare employees are some of the obstacles to blockchain technology adoption in healthcare. In order to maintain patient confidence and comply with data protection laws, it is necessary to address the unique privacy and security concerns presented by healthcare data. Moreover, the high cost and complexity of employing blockchain solutions may discourage smaller healthcare practitioners and organizations with limited resources. To address these issues, the healthcare industry, government officials, and technological specialists will need to collaborate to create a blockchain innovation environment. The difficulties that blockchain technology faces in the healthcare sector are shown in Figure 1.4.

Blockchain

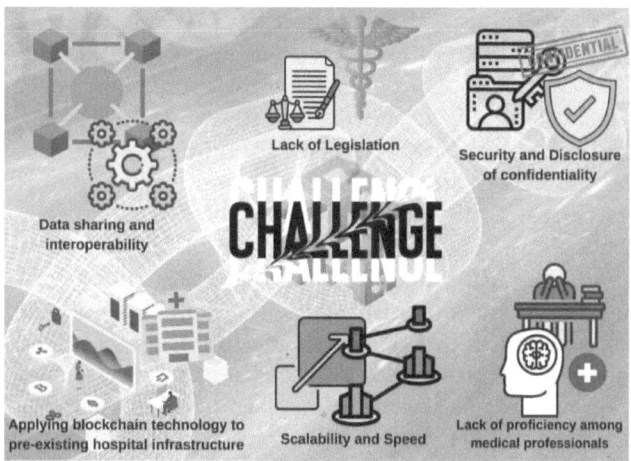

FIGURE 1.4
Healthcare and blockchain: emerging challenges.

1.4.1 Data Sharing and Interoperability

Inefficient compatibility is the cause of both patient identification issues and information obstruction, in which healthcare corporations implement an unjust restriction on the exchange of medical records or electronic health information. A lack of standardized patient IDs and the restriction of information impede healthcare efficiency significantly. In a crisis such as the coronavirus epidemic, it is also essential that systems can communicate with one another. Given the date of the epidemic, it is evident that a more comprehensive data-sharing system is required immediately to facilitate the flow of information to manage public health risks and enhance patient–provider communication. If a patient needs to see a specialist or another physician who is not their primary care provider, it is vital that they have easy access to their complete medical history. Through enhancements to the transfer of health data, physicians would also be able to conduct online consultations and remote monitoring. This provides individuals greater autonomy in communicating their health histories to physicians. As the number of confirmed cases rises, it becomes increasingly important to provide patients with timely and accurate information about the coronavirus, including how they can evaluate their own risk, exhibit symptoms, and respond to therapy. The lack of connectivity in the current system is accentuated further by public health issues [55].

Theodouli A. et al. propose a blockchain-based system architecture for managing healthcare data access and promoting the interchange of independently verified and private health information [56]. Automated procedures, client anonymization, shared data integrity, monitoring, and traceability are all features of the proposed framework's components, like characteristics and cryptographic protocols. The architecture relies on the consensus protocol, which enables off-chain verification of all network nodes. Web interfaces, cloud components, and the Ethereum blockchain are the three components that make up the proposed architecture. The registry contract (RC), the patient data contract (PDC), and the permissions contract (PC) are the three forms of smart contracts used here (PC). RC is a database that keeps track of all the devices connected to a network and a directory service that helps locate them. To create a direct connection between the encrypted healthcare data stored on the cloud service and the corresponding patient data, a PDC is utilized as a patient-specific identification. Network access control is managed by the PC since it establishes a connection between the PDC address and the requesting entity.

Mcfarlane C. et al. proposed a further investigation into the healthcare industry's twin issues of excessive expenditures and poor interoperability [57]. Owing to ineffective communication amongst EHRs institutions, the researchers developed a blockchain-based patient-oriented protocol to improve the management of ill patients. While it is essential that they have access to pertinent client records, such as imaging findings, medications, and medical history, the major emphasis of their research is on frontline medical personnel. The authors depicted the revolutionary nature of a blockchain-based healthcare data supply chain by demonstrating how blockchain technology may alleviate the strain of maintaining a vast number of present silos of patient information. Current solutions that are not blockchain-based demonstrate this problem. During the design process, the Health Insurance Portability and Accountability Act of 1996 (HIPAA) requirements for confidentiality, protection, and cloud computing were considered. In addition, it examines the limitations and disadvantages of blockchain technology in relation to HIPAA compliance. Patiotory tokens (PTOY) are necessary for blockchain functionality. These tokens determine how much space is allotted in a network, how often money is disbursed, and how thoroughly healthcare is monitored. Due to the system's inherent access control features, suppliers may anticipate minimal security breaches with this design.

1.4.2 Applying Blockchain Technology to Pre-Existing Hospital Infrastructure

Despite the fact that extensive adoption of blockchain technology for healthcare data administration would unquestionably herald in a new era of efficiency and precision, a number of obstacles must first be surmounted. Integration of cryptocurrency with existing networks is a significant obstacle. In order to implement blockchain technology, healthcare organizations will need to overhaul their current systems, which can be a time-consuming and costly process in and of itself. Numerous resources are required to ensure the successful implementation of blockchain technology in healthcare, including, but not limited to, time, money, and human knowledge. The current healthcare infrastructure may not be compatible with blockchain, requiring some institutions to acquire new systems. This can increase adoption costs and complicate matters overall. Therefore, careful consideration must be given to the impact of blockchain on existing processes and its potential interaction with existing systems. In addition, healthcare blockchain implementation must be standardized. To ensure the compatibility of diverse blockchain-based systems, data forms, security procedures, and access control must be standardized. It will enable the secure and confidential transmission of patient data between healthcare providers [58].

1.4.3 Scalability and Speed

It is widely recognized that the overwhelming volume of data poses a significant scaling challenge for blockchain-based healthcare solutions. Due to the severe performance degradation that would result from storing vast quantities of biological data on a blockchain, it is not desirable and, in some cases, may not even be possible. The issue of scaling is intrinsically attached to the working tempo. Depending on the algorithm employed, blockchain-based computing can cause significant delays, thereby limiting the system's growth. Using blockchain only as an index over healthcare data, storing only a limited amount of simplified knowledge regarding the data and how to access it, while the actual healthcare data is stored in a non-blockchain database, is one potential solution to the scalability and performance issues. This mitigation, however, eliminates the data duplication and constant accessibility that blockchain technology would otherwise provide to healthcare records. In addition, the permissioned blockchain, in which only a subset of nodes is permitted to participate in the agreement and certification processes, can ameliorate the performance issue associated with consensus methods, such as proof-of-work (PoW) employed by some public blockchains [59].

To assure scalability of data integrity and keep a transferable hash of the source information, Zhang P. et al. proposed FHIRChain, which increases the size of the data's reference pointer [60]. The complexity of the swap served as a proxy for the quantity of original data, denoted by N, while the size of the comparison signal was indicated by e. The space requirement for a hashed value of an input of variable length is fixed. A data reference pointer may expand as necessary, but actual data expands linearly. Zhang's proposal replaced constant-sized data for actual data to promote scalability. One alternative method for improving data storage is the use of a miniature blockchain. Mini-blockchains are a proposed transactional concept in [61]. To increase scalability, this solution eliminates the requirement to store the whole blockchain. By decomposing the blockchain into its component systems, even the most elementary operations may be optimized. This method reduces the size of the block by eliminating the script system and duplicate interlocking transaction data. In its place is a clearer concept of essential operations. In this case, a balance amount, taking into account all relevant transactions, was computed using an account tree. Breaking down these procedures into digestible pieces of transactions that can be put to the database at regular intervals is the key to success.

1.4.4 Security and Disclosure of Confidentiality

Consensus is what allows blockchain to function. If malicious miners control over 50% of the network's terminals, they could seize control. By denying the blocks generated by honest miners, they could then use their superior computing power to take valuable data or currency. However, the likelihood of this type of attack decreases as the magnitude of the network increases. Given that the blockchain database is open-source, the aphorism "transparency reveals confidentiality" becomes a further limitation. Due to the confidential tendency of patient data, this is particularly essential for medical data and other biological applications [62]. (Due to the open character of the blockchain, confidential data in the fields of medicine and other areas are visible to anyone.)

1.4.5 Lack of Proficiency among Medical Professionals

It can be challenging to persuade physicians and other medical professionals to switch from paper to electronic records. The transition from printed to computerized medications can be a source of frustration and confusion for many. Typically, when filling out a form, physicians disregard the optional sections. In contrast to computerized documents, physicians cannot bypass the required sections. In addition, many clinicians may have doubts about the dependability and efficacy of remote tracking systems that rely on technologies such as blockchain and IoT. The precision, swiftness, and efficacy of this technologically driven healthcare system will depend on the skill and commitment of individual physicians. Before implementing these instruments, doctors must be provided with the appropriate training and skills [63].

1.4.6 Lack of Legislation

The proposed blockchain-based healthcare system confronts difficulties in drafting appropriate laws for the administration of medical operations' ownership rights. Numerous parties have a vested interest in the outcomes of healthcare reform, making data custody and medical legislation of the current healthcare system crucial factors. Who possesses what in a blockchain, who has access to what, and how the distributed ledger is stored must be clarified in detail [64].

1.5 User Response and Acceptance

Almost every day, the media report a new incident involving the gathering, dissemination, and use of private information without consent and for detrimental purposes. As a result, individuals are less willing to use services that require them to submit personal information for risk of being hacked. This is not the case for the majority of the population, despite the fact that a personalized health service that helps individuals identify and manage their particular health concerns and promotes long-term well-being may be very beneficial for a number of individuals. For others, the answer to the privacy problems and lack of trust in sharing health data created by "databuses" is to offer individuals more control over their own data using blockchain technology (i.e., "self-sovereignty"). The usefulness of blockchain technology has been discovered to be problematic [65, 66, 67]. Blockchain is unlike other emerging technologies in that it is networked, distributed, autonomous, and global in scope, all of which have significant implications for society, government, and business. It's possible that blockchain, with the trust it can enforce, may be used to solve the problems associated with user consent. Informed consent is necessary for the ethical and legal use of health data. Although while blockchain has the potential to address some of the problems associated with patient data protection and preservation while also giving patients more control over their data, it is not without its flaws. The amount of intricacy in blockchain may be overwhelming, even for individuals who are highly well-versed in information technology. With so many people having trouble finding their way through the healthcare system as it is, it's unclear if making it even more onerous to keep track of one's own medical history and to provide appropriate permissions for the use of the information contained within will really help [68, 69].

There is a discussion of the advantages and driving force behind blockchain in light of the potential good effects it may have on societal and economic development, and they are compared to pre-existing expectations. Companies will continue to pour resources into blockchain-based technologies, according to the research, but they will take a more realistic perspective of the technology's potential in light of the widespread belief that its advantages are exaggerated. There are various barriers to widespread application of this technology, including governmental limitations, which may explain why this breakthrough has not yet lived up to its projected potential. Patients and physicians, like the general public, aren't always informed on the advantages, operation, or technicalities of blockchain technology. Concerns regarding the privacy and security of patients' data might be a major roadblock to blockchain's widespread application in healthcare. The technological limitations of the blockchain are at the heart of these concerns, and they include things like node security, the efficacy of the cryptographic features built into the architecture, and the persistence of data until requesters finish their calculations. Yet some study has highlighted larger social difficulties with the people's confidence in governments to preserve their personal information when utilizing public data sharing programs. Customers may have problems about the proposed frameworks' security owing, for instance, to their own administration or mistreatment of authorized private keys [70]. Fewer studies have examined the constraints of the social environment in which blockchain-based systems may be deployed. They acknowledge that users' access to the Internet on a national scale is crucial to the success of their proposed architecture, noting the possibility of cooperation for data falsification and the difficulty of a healthcare system to handle clinical misbehavior as examples [71].

1.6 Conclusion

Due to the combination of blockchain technology, the Internet of Things (IoT), and big data analytics, the healthcare industry might soon face a profound upheaval. To facilitate the flow of data between medical devices, physicians, and patients, blockchain technology may be linked into the Internet of Things to form an IoMT network. This has the potential to enhance patient care by enabling more precise, real-time monitoring of patients' health and the delivery of individualized medical treatment. Through the use of cryptocurrencies and big data analytics, medical providers may get even more insight into their patients and treatment strategies. Blockchain's decentralized and public nature enables researchers, healthcare professionals, and patients from all over the globe to safely and ethically exchange data. Blockchain's full potential can only be achieved with widespread adoption and use in the healthcare industry. With blockchain, patients' health information may be kept private while the system's transparency and efficiency are enhanced. Regulatory and legal obstacles, technological complexity, and incompatibility with existing healthcare systems all impede the widespread use of blockchain technology in healthcare. As the benefits of blockchain technology become more understood and its applications are recognized, it is expected that blockchain will play a significant role in the future of healthcare.

References

[1] McGhin T, Choo KK, Liu CZ, He D. Blockchain in healthcare applications: Research challenges and opportunities. *Journal of Network and Computer Applications*. 2019 Jun 1;135:62–75.
[2] Hölbl M, Kompara M, Kamišalić A, Nemec Zlatolas L. A systematic review of the use of blockchain in healthcare. *Symmetry*. 2018 Oct 10;10(10):470.
[3] Hasselgren A, Kralevska K, Gligoroski D, Pedersen SA, Faxvaag A. Blockchain in healthcare and health sciences—A scoping review. *International Journal of Medical Informatics*. 2020 Feb 1;134:104040.
[4] Vazirani AA, O'Donoghue O, Brindley D, Meinert E. Blockchain vehicles for efficient medical record management. *NPJ Digital Medicine*. 2020 Jan 6;3(1):1.
[5] Shahnaz A, Qamar U, Khalid A. Using blockchain for electronic health records. *IEEE Access*. 2019 Oct 9;7:147782–95.
[6] Leeming G, Cunningham J, Ainsworth J. A ledger of me: Personalizing healthcare using blockchain technology. *Frontiers in Medicine*. 2019 Jul 24;6:171.

[7] Harshini V, Danai S, Usha H, Kounte, MR. Health record management through blockchain technology. *Conference: 2019 3rd International Conference on Trends in Electronics and Informatics (ICOEI)*. 2019;1411–15. https://doi.org/10.1109/ICOEI.2019.8862594

[8] Azaria A, Ekblaw A, Vieira T, Lippman A. Medrec: Using blockchain for medical data access and permission management. In *2016 2nd International Conference on Open and Big Data (OBD)* (pp. 25–30). IEEE; 2016.

[9] Rghioui A. Managing patient medical record using blockchain in developing countries: Challenges and security issues. In *2020 IEEE International Conference of Moroccan Geomatics (Morgeo)* (pp. 1–6). IEEE; 2020.

[10] Musamih A, Salah K, Jayaraman R, Arshad J, Debe M, Al-Hammadi Y, Ellahham S. A blockchain-based approach for drug traceability in healthcare supply chain. *IEEE Access*. 2021 Jan 8;9:9728–43.

[11] Nakamoto S. Bitcoin: A peer-to-peer electronic cash system. *Decentralized Business Review*. 2008 Oct 31:21260.

[12] Mohana M, Ong G, Ern T. Implementation of pharmaceutical drug traceability using blockchain technology. *INTI Journal*. 2019;2019(35).

[13] Liu X, Barenji AV, Li Z, Montreuil B, Huang GQ. Blockchain-based smart tracking and tracing platform for drug supply chain. *Computers & Industrial Engineering*. 2021 Nov 1;161:107669.

[14] Reda M, Kanga DB, Fatima T, Azouazi M. Blockchain in health supply chain management: State of art challenges and opportunities. *Procedia Computer Science*. 2020 Jan 1;175:706–9.

[15] Sunny J, Undralla N, Pillai VM. Supply chain transparency through blockchain-based traceability: An overview with demonstration. *Computers & Industrial Engineering*. 2020 Dec 1;150:106895.

[16] Bali V, Soni P, Khanna T, Gupta S, Chauhan S, Gupta S. Blockchain application design and algorithms for traceability in pharmaceutical supply chain. *International Journal of Healthcare Information Systems and Informatics (IJHISI)*. 2021 Oct 1;16(4):1–8.

[17] Ahmad RW, Salah K, Jayaraman R, Yaqoob I, Ellahham S, Omar M. The role of blockchain technology in telehealth and telemedicine. *International Journal of Medical Informatics*. 2021 Apr 1;148:104399.

[18] Faruk MJ, Shahriar H, Valero M, Sneha S, Ahamed SI, Rahman M. Towards blockchain-based secure data management for remote patient monitoring. In *2021 IEEE International Conference on Digital Health (ICDH)* (pp. 299–308). IEEE; 2021.

[19] Kumar M, Chand S. MedHypChain: A patient-centered interoperability hyperledger-based medical healthcare system: Regulation in COVID-19 pandemic. *Journal of Network and Computer Applications*. 2021 Apr 1;179:102975.

[20] Pighini C. et al. SynCare: An innovative remote patient monitoring system secured by cryptography and blockchain. In: Friedewald M, Krenn S, Schiering I, Schiffner S (eds) *Privacy and Identity Management. Between Data Protection and Security. Privacy and Identity 2021*. IFIP Advances in Information and Communication Technology, vol. 644. Springer; 2022.

[21] Shaik T, Tao X, Higgins N, Li L, Gururajan R, Zhou X, Acharya UR. Remote patient monitoring using artificial intelligence: Current state, applications, and challenges. *Wiley Interdisciplinary Reviews: Data Mining and Knowledge Discovery*. 2023:e1485.

[22] Katiyar D, Singhal S. Blockchain technology in management of clinical trials: A review of its applications, regulatory concerns and challenges. *Materials Today: Proceedings*. 2021 Jan 1;47:198–206.

[23] Hang L, Chen C, Zhang L, Yang J. Blockchain for applications of clinical trials: Taxonomy, challenges, and future directions. *IET Communications*. 2022 Dec;16(20):2371–93.

[24] Malamas V, Dasaklis T, Kotzanikolaou P, Burmester M, Katsikas S. A forensics-by-design management framework for medical devices based on blockchain. In *2019 IEEE World Congress on Services (SERVICES)* (Vol. 2642, pp. 35–40). IEEE; 2019.

[25] Pane J, Verhamme KM, Shrum L, Rebollo I, Sturkenboom MC. Blockchain technology applications to postmarket surveillance of medical devices. *Expert Review of Medical Devices*. 2020 Oct 2;17(10):1123–32.

[26] Cho H, Choi J, Lee D, Lee S, Lim S, Park S. A blockchain framework for the management of medical equipment in healthcare. *Healthcare Informatics Research*. 2020;26(1):42–50. https://doi.org/10.4258/hir.2020.26.1.42

[27] Kim Y, Kim H, Park Y. Blockchain-based asset management system for medical equipment in hospitals. *Sensors* (Basel, Switzerland). 2020;20(17):4783.

[28] Lee S, Park S, Lim S. A blockchain-based medical equipment management system for enhancing patient safety in healthcare. *Journal of Medical Systems*. 2021;45(5):45.

[29] Ouyang T, Chen R, Dong J, Xie B, Zeng X. Blockchain technology for secure medical device management. *Journal of Medical Systems*. 2020;44(8):149.

[30] Haleem A, Javaid M, Singh RP, Suman R, Rab S. Blockchain technology applications in healthcare: An overview. *International Journal of Intelligent Networks*. 2021;2:130–9.

[31] He X, Alqahtani S, Gamble R. Toward privacy-assured health insurance claims. In *2018 IEEE International Conference on Internet of Things (iThings) and IEEE Green Computing and Communications (GreenCom) and IEEE Cyber, Physical and Social Computing (CPSCom) and IEEE Smart Data (SmartData)* (pp. 1634–41). IEEE; 2018.

[32] Justinia T. Blockchain technologies: Opportunities for solving real-world problems in healthcare and biomedical sciences. *Acta Informatica Medica*. 2019;27(4):284.

[33] Grishin D, Obbad K, Estep P, et al. Accelerating genomic data generation and facilitating genomic data access using decentralization, privacy-preserving technologies and equitable compensation. *Blockchain in Healthcare Today*. 2018;1:1–23.

[34] Ozercan HI, Ileri AM, Ayday E, Alkan C. Realizing the potential of blockchain technologies in Genomics. *Genome Research*. 2018;28(9):1255–63.

[35] Smith K, Caffery LJ, McInerney J, Gray K, Chatfield MD. Blockchain technology in healthcare: A comprehensive review and directions for future research. *Applied Clinical Informatics*. 2020;11(4):579–89. https://doi.org/10.1055/s-0040-1716497

[36] *Full Configuration Support End Dates Connectivity to the Microsoft 365 . . .* [Internet]. [cited 2023Mar16]. Available from: https://query.prod.cms.rt.microsoft.com/cms/api/am/binary/RE4woQm

[37] Kumar T, Ramani V, Ahmad I, Braeken A, Harjula E, Ylianttila M. Blockchain utilization in Healthcare: Key requirements and challenges. In *2018 IEEE 20th International Conference on e-Health Networking, Applications and Services (Healthcom)*. IEEE; 2018.

[38] *White Paper on Blockchain in Trade Facilitation United Nations Geneva* (pp. 128–38); 2020. Available from: chrome-extension://efaidnbmnnnibpcajpcglclefindmkaj/https://unece.org/DAM/trade/Publications/ECE-TRADE-457E_WPBlockchainTF.pdf

[39] Wutthikarn R, Hui YG. Prototype of blockchain in dental care service application based on Hyperledger Composer in Hyperledger fabric framework. In *2018 22nd International Computer Science and Engineering Conference (ICSEC)*. ICSEC; 2018.

[40] Panda S, Jena A, Swain S, Satapathy S. Blockchain technology: Applications and challenges. 2021. Springer Cham. Edition 1, ISBN: 978-3-030-69395-4. https://doi.org/10.1007/978-3-030-69395-4.

[41] Hassani H, Norouzi K, Ghodsi A, Huang X. Revolutionary dentistry through blockchain technology. *Big Data and Cognitive Computing*. 2023;7(1):9.

[42] Dajim LA, Al-Farras SA, Al-Shahrani BS, Al-Zuraib AA, Merlin Mathew R. Organ donation decentralized application using blockchain technology. In *2019 2nd International Conference on Computer Applications & Information Security (ICCAIS)*. IEEE; 2019. Available from: https://www.semanticscholar.org/paper/Organ-Donation-Decentralized-Application-Using-Dajim-Al-Farras/45f6817daa6f84324ef333e962798260ffbba9a1

[43] Hawashin D, Jayaraman R, Salah K, Yaqoob I, Simsekler MC, Ellahham S. Blockchain-based management for organ donation and transplantation. *IEEE Access*. 2022;10:59013–25.

[44] Chalissery BJ, Asha V. Blockchain based system for Human Organ Transplantation Management. *New Trends in Computational Vision and Bio-inspired Computing*. 2020:829–38.

[45] Jain U. *Using Blockchain Technology for the Organ Procurement and Transplant Network*. 2019; Master's Theses. 5065.

[46] Ranjan P, Srivastava S, Gupta V, Tapaswi S, Kumar N. Decentralised and distributed system for organ/tissue donation and transplantation. In *2019 IEEE Conference on Information and Communication Technology*. IEEE; 2019. Available from: https://www.researchgate.net/publication/340688070_Decentralised_and_Distributed_System_for_OrganTissue_Donation_and_Transplantation

[47] Adamu J, Hamzah R, Rosli MM. Security issues and framework of electronic medical record: A review. *Bulletin of Electrical Engineering and Informatics*. 2020;9(2).

[48] Agbo C, Mahmoud Q, Eklund J. Blockchain technology in healthcare: A systematic review. *Healthcare*. 2019;7(2):56.

[49] Pandey M, Agarwal R, Shukla SK, Verma NK. Security of healthcare data using blockchains. *Blockchain in Digital Healthcare*. 2021:113–50.

[50] Johari R, Kumar V, Gupta K, Vidyarthi DP. Blosom: Blockchain technology for security of medical records. *ICT Express*. 2022;8(1):56–60.

[51] Wu H, Dwivedi AD, Srivastava G. Security and privacy of patient information in medical systems based on blockchain technology. *ACM Transactions on Multimedia Computing, Communications, and Applications*. 2021;17(2s):1–17.

[52] Xi P, Zhang X, Wang L, Liu W, Peng S. A review of blockchain-based secure sharing of healthcare data. *Applied Sciences*. 2022;12(15):7912.

[53] Yaqoob S, Murad M, Talib R, Dawood A, Saleem S, Arif F, et al. Use of blockchain in healthcare: A systematic literature review. *International Journal of Advanced Computer Science and Applications*. 2019;10(5).

[54] Fan K, Wang S, Ren Y, Li H, Yang Y. MedBlock: Efficient and secure medical data sharing via Blockchain. *Journal of Medical Systems*. 2018;42(8).

[55] Attaran M. Blockchain technology in healthcare: Challenges and opportunities. *International Journal of Healthcare Management*. 2022 Jan 2;15(1):70–83.

[56] Theodouli A, Arakliotis S, Moschou K, Votis K, Tzovaras D. On the design of a blockchain-based system to facilitate healthcare data sharing. In *2018 17th IEEE International Conference on Trust, Security and Privacy in Computing and Communications/ 12th IEEE International Conference on Big Data Science and Engineering* (pp. 1374–9); 2018.

[57] Mcfarlane C, Beer M, Brown J, Prendergast N. *Patientory: A Healthcare Peer-to-Peer EMR Storage Network*. Entrust Inc.: Addison; 2017.

[58] Yaqoob I, Salah K, Jayaraman R, Al-Hammadi Y. Blockchain for healthcare data management: Opportunities, challenges, and future recommendations. *Neural Computing and Applications*. 2021 Jan 7:1–6.

[59] Agbo CC, Mahmoud QH. Blockchain in healthcare: Opportunities, challenges, and possible solutions. *International Journal of Healthcare Information Systems and Informatics (IJHISI)*. 2020 Jul 1;15(3):82–97.

[60] Zhang P, White J, Schmidt DC, Lenz G, Rosenbloom ST. FHIRCHAIN: Applying blockchain to securely and scalably share clinical data. *Computational and Structural Biotechnology Journal*. 2018;16:267–78.

[61] Bruce JD. *The Mini-Blockchain Scheme*; July 2014. Available from: http://www.cryptonite.info/

[62] Yaqoob S, Khan MM, Talib R, Butt AD, Saleem S, Arif F, Nadeem A. Use of blockchain in healthcare: A systematic literature review. *International Journal of Advanced Computer Science and Applications*. 2019;10(5).

[63] Ratta P, Kaur A, Sharma S, Shabaz M, Dhiman G. Application of blockchain and internet of things in healthcare and medical sector: Applications, challenges, and future perspectives. *Journal of Food Quality*. 2021 May 25;2021:1–20.

[64] Gökalp E, Gökalp M, Gökalp S, Eren P. Analysing opportunities and challenges of integrated blockchain technologies in healthcare. In *Information Systems: Research, Development, Applications, Education*; 2018. https://doi.org/10.1007/978-3-030-00060-8_13.

[65] Edelman. *Edelman Trust Barometer* [Internet]. Edelman; 2019 [cited 2023 Mar 16]. Available from: www.edelman.com/trust/2019-trust-barometer

[66] Eskandari S, Barrera D, Stobert E, Clark J. A first look at the usability of Bitcoin key management. 2015. https://doi.org/10.14722/usec.2015.23015.

[67] Mahula S, Tan E, Crompvoets J. With blockchain or not? Opportunities and challenges of self-sovereign identity implementation in public administration: Lessons from the Belgian case. In *DG.O2021: The 22nd Annual International Conference on Digital Government Research (DG.O'21)* (pp. 495–504). Association for Computing Machinery; 2021.

[68] Regueiro C, Seco I, Gutiérrez-Agüero I, Urquizu B, Mansell J. A blockchain-based audit trail mechanism: Design and implementation. *Algorithms*. 2021;14(12):341.

[69] Gordon WJ, Catalini C. Blockchain technology for healthcare: Facilitating the transition to patient-driven interoperability. *Computational and Structural Biotechnology Journal.* 2018; 16:224–30.
[70] Tandon A, Dhir A, Islam AKMN, Mäntymäki M. Blockchain in healthcare: A systematic literature review, synthesizing framework and future research agenda. *Computers in Industry.* 2020;122:103290.
[71] Zhang A, Lin X. Towards secure and privacy-preserving data sharing in e-health systems via consortium blockchain. *Journal of Medical Systems.* 2018;42(8).

2
Application of Blockchain in Medical Industry

Naru Venkata Pavan Saish, Vijayashree J., and Jayashree J.

2.1 Introduction

Blockchain is a type of digital ledger that enables the development and dissemination of secure, distributed databases of data. Because it is a decentralized system, there is no single point of failure or control. Instead, a network of computers maintains a common database that is regularly updated and checked. The blockchain's individual blocks each has a record of recent transactions and a distinct cryptographic hash that connects them to the block before it. Doing this forms an unbreakable chain of blocks, guaranteeing the data's accuracy [1]. It is very challenging to hack or change any of the data contained in the blockchain since it is dispersed over a network of computers. The technology behind the birth of the cryptocurrency known as "Bitcoin" might be considered blockchain, a relatively new discovery that first appeared in 2008. In general, blockchain may be considered a network organization method that combines distributed ledgers and databases. Blockchain is a technology that enables several parties engaged in communication to carry out various transactions without the involvement of a third party. These transactions and communications are verified and validated by specialized nodes known as miners [2]. The data structure known as a block contains legitimate transactions. The preceding committed transactions are necessary for the present transaction to be carried out. This technique is useful in preventing or limiting double spending in the Bitcoin system.

In this design, records are updated or maintained by a certain authority but are dispersed over all computers connected to the network so that no one node has the power to change the data that is being stored. This specific component might be useful for handling sensitive data, such as health information or financial transactions. Blockchain technology has drawn the attention of many academics, businesses, and organizations, particularly when it comes to the usage of the virtual currency Bitcoin. A peer-to-peer network's transactions can be safely recorded on a blockchain, a decentralized ledger. Moreover, it makes transactions visible and verifiable. Blockchain technology's primary goal is to enable safe two-party transactions without the need for a third-party intermediary [3]. By embracing smart technologies other than blockchain, such as machine learning, the Internet of Things, virtual reality, and artificial intelligence, many industries, and sectors, including engineering, automotive, computing and electronics, aerospace, business and accounting, banking, defense, and healthcare, have undergone a revolutionary change. From 1.0 to 4.0, the advancement of the blockchain grew tremendously. The evolution began with blockchain

1.0, which was restricted to the storage and transfer of value (e.g., Bitcoin, Ripple, Dash), followed by blockchain 2.0, whose environment is programmable via smart contracts, and blockchain 3.0, in which the technology became applications-centric and impacted daily lives by facilitating a range of sectors, including healthcare, education, agriculture, e-commerce, and more. The business blockchains mentioned here include Hyperledger, R3 Corda, and Ethereum Quorum. Next, blockchain 4.0 almost eliminates all restrictions in the prior blockchain. Blockchain 4.0, which makes use of a distributed environment, has significant problems with scalability and a low transaction rate per second [4].

Blockchain is utilized for many purposes, mainly because of its special qualities and characteristics that make it suitable for some uses. The following are some of the key causes for using blockchain:

1. *Security*. Cryptography is used by blockchain technology to safeguard data and transactions, making it incredibly impossible to hack or change any data kept there.
2. Blockchain is a decentralized system; thus, there isn't a single point of failure or control. As a result, it is more resistant to threats of all kinds, including online attacks.
3. *Transparency*. All parties involved may see and understand the transactions that are recorded on the blockchain. By doing so, fraud is deterred and accountability is raised.
4. *Efficiency*. Blockchain technology may automate procedures and eliminate middlemen, resulting in speedier and less-expensive transactions.

A secure and decentralized data storage and transmission system without the use of middlemen like banks or other financial organizations is what blockchain technology aims to build. Blockchain is a distributed ledger technology that enables several parties to keep an up-to-date database of transactions that are shared and recorded in an open and transparent manner. The main advantage of blockchain is that it enables the construction of an unchangeable, tamper-proof record of all system transactions [5]. Beyond cryptocurrencies, blockchain technology offers a wide range of uses, including voting systems, supply chain management, and digital identity verification. It is a desirable solution for a range of sectors and uses because of its decentralized structure and high level of security. As more businesses and organizations look at the possible uses of blockchain, it has grown in popularity over time. Blockchain technology has gained traction across several businesses, as seen by the expansion of the cryptocurrency industry. The worldwide blockchain market is anticipated to reach $39.7 billion by 2025, expanding at a compound yearly growth rate of 67.3% from 2020 to 2025, according to a markets analysis. Blockchain technology is becoming more and more popular, as seen by the fact that several significant businesses, like IBM, Microsoft, Amazon, and Google, have made investments in it [6]. Several nations have also begun investigating the application of blockchain technology in their own sectors.

EMR (electronic medical record) and RPM (remote patient monitoring), which are tools used by health executives, are two key areas of healthcare record management in information technology (IT). These sources generate an enormous amount of medical information. The main threat in this framework is therefore information that is extremely safe and the rise in cybercrime cases, both of which have been linked to concerns with the standard of medical information, including disordered investigation, a medical decision, and expectation. Due to the critical resource recorded being incompatible with their perspective,

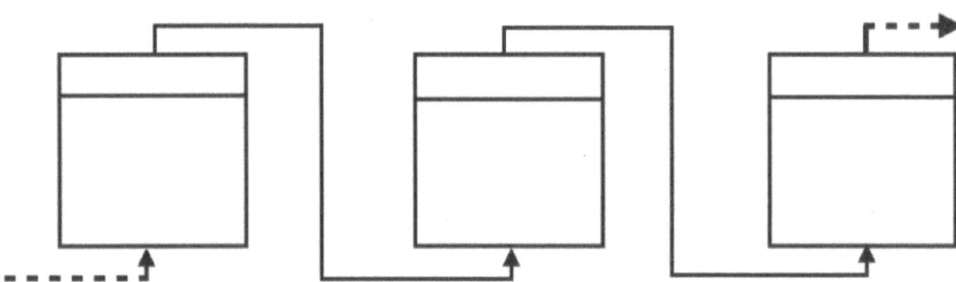

FIGURE 2.1
Structure of storing in the blockchain way.

medical records of patient history have proved the importance of uploaded documents. The demonstrative accuracy and the information repository may be enhanced by exchanging patient data among various healthcare providers via health records [7]. The healthcare industry uses blockchain technology freely in a variety of financial and insurance-related applications. The industry where resources are monitored and transactions take place serves all its intended goals: a secure network infrastructure that looks after both computerized and critical resources. Data transfers are prompted by fundamental traits, including trust, agreement, smart contracts, performance, and security.

The potential impact of blockchain on healthcare information systems is highlighted by certain research. However, the blockchain-based approach presented in this study is the first to eliminate EHR constraints brought on by patient perception. The second contribution of this study is to offer rationale and evidence in favor of using blockchain technology for information exchange. The social exchange theory, a well-known theory, is used to support the benefits of blockchain for exchanging medical information from the viewpoint of the individual (the patient). The utility of blockchain in health record systems was supported by empirical data collected using an experimental design based on the scenario [8]. In a blockchain, data may be stored in a variety of ways, including through smart contracts, transaction outputs, and external storage layers. A smart contract, which is a self-executing contract with the conditions of the agreement put directly into code, is one approach. The information can be kept in the smart contract as a variable that can be retrieved and modified using the contract's functionalities. The data can also be kept in a transaction as an output. Little pieces of data, such as the hash of a document or a digital signature, are frequently stored in this way. Finally, a reference to vast volumes of data may be maintained off-chain via an external storage layer, while the actual data itself is kept on the blockchain. Instead of putting all the data directly on the blockchain, this may be more effective and economical [9]. The type of data, its amount, and the blockchain platform being utilized are the main factors that determine how data is stored on a blockchain. Figure 2.1 shows the structure of storing in the blockchain way.

2.2 Use of Blockchain in Medical and Pharmaceuticals

Blockchain networks, as opposed to conventional centralized databases, store data in a decentralized and unchangeable way, making them the best option for storing vast volumes of data. The capacity of blockchain technology to store massive volumes of data securely and effectively is one of its main benefits. This is made feasible by the application of distributed consensus processes and cryptographic algorithms that guarantee data integrity and thwart illegal access. Blockchain networks can therefore handle massive data volumes without sacrificing security or efficiency [10]. Moreover, blockchain networks are made to be extremely scalable, which qualifies them for data storage of enormous volumes. A blockchain network's ability to store data grows together with the number of nodes in the network. Blockchain networks can handle massive volumes of data without suffering speed concerns because of its scalability feature. The immutability of blockchain technology is another advantage when utilizing it to store a lot of data. Without the agreement of the network's users, data stored on a blockchain network cannot be changed or removed. For sensitive data like bank records, medical records, and personal information that demands high levels of security and anonymity, blockchain is the perfect option.

Moreover, peer-to-peer (P2P) architecture is used in blockchain networks, which implies that data is dispersed throughout a network of nodes. This minimizes the chance of data loss or corruption by ensuring that data is duplicated across numerous nodes. In contrast, centralized databases have a single point of failure, making them susceptible to security concerns, like data leaks and cyberattacks [11]. And last, the cost-effectiveness of blockchain technology makes it ideal for storing massive volumes of data. Decentralized blockchain networks eliminate the need for intermediaries in data storage and transit. This makes it an appealing option for businesses that need to store huge volumes of data without incurring considerable costs, since it lowers the cost of maintaining and safeguarding data. In conclusion, blockchain technology provides a groundbreaking way to store massive volumes of data effectively and affordably. It is the best option for enterprises that need to store sensitive data, such as financial records, medical records, and personal information, because of its scalability, immutability, decentralization, and P2P design. Blockchain technology is positioned to be a major player in the digital transformation of organizations and sectors throughout the world as the need for data storage keeps rising.

The research, development, production, and marketing of pharmaceuticals used in the management, prevention, and treatment of illnesses make up the enormous and intricate pharmaceutical business. The sector is both difficult and extremely profitable because of its strict regulations and high investment requirements in research and development. The pharmaceutical sector manufactures a broad variety of goods, including prescription pharmaceuticals, over-the-counter medicines, vaccines, and other medical supplies [12]. Also, the sector is active in biotechnology and medical products such as prostheses, implants, and diagnostic tools. A novel medicine's development goes through several stages that might take years, including drug discovery, preclinical testing, clinical trials, regulatory approval, and post-market monitoring. Quite apart from the difficulties, the pharmaceutical sector continues to be a vital force for advancing healthcare innovation and enhancing global patient outcomes.

Since both industries play significant roles in the discovery, production, and delivery of healthcare goods and services, the pharmaceutical and medical sectors are intimately tied to one another. The pharmaceutical business is more concerned with the research, development, and manufacture of medications and other medical items than the medical sector, which primarily focuses on delivering patient care. Drugs for a variety of ailments and illnesses are developed and marketed by pharmaceutical corporations in close collaboration with healthcare professionals and medical institutes. These medications are then used by the medical sector to offer patient care and treat a range of illnesses.

There are potential advantages to pharmaceutical sectors in bringing blockchain technology. Blockchain technology has been integrated into the pharmaceutical sector for a few reasons, including the benefits it will bring to supply chain transparency, data security, efficiency, and patient outcomes [13]. The pharmaceutical business may follow the transfer of pharmaceuticals from producers to patients, confirming the legitimacy of the drugs and preventing fraud and drug diversion by utilizing blockchain's capabilities, such as its capacity to offer a transparent and tamper-proof record of transactions. Moreover, the blockchain's decentralized structure makes it the perfect tool for securely storing and exchanging sensitive data, including patient information and clinical trial findings. Blockchain technology can lessen the strain on middlemen and boost supply chain efficiency by reducing administrative procedures. Lastly, people will be able to exercise more control over their health information and safely share it with healthcare professionals, resulting in more individualized and successful treatments and improved patient outcomes [14].

Many advantages of blockchain technology make it appropriate for the medical sector. The ability to offer greater data protection is one of its most important benefits. The most sensitive information is found in medical records and health data, and blockchain technology can offer an unheard-of level of protection by encrypting the data and making it unchangeable. This lowers the risk of data breaches by ensuring that patient data is shielded from unwanted access and manipulation. By facilitating the safe sharing of health data between various providers and organizations, blockchain technology can also aid in enhancing interoperability in the healthcare industry. This is especially crucial because the healthcare sector is frequently fragmented, with data silos existing in many places and forms. All parties engaged in patient care may now have access to the same data thanks to blockchain, which lowers mistakes, enhances care coordination, and ultimately improves patient outcomes.

To provide life-saving medications and medical equipment, the medical sector primarily relies on the supply chain. Blockchain technology enables transparent and safe tracking of items from producer to a patient, which can enhance supply chain management. This can lessen the chance of diversion and assist in stopping fake pharmaceuticals from entering the supply chain. Moreover, by granting people access to their health data, blockchain technology may empower patients. People may control their health data using blockchain technology and share it with healthcare professionals, researchers, and other parties on a case-by-case basis. Better patient outcomes and more individualized treatment may result from this. Indeed, there are a lot of advantages to implementing blockchain in healthcare, such as greater interoperability, improved supply chain management, and patient empowerment.

2.3 Diseases and Outbreaks

Diseases are illnesses that impair the body's ability to operate normally and result in symptoms that might be moderate or severe. Several things, including lifestyle decisions, environmental conditions, genetic predisposition, and infectious agents, including viruses, bacteria, and parasites, can contribute to their development. Humans are susceptible to dozens of different diseases, from everyday ailments like the common cold and seasonal allergies to serious problems like cancer, heart disease, and HIV/AIDS. Diseases can have several symptoms, including fever, discomfort, exhaustion, and cognitive impairment, and they can affect different sections of the body, including organs, tissues, and cells.

Some disorders are chronic, meaning, they linger for months or even years, while others are acute, meaning, they appear quickly and continue for a short time. A person's quality of life may be significantly impacted by chronic conditions, which can often be difficult to manage. Many illnesses have been identified and treated thanks to developments in medical science and technology, improving patient outcomes and lengthening life expectancy [15]. The fact that there are several illnesses for which there are currently no viable medicines highlights the continual need for medical research and innovation. For illnesses to be prevented and treated and to ultimately improve the health and well-being of people and communities, it is crucial to understand their origins and consequences.

Significant public health risks that affect people, communities, and entire populations are diseases and epidemics. A *disease* is a condition that interferes with the body's natural function and can cause symptoms that can range in severity from moderate to severe, whereas an *epidemic* is described as a rapid rise in the number of cases of a certain illness in each geographic area or population. Infectious agents, including viruses, germs, parasites, environmental exposures, and other aspects of one's health, can all contribute to outbreaks [16]. Flu outbreaks, outbreaks of foodborne illness, and epidemics of newly developing infectious illnesses, like the COVID-19 pandemic, are typical instances of outbreaks. Outbreaks may have a big impact, causing everything from minor illness to serious illness and even death. Recovery from epidemics and illnesses is a tough process based on the sickness and its severity. The first step in healing is seeking medical treatment. Healthcare professionals can provide a diagnosis and suggest the best course of action. The suggested course of therapy, which may entail medication, rest, and a change in lifestyle, must be adhered to. Good hygiene habits, such as often washing your hands, covering your mouth and nose when you cough or sneeze, and avoiding direct contact with ill people, can help stop the spread of disease and speed up recovery.

Moreover, outbreaks can have social and economic repercussions that have an impact on travel, employment, and education. So it's essential to spot outbreaks promptly and take action to stop them in their tracks and lessen their effects. The key to controlling epidemics is prevention, and public health policies, including immunization, good hand hygiene, and infection control techniques, are crucial in lowering the likelihood of outbreaks. Public health organizations must collaborate to monitor and analyze outbreaks, determine their causes, and put control measures in place to stop their spread. Early recognition and reaction are also essential. In general, infections and outbreaks are major public health problems that need constant observation, investigation, and action to lessen their effects and enhance the health and well-being of people and communities.

Blockchain technology can change how the healthcare sector approaches ailments. The healthcare sector can promote patient empowerment, expand interoperability, and improve data security by utilizing the capabilities of blockchain [17]. Improved data security and privacy are among the most important advantages of blockchain in the treatment of illnesses. Patient data is more susceptible to data breaches and cyberattacks as electronic health records proliferate. By encrypting health data and making it unchangeable, blockchain technology can offer an unheard-of level of data protection and privacy. This lowers the risk of data breaches by ensuring that patient data is shielded from unwanted access and manipulation. Increased interoperability is an advantage of blockchain technology as well. The lack of interoperability across various organizations and providers is one of the biggest problems facing the healthcare sector. By making it possible for providers and organizations to securely share health data, blockchain technology can aid interoperability. This is crucial in the context of illness management, since successful patient care depends on healthcare practitioners having access to correct and current patient information. Blockchain technology can improve illness tracking and monitoring. Blockchain may be used by public health experts to monitor disease patterns, track epidemics, and act promptly when new health hazards arise. Blockchain can aid public health workers in making educated decisions regarding disease prevention and control strategies by supplying real-time data on the prevalence and severity of illnesses [18].

Disease outbreaks have significantly disrupted communities all around the world throughout human history. The plague of Athens, which struck the city in 430 BCE during the Peloponnesian War, was one of the first epidemics ever documented. One-third of the city's population is said to have perished because of this outbreak, which is thought to have been brought on by typhoid disease or a kindred virus. The Black Death, which started in China in the 1330s and moved to Europe in the middle of the 14th century, was another important epidemic in history. It is believed that up to 200 million people globally died because of this pandemic, which was brought on by the bacterium *Yersinia pestis*. Due to the Black Death's severe social and economic effects, feudalism declined and modern capitalism emerged. Influenza epidemics have had a significant influence on world health in the 20th century. According to estimates, the 1918 influenza pandemic, often known as the Spanish flu, infected one-third of the world population and killed up to 50 million people. Most recently, an estimated 284,000 people died globally because of the H1N1 influenza pandemic in 2009. Infectious disease outbreaks like the 2014 Ebola epidemic in West Africa and the continuing COVID-19 pandemic have brought attention to the continuous danger of infectious illnesses in the 21st century. Around 28,000 people contracted the Ebola virus, which led to an outbreak that ended in 11,000 fatalities. With over 130 million confirmed cases and 2.8 million fatalities as of early 2023, the COVID-19 pandemic, which is brought on by the SARS-CoV-2 virus, has had a huge impact on both worldwide health and the global economy. The pandemic has also brought attention to the necessity of a public health infrastructure, the need for science-based policy, and the need for international collaboration in the fight against infectious disease epidemics.

Understanding the transmission of the illness and putting effective containment measures in place depend on observations made during outbreaks. These observations might take many different forms, and studying the data can provide important details about the outbreak's characteristics [19]. During outbreaks, it's important to keep an eye out for the signs that the disease's victims display. Following the signs and symptoms can assist in spotting possible instances, tracking the disease's progression, and creating efficient treatment regimens. Moreover, symptoms can offer crucial information about the severity of the illness and its effects on certain groups. The location of verified instances is yet another finding. Identification of regions with a higher risk of infection can be aided by mapping the locations of cases. This may be helpful for putting into effect policies like travel bans or quarantines. Understanding the disease's transmission patterns can help determine the best ways to stop it from spreading further. For instance, determining high-risk behaviors or settings that encourage transmission might direct social isolation, mask use, and other treatments. It's also crucial to pay attention to the demographics of the disease's victims [20]. Populations that are more likely to contract an illness can be identified using demographic data such as age, gender, and ethnicity. This data may be used to focus interventions and give the right kind of help to individuals who need it the most. For instance, people who are older or have underlying health issues could require more intense support to recover from the illness. Finally, studying how the populace reacts to the epidemic might be helpful in figuring out the most effective ways to inform and communicate with the populace about the illness. It can also shed light on the efficacy of strategies, like social isolation and masking. Public health messages may be improved, and compliance with regulations increased, by analyzing the public's reaction. In general, diligent observation and data analysis during outbreaks can offer insightful knowledge of the illness and aid in directing efficient response actions. Public health professionals may better understand the epidemic and put effective containment measures into place by keeping track of symptoms, geographic location, mechanism of transmission, demographics, and public response.

For researchers and public health experts to learn from the past and create successful preventive, readiness, and response plans, information about previous epidemics must be stored. Finding patterns and risk factors linked to disease transmission is one of the key advantages of preserving outbreak data. Researchers can find parallels across epidemics, such as demographic characteristics, environmental factors, or mechanisms of transmission, by examining data from prior outbreaks. The development of more effective preventative efforts, such as vaccination programs or public health messages, can be aided by this knowledge. Keeping track of epidemic data can help researchers create better diagnostic tools in addition to finding trends [21]. Researchers can identify the virus causing an epidemic and create more precise diagnostic tests by reviewing previous outbreaks. Public health professionals can promptly identify patients and stop the outbreak before it spreads further with the use of more efficient testing equipment. Improving epidemic response plans is a crucial advantage of preserving outbreak data. Public health professionals can discover gaps in their response plans and strengthen them by studying prior epidemics. To better inform the public on the hazards associated with the epidemic, or to better coordinate the response among various authorities, they could identify communication gaps. Lastly, keeping track of epidemic data can help with policymaking. Policymakers may decide wisely regarding vaccine development, budget allocation, and quarantine regulations by examining the facts. With this data, policy adjustments that enhance sanitation or control animal markets may be made to stop future epidemics. In summary, keeping track of outbreak data is essential for enhancing our knowledge of infectious illnesses and strengthening our capacity to respond to epidemics in the future. Researchers can discover trends and risk factors, create better diagnostic equipment, enhance response plans, and provide policy judgments by studying previous epidemics [22]. This knowledge is essential for stopping future epidemics and guaranteeing the health and safety of people everywhere. By offering a safe and decentralized mechanism to handle patient data, the storage of medical records in a blockchain-based system has the potential to completely change the healthcare sector. Blockchain technology is a distributed ledger that records transactions in an open and secure way, making it perfect for keeping private data like medical records. Enhanced security is one of the key advantages of adopting blockchain to store medical information. Centralized databases, which are frequent targets of cyberattacks and data breaches, are used in traditional ways of keeping medical records. Blockchain makes it more challenging for hackers to access patient data since it is encrypted and stored over a dispersed network of nodes. Improved privacy is a benefit of adopting blockchain for medical records. Patients may decide who has access to their medical information in a blockchain system, and all access and changes are recorded in an immutable ledger. In this way, patient data may be protected from illegal access or manipulation [23].

Moreover, blockchain-based medical record storage can increase the precision and efficacy of healthcare services. Healthcare professionals may easily access patient data using a decentralized system from any location, eliminating the need for duplicated testing or duplicate records. Furthermore, the usage of smart contracts may automate procedures like claim processing, lowering administrative costs and enhancing payment accuracy and speed. Overall, using a blockchain-based system to store medical information has the potential to increase healthcare delivery efficiency, security, and privacy. Blockchain can assist healthcare practitioners in providing better treatment and enhancing patient outcomes by offering a safe and decentralized method to manage patient data.

By offering a safe and transparent mechanism to handle medication development, manufacture, and distribution, storing pharmaceutical data in a blockchain-based system has the potential to change the pharmaceutical business [24]. The following are some benefits of pharma data storage on blockchain:

1. Supply chain *transparency* has been increased, which is one of the key advantages of adopting blockchain to store pharmaceutical data. Blockchain can deliver a thorough, irrefutable record of every transaction along the route by following medicinal goods from the manufacturer to the end consumer. As a result, patients will obtain safe and effective drugs. This can also assist in avoiding counterfeiting, diversion, and other fraudulent actions.

2. *Enhanced security.* Placing pharmaceutical data in a blockchain-based system can help fend off cyberattacks and data breaches. Hackers find it challenging to access and alter sensitive data thanks to blockchain's secure and decentralized data storage. This can be particularly significant in the pharmaceutical sector, where data integrity and confidentiality related to drug research and clinical trials are of utmost importance.

3. *Improved data sharing.* Researchers, producers, and regulators may work together more effectively by storing pharmaceutical data in a blockchain-based system. Blockchain can hasten medication development, lessen effort duplication, and foster industry innovation by offering a safe and open platform for data sharing.

4. *Enhanced effectiveness.* Storing pharmaceutical data on a blockchain can help make the research and production of new drugs more effective and affordable. Automation of activities including clinical trial data gathering, medicine manufacture, and supply chain management using smart contracts, which are self-executing programs that run on the blockchain, lowers administrative burden and increases the speed and accuracy of these procedures.

5. *Better patient outcomes* are possible because of storing pharmacological data in a blockchain-based system. Blockchain can assist in guaranteeing that patients get the proper prescriptions at the right time, increasing their health and quality of life, by assuring the safety, effectiveness, and quality of pharmaceuticals.

Overall, the management of medication discovery, production, and distribution might be done securely, transparently, and effectively by using a blockchain-based system to store pharmaceutical data. Blockchain technology may aid in the promotion of innovation and guarantee that patients obtain safe and effective pharmaceuticals by enhancing supply chain transparency, boosting security, allowing data exchange, raising efficiency, and improving patient outcomes [25].

An "outbreak" is often described as a sudden, unanticipated rise in the incidence of a certain illness or infection in each population or geographical area. Public health experts must identify an epidemic to implement the appropriate controls and stop future transmission. These are several techniques to determine whether an epidemic is present:

- *Keep an eye on news sources.* Local and national news media frequently cover epidemics as they happen. Potential outbreaks can be discovered by routinely scanning news sources for stories about an increase in instances of a given disease or infection in a particular region.
- *Public health surveillance systems* are made to watch over and keep tabs on the spread of infectious diseases and other health-related problems. These systems gather information from a range of sources, such as public health agencies, hospitals, clinics, and labs, and then analyze the information to look for any unexpected trends or rises in the frequency of diseases.
- *Mechanisms for reporting.* Public health authorities must be notified when instances of certain infectious illnesses are reported by medical professionals and labs. Monitoring these reporting systems can aid in the detection of epidemics and offer details on the people impacted by the outbreak as well as its intensity.
- *Social media.* Social media platforms such as Twitter, Facebook, and Instagram are increasingly being utilized as a tool for public health surveillance. Researchers may monitor public opinion and spot possible epidemics in real time using data from these platforms.
- *Reports from the community.* Communities may help identify epidemics. For instance, people can alert their local health department about an increase in a certain disease in their area so that they can investigate and take appropriate action.

To sum up, a collaborative effort by public health officials, healthcare professionals, laboratories, and the community is necessary to identify outbreaks. Public health personnel may swiftly spot epidemics and take the required action to stop their spread by keeping an eye on news sources, surveillance and reporting systems, social media, and community reporting.

2.4 Analyzing Records

There are a few processes and technologies that may be utilized to assist with the study, even if it can be a difficult process to analyze patterns and outbreaks. These are some crucial actions to think about:

1. *Data collection.* Gathering pertinent information is the first stage in assessing patterns and outbreaks. This might contain details about the afflicted group, the area, the symptoms, the time frame, and other pertinent information. Data may be gathered from a variety of places, including public health organizations, hospitals, and other businesses.
2. *Visualize data.* When data has been gathered, it may be beneficial to visualize it to help with the understanding of patterns and trends. To assist in visualizing the data and see any patterns or trends, tools like graphs, charts, and maps can be employed.
3. *Data analysis.* Once the data has been visualized, it may be examined statistically to look for any noteworthy trends or patterns. This might entail tracking trends over time and across various groups, as well as computing metrics like incidence and prevalence rates.

4. *Determine probable reasons.* The following stage is to investigate potential causes when trends and patterns have been discovered. Analyzing demographic and environmental variables as well as potential risk factors and exposures might be part of this.
5. *Communicate findings.* Lastly, it's critical to let relevant parties—like public health officials, healthcare professionals, and the public—know the results of the investigation. This may be used to guide decision-making and action plans.

In general, trend and epidemic analysis necessitates a multidisciplinary strategy that includes data collection, visualization, analysis, and communication. Collaboration between several stakeholders, such as public health authorities, healthcare professionals, and researchers, is also necessary [26].

By offering a safe and decentralized platform for managing health data, enhancing patient outcomes, and cutting costs, blockchain technology has the potential to completely transform the healthcare sector. Following are some examples of blockchain's present and future uses in the healthcare industry:

- *Electronic health records (EHRs).* Health records for patients may be shared and stored securely via blockchain technology between various healthcare organizations and providers. This can boost patient safety, decrease medical mistakes, and improve care coordination.
- *Clinical trials.* Clinical trial data may be safely stored and shared via blockchain, which might hasten the medication development process and enhance patient outcomes.
- *Medical supply chain management.* Pharmaceuticals, medical equipment, and other healthcare supplies may be tracked using blockchain to increase supply chain transparency and lower the danger of fake or subpar goods.
- *Telemedicine.* Blockchain may be used to store and exchange telemedicine records in a safe manner, giving patients access to these services and raising the standard of treatment.
- *Health insurance.* Health insurance claims and payments may be managed using blockchain, which lowers administrative expenses and boosts the effectiveness of the insurance system.
- *Research and development.* Blockchain technology may be used to safely store and distribute research information, which will hasten scientific progress and enhance patient outcomes.

By establishing a secure and impartial platform for collecting and storing medical data, blockchain technology has the potential to revolutionize the way we track illnesses and epidemics [27]. We can enhance care coordination, speed up diagnosis, and ultimately save lives by utilizing the power of blockchain. Let's examine the use of blockchain technology for tracking illness and epidemic breakouts.

2.4.1 Secure Data Sharing

The capacity of blockchain technology to offer safe data transfer is among its most important advantages. We may develop a safe and decentralized platform for data exchange across various healthcare providers and organizations by leveraging blockchain to store medical data, such as patient records, test results, and epidemiological data. The likelihood of medical mistakes can be decreased, and treatment can be better coordinated as a result. For example, blockchain technology can be used to distribute and retain medical data about patients. We can guarantee that patients have access to their medical data regardless of where they seek treatment by building a blockchain network that is open to all healthcare providers. Allowing healthcare professionals to make better-informed judgments and save repeating tests or procedures can assist in enhancing the quality of treatment [28]. In a similar way, epidemiological data may be shared and stored using blockchain. In addition to information on epidemic patterns and transmission rates, this can also contain statistics on illness prevalence, incidence, and fatality rates. We can increase our comprehension of the transmission of illnesses and outbreaks and build more efficient preventive and treatment methods by developing a blockchain network that is accessible to public health organizations, researchers, and other stakeholders.

2.4.2 Real-Time Data Analysis

The capacity of blockchain technology to do real-time data analysis is another important advantage. We can develop a platform for real-time data analysis utilizing blockchain to store and process medical data, allowing healthcare professionals and public health officials to keep track of disease patterns and outbreaks immediately [29]. Cryptographic protocols, for instance, may be used to develop a real-time dashboard that shows important epidemiological data, such as prevalence, incidence, and death rates of diseases, as well as information on the patterns of outbreaks and transmission rates. Public health professionals may then be able to swiftly spot epidemics and take appropriate action to stop them, such as imposing quarantine restrictions or dispersing vaccinations or antiviral drugs. Like how it may be used to anticipate the development of illnesses and epidemics, blockchain technology can be used to develop predictive models [30]. We can examine vast amounts of medical data to find patterns and trends that can aid in forecasting the spread of illnesses and outbreaks by utilizing machine learning algorithms and other cutting-edge analytics techniques. This can make it possible for public health officials and medical professionals to take preventive steps to stop the spread of illnesses and outbreaks, such as putting in place focused vaccination campaigns or imposing quarantine restrictions in high-risk locations.

2.4.3 Improved Patient Privacy and Security

Maintaining patient protection and privacy is one of the biggest difficulties in tracking illnesses and outbreaks. We can build a platform that is extremely secure and safeguards patient privacy by leveraging blockchain technology to store and distribute medical data. Blockchain technology, for instance, may be utilized to develop a safe and secure patient identity system. We can develop a highly secure and impenetrable system that safeguards patient privacy and inhibits identity theft by utilizing blockchain to store patient identification data, such as name, date of birth, and medical history. Like this, a safe and encrypted communications system for healthcare practitioners may be developed using blockchain technology [31]. We can develop a highly secure and impenetrable system that safeguards patient privacy and averts data breaches by utilizing blockchain to store and transfer medical data and communications.

2.4.4 Reduced Costs

Ultimately, the expense of tracking illnesses and outbreaks can be decreased with the use of blockchain technology. We can lower the administrative expenses involved with storing medical data and increase the effectiveness of healthcare systems by utilizing blockchain to store and distribute medical data. Blockchain technology, for instance, may be used to automate a variety of office procedures related to handling medical data, including data entry, data verification, and data reconciliation. We can lessen the administrative strain on healthcare professionals and increase the precision and thoroughness of medical data by automating these procedures. The billing process may also be streamlined with blockchain technology. We can develop a more effective and transparent billing system that lowers the administrative costs related to billing and enhances the accuracy of billing data by utilizing blockchain to store and distribute billing information [32].

Blockchain technology has the potential to revolutionize the way we track diseases and outbreaks, providing a secure and decentralized platform for storing and sharing medical data. However, there are still challenges that need to be addressed. Nevertheless, blockchain technology is an area of interest for healthcare providers, public health officials, and researchers.

2.4.5 Algorithm to Store Data in a Blockchain Way

1. Define the data structure for the blockchain (e.g., linked list).
2. Create a new block:
   - Define the block structure (e.g., previous block hash, time stamp, data).
   - Assign the previous block hash as the hash of the previous block.
   - Set the time stamp for the new block.
   - Add the new disease/outbreak data to the block.
3. Hash the data:
   - Use a cryptographic hash function (e.g., SHA-256) to hash the data.
   - Store the hashed data in the block.
4. Add the block to the blockchain:
   - Verify that the previous block hash matches the hash of the previous block in the chain.
   - Add the new block to the end of the chain.
   - Update the hash of the current block to include the hash of the previous block.
5. Repeat the process as needed to add additional disease/outbreak data to the blockchain.
6. To query the blockchain for disease/outbreak data:
   - Start at the most recent block in the chain.
   - Verify the hash of the block to ensure it has not been tampered with.
   - If the block contains the desired disease/outbreak data, return the data.
   - If not, move to the previous block in the chain and repeat steps 2–3 until the data is found or the first block in the chain is reached.

Public health professionals and researchers can better understand, stop, and manage the spread of infectious illnesses by studying outbreaks. Early diagnosis and reaction, a better knowledge of the illness, enhanced surveillance, more focused therapies, and better resource allocation are only a few of the major advantages of outbreak analysis. The capacity to spot emerging outbreaks early and take swift action to stop disease transmission is one of the main advantages of outbreak analysis [33]. Early detection is essential for preventing the spread of infectious illnesses because it enables public health professionals to locate and treat affected people and their contacts, as well as to identify and isolate infected people. For instance, the early discovery of new cases during the COVID-19 pandemic allowed public health officials to adopt extensive testing, contact tracing, and quarantine procedures to stop the disease's spread. Analysis of outbreaks, in addition to early diagnosis and treatment, can help us learn more about the illness itself. Researchers can find trends and risk factors related to the disease, including how it spreads, its symptoms, and the best ways to treat it, by examining outbreak data. This knowledge may be applied to the creation of fresh therapies and preventative measures as well as their improvement [34].

For instance, research on the 2014 Ebola epidemic in West Africa resulted in the creation of fresh medications and vaccines. It is also possible to strengthen disease surveillance systems by analyzing outbreaks. Public health professionals may enhance their surveillance systems to better detect and handle upcoming epidemics by monitoring the disease's progress and spotting prospective outbreaks early. For instance, the development of new tools for identifying and monitoring the transmission of the disease as well as the study of prior epidemics have all contributed to major recent improvements in the worldwide surveillance network for influenza. The capacity to design more-focused measures and stop the spread of the illness is another advantage of studying outbreaks. Public health professionals can create more effective preventative and control plans by identifying high-risk people and the regions that are most affected by the illness. Public health professionals, for instance, employed outbreak analysis during the HIV/AIDS pandemic to pinpoint high-risk groups and create specialized preventive and treatment plans to stop the disease's spread. Analysis of epidemics can aid in ensuring efficient and effective resource allocation. Public health officials may direct resources, such as cash, staff, and medical supplies, to the regions most in need by identifying the places where the illness is most prevalent. This can guarantee that resources are spent wisely and that the epidemic response is as successful as it can be. It enables public health authorities and academics to identify epidemics early, enhance surveillance systems, design more focused therapies, and efficiently allocate resources. As the globe continues to encounter new and emerging infectious illnesses, the study of outbreaks will continue to be a crucial tool for preserving public health.

2.5 Building a Blockchain Network

To create a safe, scalable, and effective blockchain network, a few technological factors need to be carefully considered. Consensus methods, network design, data storage and administration, the creation of smart contracts, and security protocols are some of the key technical factors to consider while constructing a blockchain network.

- *Consensus mechanisms.* The collection of guidelines that govern how transactions are validated and added to the blockchain is known as consensus mechanisms. There are several possible consensus techniques, including Byzantine fault tolerance, delegated proof-of-stake (DPoS), proof-of-work (PoW), and proof-of-stake

(PoS) (BFT). The selection of a consensus mechanism will rely on the particular requirements of the network, and each method has strengths and drawbacks of its own.

- *Network architecture.* The blockchain network's architecture is another crucial factor. Peer-to-peer (P2P) networks and client–server networks are two possible network structures. P2P networks might be more challenging to operate and grow, but they are often more decentralized and resistant to assaults. Although more centralized, client–server networks might be simpler to run and expand [35].
- *Data management and storage.* Creating a blockchain network requires careful consideration of data management and storage. The network must be able to handle high amounts of data, while the data being stored on the blockchain must be safe and unchangeable. To guarantee that the data is kept effectively and securely, it is crucial to select the appropriate database technology. To guarantee that the blockchain can be updated over time, it is also necessary to put in place efficient data management procedures.
- *Smart contract development.* Self-executing contracts, known as "smart contracts," are kept on a blockchain. They can automate intricate business procedures and guarantee that transactions are carried out in accordance with predetermined regulations. Programming languages like Solidity, which is used to create smart contracts on the Ethereum network, are necessary for creating smart contracts. Smart contracts must be carefully tested and audited to make sure they are safe and work as intended.
- *Security protocols.* Security is an important factor in developing a blockchain network. The network needs to be built to withstand intrusions and preserve the integrity of the data kept on the blockchain. Role-based access control, multi-factor authentication, and other security methods can prevent illegal network access. Regular security audits and penetration tests are crucial to finding and fixing network vulnerabilities.
- *Scalability.* While developing a blockchain network, scalability is a crucial factor. The network must be able to manage the additional load as it expands, and new transactions are added without sluggishness or instability. Shading, off-chain transactions, and side chains are some of the scaling options that are accessible. The network's unique requirements will determine the best scaling option [36].
- *Interoperability.* Interoperability refers to the capacity of several blockchain networks to interact and communicate with one another. This is crucial for developing a more integrated and functional blockchain ecosystem. Interoperability may be achieved through the adoption of standards such as ERC-20 (Ethereum Request for Comments), which provides a common interface for tokens on the Ethereum network.

Several technological factors need to be carefully considered while developing a blockchain network. Performance, security, and usability of the network will all be significantly impacted by the consensus process used as well as network design, data storage and administration, smart contract creation, security protocols, scalability, and interoperability. Building a safe, scalable, and effective blockchain network is attainable by carefully considering certain technological factors [37]. Although connecting several blockchain networks might be difficult, doing so is crucial for the acceptance and development of the blockchain. For blockchain to realize its full potential and allow decentralized apps that can function across several networks, interoperability is essential. Many strategies exist for connecting several blockchain networks for efficient communication.

Interoperability protocols. Interoperability protocols allow various blockchain networks to connect with one another. The transmission of data and assets between multiple blockchains is made possible by these protocols, which serve as bridges between them. Protocols for interoperability include Polkadot and Cosmos, for instance. A relay chain is used by the multi-chain, sharded Polkadot network to link its several parallel chains. The relay chain offers a safe way to transport assets and data across them, and each parallel chain may be tailored to fit the requirements of a particular use case. In contrast, the hub-and-spoke architecture of Cosmos connects many separate blockchain networks, or "zones," through a single hub. Each zone has its own governance and consensus process, enabling compatibility between various blockchain networks.

Cross-chain bridges. Bridges that span various blockchain networks are known as cross-chain bridges. Using smart contracts, they enable the transfer of assets and data between several blockchains. By locking assets on one blockchain and releasing an equal representation of those assets on another blockchain, cross-chain bridges function. The assets may be unlocked and transferred back to the original blockchain because of the reversible nature of this operation.

For instance, the Polygon network employs cross-chain bridges to link up with Ethereum and Binance smart chain, among other blockchain networks [38]. This makes it possible for smooth asset transfers and blockchain interoperability.

Atomic swaps. These allow for the immediate transfer of digital assets between various blockchain networks. Atomic swaps enable the exchange of cryptocurrencies without the need for a middleman or centralized exchange by using smart contracts. For instance, a user doesn't need to go through an exchange if they wish to exchange Bitcoin for Ethereum directly via an atomic swap. Because the smart contract guarantees that both parties would get their assets simultaneously, this procedure is safe and devoid of trust. The acceptance and expansion of blockchain technology depend on the interconnection of several blockchain networks for efficient communication. It makes it possible to build decentralized applications that can run on several blockchain networks and give consumers additional alternatives for trading and transferring assets [39,40].

Blockchain is a decentralized digital ledger technology that may be applied to monitor and verify information securely and openly. Blockchain technology has several possible uses, including outbreak reporting, where it might be applied to provide a safe and impenetrable record of disease outbreaks. Here are several strategies for creating epidemic reports on blockchain:

- *Tokenization.* Tokenization can be used as a reward for reporting outbreaks. Healthcare professionals, researchers, and individuals who promptly and accurately report outbreaks can all be rewarded with tokens. These tokens may be used to pay for services connected to outbreak management and prevention, or they can be traded for other cryptocurrencies.
- *Decentralized applications (DApps).* To make outbreak reporting easier, decentralized applications may be created on top of the blockchain. These DApps may be employed to gather information from a variety of sources, including social media, news organizations, and official reports, and to provide a safe and open record of disease outbreaks. To aid academics and decision-makers in understanding how diseases spread, these DApps may be used to visualize and map epidemic data [41].

- *Permissioned blockchain.* Using permissioned blockchain, disease outbreaks may be recorded in a safe and unchangeable manner. Only authorized users have access to add, change, and remove data on a permissioned blockchain. This guarantees the reliability and accuracy of the data. A centralized outbreak reporting system that is only available to authorized individuals may be built using a permissioned blockchain.
- *Data analytics.* A lot of data on disease outbreaks may be gathered and stored using blockchain technology. Data analytics technologies may be used to examine this data and find patterns and trends in disease outbreaks. Better epidemic management and prevention methods may be created using the information provided.

Blockchain can revolutionize outbreak reporting by creating a secure and transparent record of disease outbreaks, using smart contracts, tokenization, decentralized applications, permissioned blockchain, and data analytics. This can help researchers and policymakers better understand the spread of disease and develop better outbreak management and prevention strategies [42].

There are several key disadvantages to consider even if blockchain technology has the potential to revolutionize the medical industry. Data privacy is one of the primary issues. Healthcare information is frequently delicate and private, and there is a chance that unwanted parties might obtain this information [43]. Although blockchain is intended to be safe and unbreakable, it is nevertheless feasible for users to track transactions and recognize specific users based on their activity on the blockchain. Large-scale medical applications may encounter difficulties because blockchain networks might slow down and become ineffective when they get too big. Moreover, healthcare practitioners can lack the expertise and abilities needed to deploy and manage blockchain technology due to its complexity. Lastly, the cost of integrating blockchain technology, especially for smaller healthcare providers, may prevent the technology from becoming widely used in the industry. Thus, while blockchain technology has the potential to change the medical industry, these disadvantages and limits must be carefully examined before applying it to healthcare applications [44].

2.6 Scaling Blockchain Network

The ability to detect and respond to disease outbreaks using blockchain technology has the potential to improve public health. Blockchain can help assure the accuracy and privacy of health data, promote real-time tracking of epidemics, and enable efficient response tactics because of its decentralized, tamper-proof, and transparent nature [45]. This chapter will go through how blockchain might make monitoring illness and epidemic breakouts easier. First, blockchain can enhance the security and integrity of data. Conventional healthcare systems are centralized, which implies that health information is kept in one place and managed by a small number of people or businesses [46]. This centralized system is susceptible to cyberattacks and data leaks. On the other hand, a decentralized system like blockchain distributes data among a network of computers. The blockchain's blocks are extremely hard to alter since each one has a distinct cryptographic hash. This guarantees the accuracy and confidentiality of health data, which is essential for monitoring disease outbreaks [47]. Second, blockchain can help track epidemics in real time. The manual reporting process used by traditional disease surveillance systems can be sluggish and prone to inaccuracy. Data may be captured in real time with blockchain, making it possible to identify epidemics more rapidly and precisely. Blockchain may be used, for example, to track the movement of individuals in risky places, keep track of disease outbreaks, and find probable infection origins. Public health professionals may use this real-time data to make well-informed choices about how to handle epidemics. The third benefit of blockchain is that it can facilitate better communication and coordination between public health officials and healthcare professionals [48]. Due to the fragmentation of traditional healthcare systems, many providers may use various data structures and protocol types. Sharing information and organizing epidemic responses may be challenging as a result. Public health officials, providers, and other parties may safely and openly exchange health data using blockchain. This may make it possible for collaboration and coordination to be more effective, which may speed up and improve the efficiency of epidemic containment. Lastly, blockchain can improve data ownership and privacy [49]. Patient privacy is frequently prioritized above data ownership and management in traditional healthcare systems. Patients may find it challenging to obtain their health information as a result, making it more difficult to prevent and treat disease [50]. Patients may own and control their own health data thanks to blockchain. Patients may have more choice over how their information is used and shared as a result, which may increase public confidence in the healthcare system and spur more individuals to take part in illness tracking and preventive initiatives. Blockchain has the power to completely change how we monitor and handle disease outbreaks. Blockchain can assist guarantee that epidemics are discovered and contained promptly and efficiently by strengthening data integrity and security, enabling real-time tracking, enhancing cooperation and coordination, and enhancing privacy and data ownership. Although there are still obstacles to overcome when deploying blockchain-based solutions, the advantages are obvious, and it is expected that blockchain technology in healthcare will be more widely used in the years to come.

2.6.1 Data Integrity and Usage

A critical component of preserving the quality and integrity of medical records is updating medical data on the blockchain. Medical data may be stored securely and decentralized using blockchain technology, which also makes the data tamper-proof and only accessible to authorized employees. Here are some things to keep in mind when updating medical data on blockchain:

- *Patient consent.* When it comes to updating medical data on the blockchain, patient consent is the most important factor to consider. Prior to having their medical information published on the blockchain, patients must give their express approval. A clear understanding of how the data will be used, who will have access to it, and how long it will be held should be included in the consent.
- *Data quality.* When it comes to updating medical data on the blockchain, data quality is still another crucial factor. The information must be true, full, and current. By offering a safe and transparent mechanism to trace the data's beginnings and history, blockchain technology can guarantee the quality of the data.
- *Audit trail.* An audit trail is a record of every transaction that has ever taken place on a blockchain. An audit trail can give a thorough account of who has accessed the data, when they did so, and what modifications have been done. The medical data saved on the blockchain may benefit from an additional degree of security and accountability provided by an audit trail.

Patient permission, data privacy, interoperability, data quality, and audit trail are important factors to consider while updating medical data on a blockchain. Blockchain technology can transform the healthcare sector by enhancing patient outcomes, lowering costs, and boosting efficiency. It offers a safe and transparent means to store and communicate medical data [51].

The way we identify and monitor disease epidemics might be completely transformed by blockchain technology. Blockchain can speed up the detection and containment of epidemics by supplying a decentralized, open, and unchangeable record of health data. The capacity of blockchain technology to store and distribute data transparently and securely is one of the major advantages it has for illness diagnosis. Healthcare providers and academics may safely exchange health data on a blockchain network without worrying about data loss or unwanted access [52]. As a result of healthcare practitioners being able to communicate and work together more readily, illnesses and epidemics may be detected quicker and with greater accuracy. In general, blockchain technology has the power to completely change how we identify and address disease epidemics. Blockchain can enable quicker and more accurate epidemic detection, as well as a more efficient and effective response, by offering a secure, open, and decentralized platform for health data. Although there are still issues to be resolved, such as protecting privacy and data security, blockchain technology has the potential to be very beneficial. In addition, a decentralized system for disease surveillance can be developed using blockchain technology [53]. Healthcare providers may track epidemics in real time using a blockchain-based network of linked devices, enabling early identification and response. This may be especially helpful in regions with few resources and insufficient traditional disease surveillance systems. The usage of smart contracts is another possible blockchain use in the field of illness diagnosis. With smart contracts, the details of the agreement between the buyer and the seller are directly encoded into lines of code [54]. These contracts self-execute. Smart contracts may be used to automate data collection, analysis, and reaction in the context of illness detection. A smart contract might be set up, for instance, to automatically give resources to afflicted areas or to send out an alarm once a particular threshold of illness cases is achieved.

2.7 Conclusion

In conclusion, using blockchain technology to track outbreaks has the potential to completely transform how diseases are monitored and dealt with. The accuracy and transparency of data pertaining to epidemics may be helped to assure by the decentralized and irreversible nature of blockchain, which lowers the chance of fraud, mistakes, and manipulation. Information exchange across different stakeholders, such as public health authorities, healthcare providers, and individuals, may be made more efficient and safer. Blockchain can also facilitate the creation of decentralized contact tracking systems, which can aid in the identification and isolation of affected people and stop the spread of the illness.

References

[1] Hasselgren, A., Kralevska, K., Gligoroski, D., Pedersen, S. A., & Faxvaag, A. (2020). Blockchain in healthcare and health sciences—A scoping review. *International Journal of Medical Informatics, 134*, 104040.

[2] Yaqoob, I., Salah, K., Jayaraman, R., & Al-Hammadi, Y. (2021). Blockchain for healthcare data management: Opportunities, challenges, and future recommendations. *Neural Computing and Applications*, 1–16.

[3] McGhin, T., Choo, K. K. R., Liu, C. Z., & He, D. (2019). Blockchain in healthcare applications: Research challenges and opportunities. *Journal of Network and Computer Applications*, 135, 62–75.

[4] Fusco, A., Dicuonzo, G., Dell'Atti, V., & Tatullo, M. (2020). Blockchain in healthcare: Insights on COVID-19. *International Journal of Environmental Research and Public Health*, 17(19), 7167.

[5] Tandon, A., Dhir, A., Islam, A. N., & Mäntymäki, M. (2020). Blockchain in healthcare: A systematic literature review, synthesizing framework and future research agenda. *Computers in Industry*, 122, 103290.

[6] Chukwu, E., & Garg, L. (2020). A systematic review of blockchain in healthcare: Frameworks, prototypes, and implementations. *IEEE Access*, 8, 21196–214.

[7] Chen, H. S., Jarrell, J. T., Carpenter, K. A., Cohen, D. S., & Huang, X. (2019). Blockchain in healthcare: A patient-centered model. *Biomedical Journal of Scientific & Technical Research*, 20(3), 15017.

[8] Ismail, L., Materwala, H., & Zeadally, S. (2019). Lightweight blockchain for healthcare. *IEEE Access*, 7, 149935–51.

[9] Soltanisehat, L., Alizadeh, R., Hao, H., & Choo, K. K. R. (2020). Technical, temporal, and spatial research challenges and opportunities in blockchain-based healthcare: A systematic literature review. *IEEE Transactions on Engineering Management*, 70(1), 353–368. https://doi.org/10.1109/TEM.2020.3013507.

[10] Singh, A. P., Pradhan, N. R., Luhach, A. K., Agnihotri, S., Jhanjhi, N. Z., Verma, S., . . . & Roy, D. S. (2020). A novel patient-centric architectural framework for blockchain-enabled healthcare applications. *IEEE Transactions on Industrial Informatics*, 17(8), 5779–89.

[11] Abdellatif, A. A., Al-Marridi, A. Z., Mohamed, A., Erbad, A., Chiasserini, C. F., & Refaey, A. (2020). ssHealth: Toward secure, blockchain-enabled healthcare systems. *IEEE Network*, 34(4), 312–19.

[12] Jaiman, V., & Urovi, V. (2020). A consent model for blockchain-based health data sharing platforms. *IEEE Access*, 8, 143734–45.

[13] El-Gazzar, R., & Stendal, K. (2020). Blockchain in health care: Hope or hype? *Journal of Medical Internet Research*, 22(7), e17199.

[14] Prokofieva, M., & Miah, S. J. (2019). Blockchain in healthcare. *Australasian Journal of Information Systems*, 23.

[15] Chen, M., Malook, T., Rehman, A. U., Muhammad, Y., Alshehri, M. D., Akbar, A., . . . & Khan, M. A. (2021). Blockchain-enabled healthcare system for detection of diabetes. *Journal of Information Security and Applications*, 58, 102771.

[16] Agbo, C. C., & Mahmoud, Q. H. (2020). Blockchain in healthcare: Opportunities, challenges, and possible solutions. *International Journal of Healthcare Information Systems and Informatics (IJHISI)*, 15(3), 82–97.

[17] Capece, G., & Lorenzi, F. (2020). Blockchain and healthcare: Opportunities and prospects for the EHR. *Sustainability*, 12(22), 9693.

[18] Onik, M. M. H., Aich, S., Yang, J., Kim, C. S., & Kim, H. C. (2019). Blockchain in healthcare: Challenges and solutions. In *Big data analytics for intelligent healthcare management* (pp. 197–226). Academic Press.

[19] Azbeg, K., Ouchetto, O., Andaloussi, S. J., & Fetjah, L. (2021). *A taxonomic review of the use of IoT and blockchain in healthcare applications*. IRBM.

[20] Jennath, H. S., Anoop, V. S., & Asharaf, S. (2020). Blockchain for healthcare: Securing patient data and enabling trusted artificial intelligence. *International Journal of Interactive Multimedia and Artificial Intelligence*, 6(3), 15–23. https://doi.org/10.9781/ijimai.2020.07.002.

[21] Rajora, N. (2022). Blockchain technology—A basic need of the pharmaceutical industry. *International Journal*, 10(4).

[22] Bhatia, D., Mishra, A., & Prasad, A. K. (2022). Blockchain technology for biomedical engineering applications. In *Applications of blockchain and big IoT systems* (pp. 245–66). Apple Academic Press.

[23] Ghazal, T. M., Hasan, M. K., Abdullah, S. N. H. S., Bakar, K. A. A., Taleb, N., Al-Dmour, N. A., . . . & Alshurideh, M. (2023). An integrated cloud and blockchain enabled platforms for

[24] Saddikuti, V., Galwankar, S., & Akilesh Sai, S. V. (2023). Application of blockchain technology in healthcare supply chains. In *Blockchain in healthcare: From disruption to integration* (pp. 215–23). Springer International Publishing.

[25] Elangovan, D., Long, C. S., Bakrin, F. S., Tan, C. S., Goh, K. W., Yeoh, S. F., . . . & Ming, L. C. (2022). The use of blockchain technology in the health care sector: Systematic review. *JMIR Medical Informatics*, 10(1), e17278.

[26] Kumari, M., Gupta, M., & Ved, C. (2022). Decentralized and secured applications of blockchain in the biomedical domain. In *Applications of blockchain and big IoT systems* (pp. 267–82). Apple Academic Press.

[27] Khan, D., Low, T. J., & Dang, V. T. B. (2022, December). Challenges and application of blockchain in healthcare systems. In *2022 international conference on digital transformation and intelligence (ICDI)* (pp. 15–20). IEEE.

[28] Sai, S., Chamola, V., Choo, K. K. R., Sikdar, B., & Rodrigues, J. J. (2023). Confluence of blockchain and artificial intelligence technologies for secure and scalable healthcare solutions: A review. IEEE Internet of Things Journal, 10(7), 5873–5897. https://doi.org/10.1109/JIOT.2022.3232793.

[29] Jyothilakshmi, K. B., Robins, V., & Mahesh, A. S. (2022). A comparative analysis between hyperledger fabric and ethereum in medical sector: A systematic review. In *Sustainable communication networks and application lecture notes on data engineering and communications technologies*. Springer. https://doi.org/10.1007/978-981-16-6605-6_5.

[30] Abdallah, S., & Nizamuddin, N. (2023). Blockchain based solution for Pharma Supply Chain Industry. *Computers & Industrial Engineering*, 108997.

[31] Xu, X., & He, Y. (2022). Blockchain application in modern logistics information sharing: A review and case study analysis. *Production Planning & Control*, 1–15.

[32] Mhamdi, H., Othman, S. B., Zouinkhi, A., & Sakli, H. (2022). Blockchain technology in healthcare: Use cases study. In *Intelligent healthcare: Infrastructure, algorithms and management* (pp. 261–79). Springer Nature Singapore.

[33] Rahman, M. S., Islam, M. A., Uddin, M. A., & Stea, G. (2022). A survey of blockchain-based IoT eHealthcare: Applications, research issues, and challenges. *Internet of Things*, 19, 100551.

[34] Bhushan, S., Kumar, P., Garg, A. K., & Nair, S. (2022). Blockchain powered vaccine efficacy for pharma sector. *Computational & Mathematical Methods in Medicine*, 2022, 4862742. https://doi.org/10.1155/2022/4862742.

[35] Awotunde, J. B., Chakraborty, C., & Folorunso, S. O. (2022). A secured smart healthcare monitoring systems using blockchain technology. In *Intelligent Internet of Things for healthcare and industry* (pp. 127–43). Springer International Publishing.

[36] Hang, L., Chen, C., Zhang, L., & Yang, J. (2022). Blockchain for applications of clinical trials: Taxonomy, challenges, and future directions. *IET Communications*, 16(20), 2371–93.

[37] Mhamdi, H., Soufiene, B. O., Zouinkhi, A., Almalki, F. A., & Sakli, H. (2022). Blockchain technology in healthcare: A systematic review. *Blockchain Technology in Healthcare Applications*, 199–214.

[38] Rajawat, A. S., Bedi, P., Goyal, S. B., Shaw, R. N., Ghosh, A., & Aggarwal, S. (2022). Ai and blockchain for healthcare data security in smart cities. *AI and IoT for Smart City Applications*, 185–98.

[39] Ramzan, S., Aqdus, A., Ravi, V., Koundal, D., Amin, R., & Al Ghamdi, M. A. (2022). Healthcare applications using blockchain technology: Motivations and challenges. *IEEE Transactions on Engineering Management*, 70(8), 2874–2890. https://doi.org/10.1109/TEM.2022.3189734.

[40] Mamun, Q. (2022). Blockchain technology in the future of healthcare. *Smart Health*, 23, 100223.

[41] Deshmukh, A., Tyagi, A. K., Hansora, H., & Menon, S. C. (2023). Applications of distributed ledger (blockchain) technology in e-healthcare. In *The Internet of Medical Things (IoMT) and telemedicine frameworks and applications* (pp. 248–61). IGI Global.

[42] Poongodi, T., Ilango, S. S., Gupta, V., & Prasad, S. K. (2022). Influence of blockchain technology in pharmaceutical industries. In *Blockchain technology for emerging applications* (pp. 267–96). Academic Press.

[43] Dashtizadeh, M., Meskaran, F., & Tan, D. (2022, October). A secure blockchain-based pharmaceutical supply chain management system: Traceability and detection of counterfeit COVID-19

vaccines. In *2022 IEEE 2nd Mysore sub section international conference (MysuruCon)* (pp. 1–5). IEEE.
[44] Yakubu, A. M., & Chen, Y. P. P. (2022). A blockchain-based application for genomic access and variant discovery using smart contracts and homomorphic encryption. *Future Generation Computer Systems*, 137, 234–47.
[45] Ghosh, P. K., Chakraborty, A., Hasan, M., Rashid, K., & Siddique, A. H. (2023). Blockchain application in healthcare systems: A review. *Systems*, 11(1), 38.
[46] Jayaraman, R., Srivastava, A., & Kumar, M. (2022). Blockchain technology for protection of biomedical documents in healthcare society. *International Journal of Internet Technology and Secured Transactions*, 12(6), 566–82.
[47] Fiore, M., Capodici, A., Rucci, P., Bianconi, A., Longo, G., Ricci, M., . . . & Golinelli, D. (2023). Blockchain for the healthcare supply chain: A systematic literature review. *Applied Sciences*, 13(2), 686.
[48] Sravanthi, C., & Chowdary, S. (2022). Deep learning and blockchain for electronic health record in healthcare system. In *Intelligent system design: Proceedings of INDIA 2022* (pp. 429–36). Springer Nature Singapore.
[49] Vîrgolici, H. M., Ceban, D., Răducu, R. C., & Purcărea, V. L. (2021). Blockchain technology used in medicine. A brief survey. *Romanian Journal of Military Medicine*, 125(3), 506.
[50] Bennacer, S. A., Sabiri, K., Aaroud, A., Akodadi, K., & Cherradi, B. (2023). A comprehensive survey on blockchain-based healthcare industry: applications and challenges. *Indonesian Journal of Electrical Engineering and Computer Science*, 30(3), 1558–71.
[51] Xi, P., Zhang, X., Wang, L., Liu, W., & Peng, S. (2022). A review of blockchain-based secure sharing of healthcare data. *Applied Sciences*, 12(15), 7912.
[52] Ali, O., Jaradat, A., Ally, M., & Rotabi, S. (2022). Blockchain technology enables healthcare data management and accessibility. *Blockchain Technologies for Sustainability*, 91–118.
[53] Rawat, R. (2022). A systematic review of blockchain technology use in e-supply chain in internet of medical things (IOMT). *International Journal of Computations, Information and Manufacturing (IJCIM)*, 2(2).
[54] Attaran, M. (2022). Blockchain technology in healthcare: Challenges and opportunities. *International Journal of Healthcare Management*, 15(1), 70–83.

3

Blockchain: A Decentralized, Persistent, Immutable, Consensus, and Irrevocable System in Healthcare

Dipa K. Israni and Mansi K. Shah

3.1 Introduction

After the October 2008 publication of the Bitcoin white paper, blockchain became a distributed ledger system that was widely recognized. The primary benefit of blockchain, which serves as the foundational technology for Bitcoin, is that it enables the interchange of digital currency among users in a dispersed manner, without the need for a centrally controlled, trustworthy third-party network. The implementation of the Bitcoin cryptocurrency included the publication of the code as open-source, allowing others to alter and enhance it to produce subsequent versions of blockchain-based technologies [1].

The early uses of blockchain-based coins like Bitcoin make up blockchain 1.0, the first version of the technology. To mention a few, other blockchain 1.0 platforms include Litecoin, Monero, and Dash. With blockchain 2.0, smart contracts and smart assets were released, the second iteration of the technology. Digital characteristics or assets that can be managed via a blockchain-based network are referred to as smart properties. The software programs known as smart contracts include the regulations and procedures for handling and governing smart properties. The coins Ethereum, Ethereum Classic, NEO, and QTUMare examples of blockchain cryptocurrencies [1].

Adding to what was said earlier, blockchain 3.0, the third iteration of technological innovation, is now focused on uses outside of the banking sector. In order to achieve this, efforts have been made to broaden the scope of science by possible applications outside of the financial industry, enabling various industries to utilize the exciting features from blockchain. Healthcare has become a prominent business where many use cases have been established for the application of blockchain due to the growing relevance in blockchain technology and its acceptance by many organizations and sectors [1].

Blockchain is a decentralized ledger technology (DLT) that uses cryptographic codes to connect an increasing sequence of immutable blocks to safely store data on a P2P network. A decentralized record of events, called a distributed ledger, is shared and synchronized by numerous peers. When new information is added, records are immediately changed, and each node has an exact duplicate of each record. Consensus is a crucial idea in blockchain technology. All participants in the blockchain have access to new data and can approve or refuse it by reaching a consensus. Data is entered into the logbook as a series of "blocks" and is unchangeable once it has been authorized. This is one of the greatest advantages of ledger technology. Smart contracts, which are self-executing contracts built on blockchain technology and autonomously initiate actions or payments once conditions are met, are another noteworthy feature introduced by blockchain [2].

Upcoming innovations will involve using real-time data, such GPS data, to start operations like the transfer of money and control. The technology has the ability to drastically change corporate strategies by shifting them from a concentrated to a decentralized strategy, even if it is still under development and validation. The top five industries now employing blockchain technology are oil and gas, finance, healthcare, logistics/supply chain, legal, and government [2].

However, it is believed that blockchain science has the ability to greatly enhance healthcare data networks. In the present review, working of blockchain technology, its applications, constraints, and healthcare challenges will be discussed.

3.2 Type of Blockchains

When creating a blockchain-based solution, we would first determine which form of blockchain is best suited to the project. As a result, it is critical to have a thorough grasp of the blockchain structure choices.

Blockchain can be un-permissioned (public blockchain), permissioned (private blockchain), or both (hybrid blockchain) [3].

3.2.1 Un-Permissioned or Public Blockchains

When nodes linked to the network have the ability to access the Internet, the record is referred to as an un-permissions database or a public blockchain. An *un-permissioned blockchain* is a decentralized network that allows everyone to connect and verify transactions [3]. As a consequence, using a consensus algorithm like PoW, or proof-of-stake, any network member can confirm a transaction and take part in the approval process. The main goal of a blockchain is to do away with centralized control in the trade of digital assets. P2P transactions generate a chain block, which ensures decentralization. Before being recorded in the system's unchangeable database, each transaction is connected to the preceding transaction via the cryptographic hash Merkle tree as a part of the chains.

As a result, the blockchain operation record is compatible with and synchronized with all network servers. Everyone with a laptop and a cyberspace connection can register as a node and gain access to the entire blockchain database. The technique is entirely secure because every server in the network repeats synchronized un-permissioned blockchains. However, the process of verifying transactions on this form of blockchain has been slow and inefficient. Each transaction requires a substantial amount of electrical power, and this power should grow considerably as each node is integrated into the network [4]. For example, Bitcoin, Ethereum, and Litecoin [5,6].

3.2.2 Permissioned or Private Blockchains

A permissioned blockchain is a restricted or limited blockchain that only works within a specific network. It is most commonly used within a company where only a subset of employees participates in a blockchain network [3]. This type of limited blockchain allows for the reintroduction of a middleman. Commercial blockchains strictly control network data access authorization. Nodes in the P2P network cannot perform transaction verification and validation without authorization. It is most commonly used within a company where only a subset of employees participates in a blockchain network. This type of restricted blockchain allows for the payback of a middleman. Commercial blockchains rigorously regulate network data access authorization [7]. For example, Ripple, Hyperledger [5,6].

3.2.3 Hybrid Blockchain

A mixed blockchain combines the advantages of private (permissioned) and public (permissionless) blockchains. Hybrid blockchain is tailored to specific industries and is designed to meet a variety of company requirements. It allows organizations to set up a restricted, approval-based system alongside a community, approval-less system, giving them control over who has ability to view blockchain data and what data is made public. For example, IBM Food Trust [5].

3.2.4 Consortium or Federated Blockchain

To complete transactions, consortium blockchain makes use of both permissioned and un-permissioned blockchains. They are governed by a small group of individuals and forbid outside parties from confirming transactions. Viewing transactions is available to anybody, while writing transactions requires membership in a particular group [8]. A consortium is a combination of permissioned and un-permissioned blockchains that is partly decentralized. In a blockchain network, every data exchange has the option to be either open or confidential, and nodes have the authority to select them beforehand. Permissioned blockchains and consortiums are not the same entity. Consortium blockchains, in general, are hybrid models that combine highly trusted permissioned blockchains with untrustworthy, un-permissioned blockchain entity models. Permissioned blockchains are conventional controlled systems with a powerful encoding model to check and confirm network transactions. The consortium blockchains' development in terms of dependability, authenticity, and precision is still being defined [9]. For instance, Hyperledger Fabric [5,6].

3.3 Advantages of Utilizing Blockchain Technology in Healthcare

Traditional tasks like tracking things, keeping track of orders, receipts, invoicing, payments, and so on can be completed quickly with a blockchain-based medical supply chain [10]. In addition, blockchain offers the advantages, capabilities, and ability to address a number of problems, some of which are described in what follows and illustrated in Table 3.1.

3.3.1 Immutability and Data Integrity

Immutability means that once every transaction has been documented on the blockchain, nobody will be able to insert, erase, or amend any information. Because every action is time- and date-stamped, the blockchain is a permanent repository [11].

3.3.2 Decentralized Technology

Because the network is decentralized, there is no governing body or singular point of contact. Instead, a group of nodes manages the system, making it distributed [5].

3.3.3 Enhanced Speed and Efficiency

A blockchain-based system aids in completing deals in a timely manner. There is no need for paper labor, because the blockchain system stores all transactional information and user password [11].

3.3.4 Transparency

Each participant has a duplicate of all the info. Without the consent of the plurality of nodes, no one is permitted to add any transaction entries to the ledger. This makes the system more transparent and prevents scams by enabling companies to monitor every aspect of it [5].

3.3.5 Scalable and Dispersed

A distributed ledger system's backend is made up of a network of processors, each of which contains apps and data. This department makes ensuring that the system is easily accessible and efficient [2].

3.3.6 Security and Privacy

Because blockchain saves data over a network and inhibits undesired activities, which helps avoid data breaches, encryption from end to end is made for the purpose of maintaining archives of data and interactions forever [11].

3.3.7 Distributed Ledgers

These are a class of databases that are shared, copied, and synced among the users of a decentralized network. An exact duplicate of a ledger will be stored on each collaborating node [5].

3.3.8 Consensus

Consensus is an algorithmic procedure that makes sure each server only has access to one duplicate of each document. Agreement methods guarantee accurate and truthful records [5].

3.3.9 Open Source

Blockchain gives everyone in the network access to open source with a feeling of order [12].

3.3.10 Anonymity

As data is transferred between nodes, the individual's name stays hidden [12].

TABLE 3.1

Characteristics and Advantages of Blockchain in Healthcare System

Characteristics of Blockchain	Advantages of Blockchain
Accurate Data	Deterministic patient data available
Safety and Transparency	Transparency in data availability to various medical practitioners
Data Security and Privacy	Cryptography and dual public/private key
Efficiency	Low cost of transactions between agents
Interoperability	Harmonized between healthcare datasets through the exchange of data regarding health

3.3.11 Uniqueness and Ownership

Every document that is traded on the blockchain maintains ownership information with a distinct hash number [12].

3.3.12 Provenance

Every object in the blockchain has a digital record document that demonstrates its validity and origin [12].

3.3.13 Smart Contracting

In smart contracting, each node is given a unique address, so the information saved in the network is only available to the nodes that are participating and not to the other nodes [13].

3.4 Blockchain Technologies

3.4.1 Ethereum

Ethereum is a decentralized program that allows for the use of smart contracts. Smart contracts allow parties to trade money, shares, and other assets. Peer-to-peer (P2P) transfers are also possible on the Ethereum network [11].

3.4.2 Smart Contract

Other parties are not needed to validate transactions in smart contracts because they run on the blockchain and contain all relevant information. Implementation is simple, economical, and secure [11].

3.4.3 Solidity

Smart contracts are executed using Solidity. It uses a complex computer language. The Ethereum network for the blockchain's smart contracts is developed using the object-oriented computer language Solidity [11].

3.4.4 Express.js

The application program interfaces (APIs) of the Node.js web server can be streamlined, and new capabilities can be added with the help of the little framework called Express. By the use of middleware and navigation, it streamlines the arrangement of the features in your application [11].

3.4.5 Ganache

In a permissioned Ethereum blockchain called Ganache, users can test out and freely employ smart contracts. With Ganache, we can create, distribute, and test our applications throughout the entire development cycle in a safe and controlled setting [11].

3.4.6 React

The development of dynamic user interfaces is made easier with React. At each phase of your application, create straightforward views, and React will update and show only the pertinent elements when your data changes [11].

3.4.7 MetaMask

In the same way you would load any other piece of software, a browser extension called MetaMask functions as an Ethereum wallet. By holding Ethereum and other ERC-20 coins, users can transfer them to any Ethereum account after deployment [11].

3.5 Blockchain Technology Components

The blockchain platform is made up of three primary components: data blocks, global ledgers, and consensus algorithms. Each component is described in detail in what follows.

3.5.1 Data Block

It is made up of a collection of blocks that, in order to form a secure chain, connect each freshly modified block to its predecessor block before linking it back to its original block. This completely excludes the possibility of alteration as a result of the fact that each block's hash number closely links it to the block before it [14].

3.5.2 Distributed Ledger

It is also referred to as a databank because it records and saves user-generated transactions. The record cannot be altered because each transaction has a distinct encryption signature that is unconnected to a date. Furthermore, this ledger is distributed simultaneously across all network participants, allowing users to be updated in real time [14].

3.5.3 Consensus Algorithm

To prevent security flaws like double-spending, no organization should be allowed to regulate how a block is transacted across the network, where each block is managed by all participants with equal rights. To do this, the agreement approach is employed. According to the blockchain, organizations come to an agreement on the authentication of each data block through the consensus process. This is accomplished by nodes competing with one another during the mining process to validate the block in order to profit from their labor.

To manage transfers, Bitcoin, for example, employs a proof-of-work (PoW) algorithm, whereas Ethereum employs a proof-of-stake (PoS) mechanism. The Byzantine defective tolerant (BFT) method is one of many others [14]. In contrast to conventional database systems, blockchain technology makes use of its built-in characteristics to guarantee transparency, immutability, and correctness throughout the data gathering and management processes.

Blockchain also makes it possible for two or more parties to conduct business and interact digitally without the need for a single authority. By facilitating value exchange, openness, and confidence across corporate networks, blockchain is revolutionizing numerous sectors in a variety of ways. Supply chain management, law, tourism, energy, banking, and healthcare are just a few of the sectors that use it. It has shown to be particularly helpful in the medical industry, where it helps improve healthcare data protection and safe data administration. It is therefore perfect for handling healthcare problems caused by the coronavirus [15].

3.6 Working of Blockchain

Blockchain, as previously stated, is used to ensure that documents have not been tampered with; it saves data in the format of blocks. Each block typically consists of three components: data, the block's hash, and the hash of the block before it. The information kept within a block varies according to the blockchain type; for example, a Bitcoin contains financial data (transaction details) recorded in its blocks. When a block is formed, its hash value is generated; its value will not be the same if the block's data is changed, and it also includes the prior block's hash value. A genesis block represents the initial block in a blockchain, and it will not have the hash value of any prior block; instead, it will begin from zero, as shown in Figure 3.1.

When a new transaction occurs, a block with the associated data is appended. As a result, a new block is connected, forming a chain in the process, hence the term *blockchain*. The info in the blockchain cannot be changed because it is unchangeable [16].

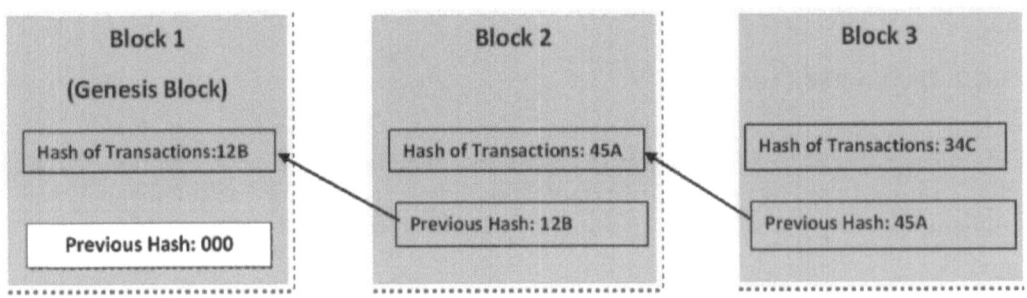

FIGURE 3.1
Schematic diagram of a genesis block.

When data in a block is changed, the hash value of the information modifies as well. As a result, this block's hash value and the previous hash value of the next blocks will not be the same, breaking the chain and rendering it invalid; however, there is a possibility of recalculating the remaining block's hash values to make it valid again using advanced supercomputers; to avoid this, we employ the concept of proof-of-work.

Proof-of-work (PoW) is the original agreement method in a blockchain network. PoW is performed by individuals known as miners to guarantee that transfers are authentic. This technique of transaction confirmation is known as mining; once transactions are validated, they can be added to the blockchain. A smart contract is a software that can function as a protocol or an arrangement that cannot be changed [16]. In the case of Bitcoin, these are extremely important. Once installed on the network, these can be called or initiated using a unique identifier given to them. As a result, when a smart contract is implemented, the info is saved on the network and is available to the collaborating nodes. The particulars of the smart contract cannot be changed by the other peers on the network. The smart contract has numerous applications. For example, if we want to sell a specific item (car, home, etc.), we can find a prospective customer on the network, excluding the requirement for a third party. As a result, smart contracts can be self-verified. Solidity is a popular computer language for creating and executing code. The Solidity computer language is used by Ethereum and Zeppelin, two blockchain systems [13].

3.7 Blockchain Structure

It has five components that build standards and manage different processes for blockchain apps [17,18].

3.7.1 Module for Data Source

In the "distributed and shared systems," it aids in the development of the blockchain. It makes sure that users' info on blockchains is not compromised or changed. Key elements of blockchain include data security, tamper-proof storing in any format, and a common information ledger accessible through a "application programming interface (API)" [12].

3.7.2 Transaction Module

It monitors, regulates, approves, and promotes "a transaction's journey in blockchain." It aids in the validation and facilitation of blockchain additions. Data is transmitted via smart contracting transaction barriers. Along with common transaction visibility, the blockchain facilitates the movement of information across the SC. Transactions are combined and transmitted in the shape of a block to each server. It should be noted that once a transaction has been completed, it is extremely difficult to remove or return in blockchains [12].

3.7.3 Module for Block Creation

Blocks are considered to be data structures created by miners. They keep data and information that is copied among all network components. By giving a hash code and connections from the preceding block, the block creation module enables you to add new blocks to an existing SC. "Chronological blocks" used to store transaction patterns make it simple to identify and monitor erroneous transactions [12].

3.7.4 Consensus Module

Algorithms for PoW and proof-of-stake are utilized to prove and verify transactions, all exchanges, in order to prevent data tampering. The meticulously developed "consensus algorithms" ensure data integrity in the dispersed network. Distributed consensus aids in both the verification of transaction legitimacy and the construction of links between nodes in the blockchain system [12].

3.7.5 Module for Connection and Interface

It aids in providing current information on smart contracts and keeps track of transaction history. This part coordinates all the platforms, protocols, and tools needed for blockchain apps. Various distributed ledger systems that offer agreement mechanisms for the blockchain system, whether it is permissioned or un-permissioned, may be introduced to the market, depending on the use cases. [12].

3.8 Applications of Blockchain in Healthcare

Healthcare organizations are having difficulties merging information at several places, such as preserving a central record of all documents, building confidence, keeping data at a cheap cost, and so on. BcT solves these issues by keeping confidence among partners, reducing costs, and ensuring a tryout for anyone with access to the data [19]. Blockchain technology has the potential to significantly alter the business. It could contribute to the development of a global healthcare system with the digital infrastructure to handle today's problems and confidently confront tomorrow's challenges. Various sectors where blockchain technology is utilized are shown in Figure 3.2.

It could contribute to more equitable patient care, competent medical study, and cost-effective professional processes [20]. The options are genuinely endless. The following are a few of the extensive possible uses of blockchain in healthcare [21].

3.8.1 Patient Consent Management

Electronic health records (EHRs), which include a patient's health history, prognosis, medications, and disease management plans, must be accurate for virtual care and health tracking to be effective. EHRs must be safely shared among peers, including hospitals, pharmacies, and health authorities, in order to keep a patient's medical information accurate and up-to-date [22].

The telemedicine healthcare law has given individuals the authority to control and regulate their clinical data through the creation of information guidelines for utilization and accessibility. The problems with conventional consent management methods are numerous, including lengthy integration periods when sharing EHR with experts, hostility towards servers from third parties that offer consent from patient's management services, and a failure to perform objective audit trials. Participants in telemedicine can activate blockchain services.

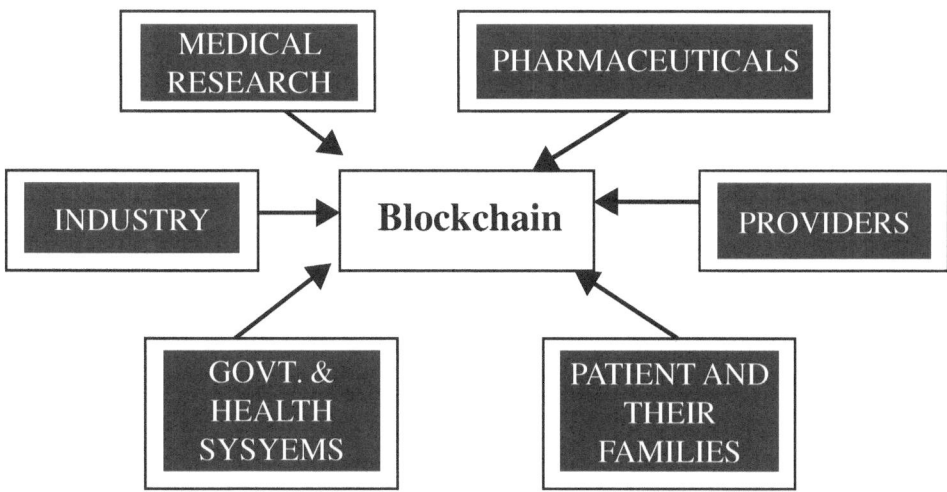

FIGURE 3.2
Blockchain in various sectors.

Blockchain technology can assist in maintaining trust because there are no intermediaries. Blockchain ensures and defends consent management by utilizing several peers from numerous participating groups [23–25]. Furthermore, the inherent immutability, tracking, and openness of blockchain can help perform audit trials to ensure conformance with consent management policies [26].

3.8.2 Remote Treatment Traceability

Telehealth and telemedicine require an online audio-video interaction between patients and experts for successful distant patient well-being evaluation. Following direct-to-consumer (D2C) and business-to-business (B2B) methods, telehealth services are provided.

Thanks to technology that enables audiovisual conferencing, carers in the more recent model remotely can engage virtually in discussions and medical training services (such as patient surgery), whereas patients in the previous scenario can communicate online with doctors to discuss their health. Asynchronous transmission of videos and images, such as X-rays or other examination, can help caretakers correctly identify the patients' health conditions during an electronic face-to-face consultation [27].

Health groups cannot monitor patient health information structures due to current telemedicine systems' restricted data sharing between one another. Blockchain technology solves this problem by giving all involved parties access to a unified and consistent picture of the patient's electronic health record (EHR). The linked participating organizations are able to track a patient's medical past and suggest an appropriate course of therapy thanks to the visibility and transparency of health data. For instance, checks can be conducted using blockchain technology to determine who viewed and precisely what trades were made on electronic documents [26].

3.8.3 Remote Monitoring IOT Security

One of the most substantial advances in digital health is the use of faraway nursing solutions, in which various sensors that sense patients' vital signs are used to give new healthcare consultants greater insight into patients' well-being, allowing for more preventative care [28]. Even so, patient data security and privacy, as well as preventing its manipulation to produce misleading data, remain critical issues in the health IoT. It is also crucial that the enabling systems are resistant to DDoS and other assaults that could disrupt service when a linked device is needed in an emergency, such as notifying the carer of an old person who collapsed or encountered a cardiac arrest. Blockchain technology may benefit in-field secure IoT device monitoring:

1. Blockchain cryptography guarantees that only authorized parties can access confidential information, because it is stored on the blockchain as a distinct hash function (a user requires a particular set of cryptographical keys to decrypt the hash function into the information sources because every modification to the source data generates a new hash function).
2. It is nearly impossible to change patient data once it has been documented on the blockchain database (as a hash function), as doing so generates a new hash function

3.8.4 Managing and Maintaining Patients' Health Records

Many scholars have raised the idea of using blockchain application authentication to protect EHRs after realizing the urgent need for a novel approach to handling EHRs that enables patients to participate in both their modern and traditional health data. A "MedRec" version makes use of unique blockchain benefits to handle security, honesty, and quick data exchange [29]. It maintains data and claims on a dispersed basis and gives patients access to their specific clinical records quickly and easily through a variety of clinicians and care facilities. It also gives patients a full, lasting background [30]. Medical records would not be preserved by "MedRec" or cause a transition period to start. It notifies the patient who is responsible for where the form will go and saves a record mark on a blockchain.

When it comes to the deployment of EHR, medical data sharing has significant disadvantages, such as losing authority over data, data origins, tracking, and safety monitoring. MeDShare was introduced as a safe blockchain system with some restrictions for exchanging medical data with unknown parties. MeDShare can be used by cloud service providers, doctors, and healthcare study organizations to exchange medical information and keep virtual medical data with highest data accuracy, tailored audit authority, and minimal possible threats to data security and privacy. EHR typically contains extremely permissioned and crucial patient information that is shared for effective diagnosis and therapy by doctors, neurosurgeons, healthcare providers, and scientists [31].

When a hospital appointment begins, the majority of the professionals treating that patient have seemed to notice things right away. Medical errors, allergy symptoms, and medication solutions could be handled across blockchain archives by helpful patient-caring algorithms, eradicating the need for time-consuming medical management methods. As a result, implementing blockchain invention will improve patient treatment accessibility, medical data oversight, faster verification of clinical expertise, increased surveillance, and more effective care organization [32].

All types of information can be stored in this database, including information on hypertension, cardiac diseases, and demographic records, as well as the cost of different consultations and insurance fees. Data from both physical and virtual meetings, applications, used medications, etc. will be combined. In order to suggest individualized care, it will be simpler for physicians to comprehend the patient's history and prior treatments. The patient will not have to spend time trying to recall past information for the doctor, and it won't matter if they neglect important details. With its multiple levels of security and unpermissioned and private keys, blockchain will keep the patient's info secure [21].

3.8.5 Managing the Supply Chain

Even though the majority of countries have laws in place to control and safeguard the sanctity of the supply chain, fake medications still find their way onto the market.

These medications are detrimental to the general populace and can make users allergic or develop serious health problems. If a blockchain is utilized to regulate the flow of medications from the producer to the end user, it will be simple to locate the site where a fake drug was used in place of the authentic one. It will assist in halting the spread of fake medicines. Another use involves following the movement of the medications in actual time in order to precisely calculate the "time of arrival" [21].

3.8.6 In-Home Medical Gadgets and Kits for Patient Monitoring

Medical tools and equipment that patients can use at home can help them diagnose themselves in a setting away from a facility. The use of widely accessible test kits and devices to monitor particular biomedical responses for self-examination and early disease discovery can aid in lowering total healthcare expenses [33]. The absence of medical equipment openness, visibility, and data provenance within conventional centralized telehealth-based systems makes it hard for physicians and patients to purchase trustworthy medical kits.

In this scenario, the distributed database can be used to permanently and publicly record ownership and performance-related activities involving testing equipment custody. Based on performance evaluations, the smart contracts can be used to compile image ratings for every medical test kits and gadgets used for residential care facilities. Thus, patients, doctors, and laboratory engineers can benefit from the smart contracts in order to obtain extremely accurate and dependable medical equipment from reputable makers [26].

3.8.7 Access to Private Health Data in a Secure Manner

A person's private medical record contains information on their medical history, their confidentiality, and other information about their care. The personal health record entries are created, managed, and maintained by the data owner. Yet the EHR has more detailed health data because it is formed, sustained, and controlled by healthcare practitioners.

Because they are handled by a single organization, the overwhelming majority of conventional agreements used to offer online medical services are built on less-reliable cloud platforms. Also, the PHRs' truthfulness is threatened by typical cloud-based systems. Because decentralized blockchain technology is inherently anonymous, the proprietor of the health information can keep the data's secrecy [26].

The smart contracts can be utilized to authorize users and grant them access to patient data in line with the individual's authorization rule. Furthermore, the versatility of blockchain-based technology allows the information proprietor to manage and share the information with authorized individuals while adhering to their own terms and conditions [26].

3.8.8 Payments on Automatic Basis

Existing healthcare structures heavily depend on central third-party providers to resolve payments for services used by subjects, caretakers, and insurance companies. The central money clearance methods, however, are opaque, possibly hacker-prone, and comparatively slow. Additionally, micropayments are not available in central financial managing platforms or do so at a very high cost. The blockchain network provides coin token-based payment to enable micropayments in the telehealth industry.

Therefore, the direct transmission of digital currencies to the wallet of the solution supplier provides a rapid, safe, visible, and accountable system that eliminates the need for a centralized dispute settlement service to resolve payment disputes [30]. Furthermore, the ability of customers and healthcare providers to retract transactions in the future is guaranteed by digitally signed payment–settlement transactions. Cash-on-delivery services can be implemented with the help of blockchain technology, reducing the likelihood of payment-related scams. For instance, smart contracts can be planned to retain cryptocurrency coins and send them to pharmacists' wallets only after the medications are effectively distributed to the distant patient when deploying a remote medication delivery service for telepharmacy [26].

3.8.9 Dependable Supervision of Elderly Patients

The telehealth industry can benefit from the Internet of Things (IoT) technical developments by using accurate biomedical devices to virtually watch a patient's health [34–36]. In order to assess a patient's health, the biomedical devices can constantly watch and record health data on a high-performance edge computer. Vital indicators like arterial pressure and bodily temperatures can be linked to health information.

Medical mistakes, however, can result from inaccurate data that a malfunctioning gadget collects. In order to effectively address this problem, autonomous blockchain technology utilizes smart contracts to authorize and confirm the rights granted to users of biomedical devices to record the electronic health record (EHR) on the database [37].

Smart contracts have the ability to promptly send warnings to medical professionals and treatment facilities in the event of an unexpected disaster. Blockchain-enabled IoT systems can effectively alert the patient to the need for medicine refills for in-home care services. It guarantees that only approved users who comply with the patient consent document may view a patient's electronic health record [26].

3.8.10 Traceability of Medication Distribution and Pharmacy Fill-Ups

In order for the online consultancy-based medical system to exchange a prescription for drugs with the neighboring pharmacy, the doctors must conduct transactions on the blockchain. Blockchain technology can help reduce the possibility of prescription mistakes and documents manipulation by utilizing its hash functions [38]. Authorized pharmacies have access to the blockchain-stored medicine prescriptions for the purposes of validating, preparing, and delivering pharmaceuticals to patients.

In return, the shipper can update the blockchain with the cargo's current location so that patients and pharmacists can more easily track down the shipment. Patients and medical experts can also verify the legitimacy of medication by looking at the source of its data, because blockchain transactions are transparent and traceable. A smart contract has the ability to immediately order (intermittent) prescription fill-up for the drug from the pharmacy once a preset condition is met. The pharmacist can then verify and confirm the order to grant a refill in response. After a successful prescription renewal, the patient receives their medication, and the records are updated as necessary [26].

3.8.11 Trustworthy Health Insurance Services

Due to the lack of financial rewards and stringent privacy protection laws, many people are typically least interested in providing insurance companies with information about their medical history. As a result, patients frequently choose an insurance policy that is not suitable, which can result in the denial of legitimate demands for insurance.

Online medical legislation secures patients' rights to compensation at the identical amount as in instances of real medical care networks. When it comes to insurance-related fraud, it takes a couple of days to ascertain the actuality from the data that has been given (such as when an incorrect medical claim is submitted to an insurance company).

By giving them access to a patient's medical data, blockchain technology can assist insurance companies in lowering insurance scams (consent-based). Patients may receive rewards for permitting insurance firms to utilize their health information. Additionally, a lot of insurance providers give premium users rewards in the form of Bitcoin tokens for having a hale and hearty life, like keeping track of their gym trips. The patient's smart gadgets can conduct transactions on the blockchain to build confidence [26].

3.8.12 Reputation-Aware Specialist Referral Services

The key players in telemedicine-based cross-regional and disciplinary finding and therapy include patients, sending healthcare professionals, and consulting healthcare experts.

During remote patient care, medical recommendations and expert views are sought through healthcare alliances and smart contracts. Using a blockchain-created explanation, the suggesting medical professional can keep the reference materials on an IPFS server, which creates an IPFS hash of the file and stores it on the blockchain so that it can be accessed by traveling medical professionals [39,40].

It is possible to determine whether or not the document is changed by using the IPFS hash recorded on the network. The patient's health report can be examined by the consulting healthcare professional, who can then record the results of their examination on the blockchain database. Based on the advising health expert's overall service time and satisfaction ranking, the suggesting healthcare professional can refresh the reputation score on the blockchain [26].

3.8.13 Automated Patient Follow-Up Service

After therapy is finished, a patient's health can be carefully monitored thanks to follow-up care services. In some instances, the patient must register for a video meeting before sending the outcomes of blood and urine samples to the practitioners as part of the follow-up service. Through the use of smart contracts, blockchain technology allows the systematization of the patient's follow-up service.

To instantly notify the patient, doctor, and hospital staff of impending follow-up visits, the smart contracts can transmit messages to all three parties [41]. The doctor can verify the patient's health status as reported during the most recent follow-up appointment by accessing the patient's visible and immutable EHR (virtual). The user can also use a smart contract to trade the IPFS hash with the doctor using IPFS servers that can keep test results in order to obtain health data [26].

3.8.14 Pharmaceutical Research and Development

The rate of scientific advancement in the medicinal sector is astounding. The search for treatments for the new coronavirus and other illnesses is a race against time for businesses. Every time a discovery is made, it is reported in the media, etc.

However, no data or studies are shared while researching to make a success. Here, BC enables the spreading of new medications, hastening the discovery of a cure as businesses can communicate their developments. Additionally, BC supports the publication of medical research to ensure that each piece of study is validated.

The BC is also used in the medication manufacturing process. Every medication has a production recipe. BcT is able to assess, monitor, and confirm that the medications are being produced precisely as outlined in the process [26].

3.8.15 Medical Staff Credential Verification

Similar to how they can be used to trace the origins of a medical product, cryptographic protocols can be used to monitor the experience of medical practitioners. The credentials of staff members can be logged by reputable medical facilities and healthcare organizations, which streamlines the recruiting procedure for those organizations.

ProCredEx, a company located in the United States, has developed a medical identity verification system based on R3 Corda blockchain technology [42,43]. The primary benefits of blockchain technology are as follows:

1. Healthcare administrations will be able to obtain credentials more rapidly throughout the hiring procedure.
2. An opportunity for healthcare organizations, insurers, and medical facilities to benefit from their current qualifications information on former and current workers.
3. Through openness and security for associates, such as firms that subcontract locum tenens or cutting-edge online well-being delivery models, patients can learn about the knowledge of the medical staff [32].

3.8.16 Supply Chain Transparency

Healthcare, like many other industries, places a premium on the guarantee of medicinal goods' provenance to establish their legitimacy. Using a blockchain-based system, consumers can monitor products from the point of manufacture to every step of the supply chain, providing them with full visibility and transparency over the things they are purchasing [43]. This is a major issue for the sector, particularly in developing nations, where fake prescription medicines result in tens of thousands of deaths each year. It is also getting more important for medical apparatus, which is growing quickly, as more remote health tracking is adopted and piquing the interest of dishonest actors. A well-known blockchain platform called MediLedger enables companies in the prescribed medication supply chain to verify the legitimacy of drugs, as well as their expiry dates and other important details [32].

3.8.17 Tracking Clinical Trials and Pharmaceuticals

A medical strategy used to identify and avoid illness are clinical trials. To avoid and identify diseases, numerous methods have been developed in recent years. Data integrity, record-sharing, data protection, and patient registration are some of the faults in these systems, which blockchain technology can address. The clinical healthcare platforms listed in the following offer data security and anonymity. Monitoring data on, among other things, insurance companies, hospitals, doctors, and health programs is done using healthcare, token-based money.

Using smart contracts, the FHIRChain smart health system [44] enables the sharing of clinical healthcare data. The blockchain-based record-sharing tool Connecting Care is similar and is available in several English towns. Connecting Care is used in a diverse healthcare company to protect information about hospitals as well as medical record data.

To guarantee that only individuals with permission can view the clinical system, it offers an access control list. The blockchain's smart contract functionality is implemented using an Ethereum-based architecture. The system uses an enrolment method to sign up a user for the healthcare system. The patient can input their confidential data into the system, and the authorities can view the patient's medical information [45].

Blockchain-based clinical settings will surely create new scientific possibilities for the advancement of a medical study. However, the reliable, secure, and adaptable collection, archival, and recovery of these clinical investigations in apps for precision medicine will aid in the development of enticing possibilities for the identification and management of maladies. An online library could be used for cognitive strategies. Blockchain technology may be used to handle a computerized brain, and neurotechnologies are still in the experimental phase. Few businesses have actually announced a stance for blockchain technology [32].

3.8.18 Disease Surveillance at the Community Level

"Some meanings of surveillance include systematic, continuous data collection, collation, and analysis, as well as the quick dissemination of data to people who require it in order that steps can be taken" are some of the definitions used to describe *surveillance* [46].

It is done for both contagious diseases and noncommunicable diseases in line with state goals and the WHO's Worldwide Healthcare Regulations. For instance, a fatal virus like Nipah can spread throughout the world in less than 36 hours and start an epidemic by jeopardizing health security as a result of unchecked development and globalization [47]. Because so many self-regulatory groups submit reports to a single information system, communicable disease surveillance is a continuous, complicated, and ineffective process. Keeping the information flowing smoothly and on schedule is therefore a difficult job [48].

Additionally, there are no rewards provided for regular employees. These independent groups may be able to handle data more effectively during pandemics with the aid of blockchain [49]. Additionally, it might aid in monitoring data for current un-permissioned health crises, such as traffic crashes, substance abuse, opioid misuse, and so forth [50]. When blockchain technology is used in the un-permissioned health sector, these systems may be capable of managing safe data exchange and the preservation at different levels within medical institutions.

By detecting possible outbreaks or bioterrorism, this technology can deliver real-time information. Therefore, it is likely to avoid significant fatalities if vaccines, anti-microbial agents, and other illness control methods are implemented quickly.

For instance, in recent years, false information on social media opposing immunization has seriously harmed un-permissioned health [51]. In order to trace the sources of such damaging content and pinpoint the group most at risk in digital communication, Huckle et al. reported using a blockchain-based method [52].

This illustrates how, in the era of automation, blockchain technology has the possibility for advancement un-permissioned health surveillance. Nowadays, the majority of nations employ machine learning methods for monitoring. Blockchain technology has some special and extra benefits over machine learning methods. The blockchain primarily prevents illegal activities, such as data theft and replication. The inclusion of blockchain technology and artificial intelligence (AI) is a perfect combination for the field of medical study and healthcare industry advancement [53].

Additionally, there is a ton of room for merging with geographic information systems (GIS) to speed up regular epidemic inquiries and supply chain management for medications and vaccines. The blockchain also removes the limitations of the district health information systems by assuring openness and accurate reporting, such as when revealing deaths from a specific outbreak. The improvement of attempts to ensure patient security comes from the usage of blockchain in surveillance systems. There is a lot of potential for real-time monitoring for the finding of non-communicable diseases (NCD) under these three general groups of disease control action phases, namely, prevention, detection, and response. The Global Health Security Agenda (GHSA) action packages address this as well. The early risk factor identification for NCDs can be ensured through real-time tracking. Effective supply chain systems can also aid in disaster response by improving the abilities of medical and healthcare staff [54,55].

3.8.19 Treatment Optimization

Targeted therapy and telemedicine are two factors for treatment improvement. In many countries, the quantity of medical patients has sharply increased, causing it to be more and more challenging for patients to receive immediate assistance from physicians or nursing personnel [56].

The technology used in telemedicine is viewed as a means of providing medical treatment that is both fair and economical [57].

There are security dangers in the transmission and logging of data exchanges as a result of the creation and widespread use of Internet of Things devices and other types of remote patient tracking systems. The blockchain's intelligent contract can be used to support security research and administration of medical devices because it is tamper-proof, anonymous, and transparent [37].

For instance, Medicalchain has introduced a smart contract that enables patients to allow doctors to virtually evaluate health cases and offer recommendations or second views [58].

Additionally, organizations for drug research and development can categorize the data with user approval to carry out drug-focused research and development, and the data can be transmitted safely using blockchain asymmetry cryptography encoding [59,60].

3.8.20 Doctor Management

Three factors are used in doctor management: client selection, staff screening, and identification. Blockchain technology allows healthcare professionals, patients, and managers for large-scale data exchange, patient tracking, identity security, and validation. Additionally, blockchain can be used to track medical interventions made by physicians, preventing medical conflicts and assisting both patients and medical organizations in making informed physician selections. For instance, the blockchain-based project MedicoHealth enables totally private and safe customer contact with the top doctors in the world. Only one allocated doctor may access patient information in confidence at a given moment, and information regarding the status of a doctor's certificates and licenses is updated in an unalterable decentralized data [58,60].

3.9 Barriers in Leveraging Blockchain Technology in Healthcare

There are some obstacles with applying blockchain technology that must be overcome before it can be used in digital healthcare. Each healthcare practitioner maintains their own set of patient notes, and frequently they do not share this information with patients or other medical systems. Additionally, healthcare data comes from a range of resources, such as health records and therapy histories, investigations, and health data gathered from wearable devices or sensors that track patients' health [2,61]. The healthcare industry has long-standing issues with the following.

3.9.1 Regulation, Both Internal and External

Internal oversight primarily refers to the ongoing monitoring by medical organizations of supplies, tools, and medications. The administrative authority is the regulating body, and healthcare transportation network control, entire healthcare procedure legislation, and healthcare trash removal operation governance are the three factors for external regulation. Individuals, organizations, activities, information, and resources comprise the application chain, which includes the distribution of sellers' goods or services to consumers. Its aim is to ensure the integrity of fragile products throughout the transportation process.

Drug distribution chain management is essential for keeping track in terms of basic substance supply, the production process, and the distribution of finished items [62]. Drug supply networks are susceptible to manipulation, fraud, and corruption [63]. A good distribution chain management strategy is especially vital in the healthcare sector, since a disrupted drug distribution chain has a direct impact on patient protection and medical results.

Blockchain technology is one method for improving the safety, stability, sources of data, and utility of a reliable drug distribution chain. Blockchain technology transactions in the distribution chain are safe, are transparent, and can be continuously watched and documented, significantly decreasing the amount of time needed and the chance of human error [58]. Furthermore, the usage of blockchain knowledge can improve the protection of medical instruments and materials. Blockchain technology can be applied by keeping exclusive device IDs for each health device and using smart contracts to track and distribute software updates. Invariance can be combined with blockchain-based healthcare equipment monitoring to avoid gadget loss, theft, and malicious manipulation [60].

3.9.2 Challenges in Medical Care Information Transfer and Lack of Interoperability

The lack of interoperability between institutions and suppliers of medical services is currently a major problem. As a result, medical data are dispersed, fragmented, and challenging to trade. As a result, a patient's medical records are ultimately saved in various places: medical inquiries are kept in the systems of the providers, prescription information is kept locally with different pharmacies, etc. Patients and carers encounter significant obstacles when trying to start data retrieval and sharing because of this absence of interoperability [64].

Thus, in the present situation, where the amount of medical data produced is quickly growing, defining a universal norm to combine medical records to collect information from numerous sources and improve data sharing throughout the entire value chain becomes essential [2].

3.9.3 Interoperability Assistance for Cross-Platform Transactions

The healthcare participants, including doctors and patients, require that the patient health referral services safely trade across the blockchain platforms. Blockchain platforms' interoperability support enables users to interact with one another without the need for middlemen for transaction processing and sending [26]. For example, a stage that supports interoperability can help medical professionals use Bitcoin coins for deals on the Ethereum blockchain network.

However, it is challenging to design interoperable blockchain systems due to a number of issues, such as differences in the recognized languages and consensus methods of the platforms on the blockchain [65].

To safeguard telehealth users' privacy, compatible systems should ideally be fast, private, and fault-tolerant [26].

3.9.4 Challenges to Blockchain Adoption in Institutions

Conventional telemedicine platforms generally rely on outmoded methods to preserve and safeguard patient information, which might limit prospects for association between healthcare consumers and professionals. This increases system expenses, which have an important bearing on how successfully a patient receives therapy. By establishing permanent records of transactions and medical data, by using blockchain technology, it is possible for authorized people to maintain and watch a patient's full and authentic health data [66]. Blockchain technology has a lot of potential, but telehealth consumers can't fully take use of it because they don't know enough about it, the technology is in its infancy, and there are no security or privacy rules in place. Therefore, more study is required on blockchain technology to create guidelines and laws for its broad usage in telehealth, and organizations that want to switch to blockchain technology should be investigated [26].

3.9.5 Difficulties in Ensuring Data Confidentiality and Privacy

Private medical information lacks a secure foundation, which leads to frequent data breaches.

About 13 million pieces of overall health information were made un-permissioned as a result of data leaks that the Office for Civil Rights (OCR) of the Department of Health and Human Services (USA) reported in 2018. To achieve full interoperability, healthcare stakeholders must communicate data while safeguarding confidential data and limiting access to authorized people. Data exchange and sharing on the road to interoperability offer a fantastic opportunity to enhance the healthcare environment, but it also raises one of the biggest privacy concerns [2].

3.9.6 Safety Susceptibilities of Smart Contracts

The alteration and interruption of a patient's health records are possible due to smart contract faults and vulnerabilities, which can significantly change their typical behavior [67].

For instance, using a re-entrancy vulnerability attack, a smart contract with restricted access to another contract may be able to alter a patient's electronic health record or withdraw funds from an actual user's pocket [61]. The testing tools that the professionals advise are ZeppelinOS, SolCover, and Oyente. These tools assist developers in recommending protections against external threats by locating the weak places in smart contracts [67]. However, the proposed fixes fall short of identifying all weak points and faults in smart contracts. Hence, before they are implemented, care must be made to properly examine smart contracts for possible flaws, by utilizing a variety of test scenarios and a number of tools [26].

3.9.7 Data Ownership

The inability of individuals to fully manage their own medical information is another issue with data ownership in today's healthcare system. The importance of this element has increased as wearable technology and customized therapy have advanced [68]. To make the procedure obvious, the patient's authorization is required in the framework of data exchange [69]. Giving patients accessibility to their information will allow them to determine who has the authorization to access it and with what rights, which is a necessary step toward creating a completely integrated and open healthcare system. The administration of health data would become more adaptable and secure as a result. In reality, all the current systems share the issue of having a lack of adequate security measures for people viewing or exchanging data [70], as there are significant concerns with regard to user privacy and, consequently, restrictions on privileged access to personal information [2].

3.9.8 Patient Data Overload

Despite advancements in health information technology (HIT), a complete viewpoint of a patient's medical past record is still lacking [71,72]. One of the most recent techniques for keeping own medical records focuses on merging medical data received from various sensors, monitors, and wearable technology, like smartwatches, fitness trackers, or technology that measures medical metrics (heart rate, blood sugar level, etc.) [2]. A hurdle in this situation is the massive quantity of data produced that must be managed, assessed, and archived. Thus, new techniques for managing and storing data must be created. A strong user interface (UI) becomes crucial for giving information to healthcare professionals in a way that is both aesthetically pleasing and intelligible. To meet this demand, healthcare organizations are increasingly putting a concentration on user interface designers being involved in the workflow and customer experience [73]. The goal of our study was to create a dispersed and compatible PHR system using blockchain technology to provide patients with access to a singular, interoperable version of their medical information that can be distributed to medical professionals throughout the healthcare value chain [2].

3.10 Conclusion

The worldwide healthcare industry is noticing the current pattern in research on blockchain's application in healthcare. Healthcare organizations are in urgent need of new and better trust-preserving solutions because it is crucial to uphold confidence while satiating the ever-increasing demand for data exchange within the healthcare ecosystem. Blockchain technology's advantages of decentralization, tamper-proofness, traceability, immutability, audibility, and security make it appropriate for use in the healthcare industry. The state of research, as illustrated in this study, indicates that a few EHR, PHR, and clinical trial system use cases are presently investigating blockchain-based solutions. Other areas of health information systems, such as community-level disease surveillance, insurance claim resolution, remote patient monitoring of elderly patients, therapy optimization, population health management systems, and pharmaceutical supply networks, are understudied. Few businesses have used blockchain technology, despite its potential to dramatically improve the storage and retrieval of data about supply networks and individuals' health information. With the help of this technology, medical professionals can securely and instantly update patient data whenever it is required across a variety of facilities and locations. This would be very helpful in the modern era, when the healthcare system is already overburdened, as it would cut down on administrative time and free up resources for patient treatment. Blockchain technology can simplify and enhance the way that vaccines and medications are currently administered. Blockchain technology has the potential to significantly increase the supply of drugs' openness, efficiency, and dependability while preventing the entrance of counterfeit medications wherever along the complete process. Blockchain technology would be helpful by keeping track of the vaccinations' cold chain supply. Blockchain technology, like all other technologies, has some limitations, but they are not insurmountable. Adoption and execution are pricey because blockchain technology uses a lot of electricity. Newer technologies are, however, emerging so that more businesses can utilize them. It takes a lot of energy and processing capacity to provide the protection layer that "proof-of-work" does. The less costly "proof-of-spike" and "proof-of-fire" are used in more recent iterations of blockchain technology. This device was made to record transactions as well. It will need more storage space as its use spreads because it will retain more data. Blockchain technology will have to become more resilient and flexible as more transactions and data are recorded and stored. To successfully implement blockchain technology in healthcare, international standardization bodies will need to be involved in establishing standards. The advantages of blockchain technology have been discussed in this chapter, and they include its decentralized, unchangeable, private, and auditable nature. The likelihood of perpetrating deception is very low. In the long term, operating and maintaining this technology will be less expensive and quicker. In order to establish up, businesses will need to train staff and alter mindsets, just like with any new tool. However, they can save money, and it is a tiny price to pay for the enormous advantages that blockchain technology offers. It is obvious that the time for blockchain technology is now, given the more than 17 healthcare organizations that have adopted this technology.

References

1. Agbo CC, Mahmoud QH, Eklund JM. Blockchain technology in healthcare: A systematic review. *Healthc.* 2019;7(2).
2. Cernian A, Tiganoaia B, Sacala IS, Pavel A, Iftemi A. Patientdatachain: A blockchain-based approach to integrate personal health records. *Sensors* (Switzerland). 2020;20(22):1–24.
3. Solat S, Calvez P, Naït-Abdesselam F. Permissioned vs. permissionless blockchain: How and why there is only one right choice. *J Softw.* 2021;16(3):95–106.

4. Anoaica A, Levard H. Quantitative description of internal activity on the ethereum public blockchain. In *2018 9th IFIP Int Conf New Technol Mobil Secur NTMS 2018—Proc.* 2018;2018:1–5.
5. Jadhav JS, Deshmukh J. A review study of the blockchain-based healthcare supply chain. *Soc Sci Humanit Open* [Internet]. 2022;6(1):100328. https://doi.org/10.1016/j.ssaho.2022.100328
6. Hussien HM, Yasin SM, Udzir SNI, Zaidan AA, Zaidan BB. A systematic review for enabling of develop a blockchain technology in healthcare application: Taxonomy, substantially analysis, motivations, challenges, recommendations and future direction. *J Med Syst*. 2019;43(10).
7. Feng L, Zhang H, Tsai WT, Sun S. System architecture for high-performance permissioned blockchains. *Front Comput Sci*. 2019;13(6):1151–65.
8. Xiao Y, Xu B, Jiang W, Wu Y. The healthchain blockchain for electronic health records: Development study. *J Med Internet Res*. 2021;23(1):1–13.
9. Khan C, Lewis A, Rutland E, Wan C, Rutter K, Thompson C. Blockchain technology in finance a distributed-ledger collaborative innovation. *IEEE Comput*. 2017;50(9):29–37.
10. Tijan E, Aksentijević S, Ivanić K, Jardas M. Blockchain technology implementation in logistics. *Sustain*. 2019;11(4).
11. Rai BK. BBTCD: Blockchain based traceability of counterfeited drugs. *Heal Serv Outcomes Res Methodol* [Internet]. 2022;(October). https://doi.org/10.1007/s10742-022-00292-w
12. Dutta P, Choi TM, Somani S, Butala R. Blockchain technology in supply chain operations: Applications, challenges and research opportunities. *Transp Res Part E Logist Transp Rev* [Internet]. 2020;142(July):102067. https://doi.org/10.1016/j.tre.2020.102067
13. Kakarlapudi PV, Mahmoud QH. A systematic review of blockchain for consent management. *Healthc*. 2021;9(2).
14. Zheng Z, Xie S, Dai H, Chen X, Wang H. An overview of blockchain technology: Architecture, consensus, and future trends. *Proc—2017 IEEE 6th Int Congr Big Data, BigData Congr 2017*. 2017;(June):557–64.
15. Marbouh D, Abbasi T, Maasmi F, Omar IA, Debe MS, Salah K, et al. Blockchain for COVID-19: Review, opportunities, and a trusted tracking system. *Arab J Sci Eng* [Internet]. 2020;45(12):9895–911. https://doi.org/10.1007/s13369-020-04950-4
16. Szabo N. View of formalizing and securing relationships on public networks | First Monday. *First Monday* [Internet]. 1997;1–21. Available from: https://firstmonday.org/ojs/index.php/fm/article/view/548/469
17. Choi TM. Innovative "bring-service-near-your-home" operations under Corona-Virus (COVID-19/SARS-CoV-2) outbreak: Can logistics become the Messiah? *Transp Res Part E Logist Transp Rev* [Internet]. 2020;140(March):101961. https://doi.org/10.1016/j.tre.2020.101961
18. Min H. Blockchain technology for enhancing supply chain resilience. *Bus Horiz* [Internet]. 2019;62(1):35–45. https://doi.org/10.1016/j.bushor.2018.08.012
19. Krawiec RJ, Housman D, White M, Filipova M, Quarre F, Barr D, et al. Blockchain: Opportunities for health care. *Deloitte Insights* [Internet]. 2020;14. Available from: www2.deloitte.com/us/en/pages/public-sector/articles/blockchain-opportunities-for-health-care.html
20. Kassab M, Defranco J, Malas T, Laplante P, Destefanis G, Neto VVG. Exploring research in blockchain for healthcare and a roadmap for the future. *IEEE Trans Emerg Top Comput*. 2021;9(4):1835–52.
21. Arumugam SK, Sharma AM. Blockchain: Opportunities in the healthcare sector and its uses in COVID-19 [Internet]. *Lessons from COVID-19: Impact on Healthcare Systems and Technology*. 2022:61–94. http://doi.org/10.1016/B978-0-323-99878-9.00002-9
22. Dubovitskaya A, Xu Z, Ryu S, Schumacher M, Wang F. Secure and trustable electronic medical records sharing using blockchain. AMIA. *Annu Symp Proceedings AMIA Symp*. 2017; 2017:650–9.
23. Genestier Jotisftae. Blockchain for consent management in the ehealth environment: A nugget for privacy and security challenges introduction and use case. *J Int Soc Telemed Ehealth*. 2017;5:24–5.
24. Zhang X, Poslad S, Ma Z. Block-based access control for blockchain-based electronic medical records (EMRs) query in eHealth. *2018 IEEE Glob Commun Conf Globecom 2018—Proc*. 2018:1–7.
25. Zhang X, Poslad S. Blockchain support for flexible queries with granular access control to electronic medical records (EMR). *IEEE Int Conf Commun*. 2018;2018:1–6.

26. Ahmad RW, Salah K, Jayaraman R, Yaqoob I, Ellahham S, Omar M. The role of blockchain technology in telehealth and telemedicine. *Int J Med Inform* [Internet]. 2021;148(June 2020):104399. https://doi.org/10.1016/j.ijmedinf.2021.104399
27. Mannaro K, Baralla G, Pinna A, Ibba S. A blockchain approach applied to a teledermatology platform in the Sardinian Region (Italy). *Information*. 2018;9(2).
28. Khan PW, Byun Y. A blockchain-based secure image encryption scheme for the industrial internet of things. *Entropy*. 2020;22(2).
29. Wang C, Zhang Y. Improving scoring-docking-screening powers of protein—ligand scoring functions using random forest. *J Comput Chem*. 2017;38(3):169–77.
30. Scekic O, Nastic S, Dustdar S. Blockchain-supported smart city platform for social value co-creation and exchange. *IEEE Internet Comput*. 2019;23(1):19–28.
31. Cyran MA. Blockchain as a foundation for sharing healthcare data. *Blockchain Healthc Today*. 2018.
32. Tagde P, Tagde S, Bhattacharya T, Tagde P, Chopra H, Akter R, et al. Blockchain and artificial intelligence technology in e-Health. *Environ Sci Pollut Res*. 2021;28(38):52810–31.
33. Weissman SM, Zellmer K, Gill N, Wham D. Implementing a virtual health telemedicine program in a community setting. *J Genet Couns*. 2018;27(2):323–5.
34. Kazmi HSZ, Nazeer F, Mubarak S, Hameed S, Basharat A, Javaid N. *Trusted remote patient monitoring using blockchain-based smart contracts* [Internet]. Vol. 97, Lecture Notes in Networks and Systems. Springer International Publishing; 2020. 765–76 p. http://doi.org/10.1007/978-3-030-33506-9_70
35. Rehman MHU, Ahmed E, Yaqoob I, Hashem IAT, Imran M, Ahmad S. Big data analytics in industrial IoT using a concentric computing model. *IEEE Commun Mag*. 2018;56(2):37–43.
36. Alblooshi M, Salah K, Alhammadi Y. Blockchain-based ownership management for medical IoT (MIoT) devices. *Proc 2018 13th Int Conf Innov Inf Technol IIT 2018*. 2019;151–6.
37. Griggs KN, Ossipova O, Kohlios CP, Baccarini AN, Howson EA, Hayajneh T. Healthcare blockchain system using smart contracts for secure automated remote patient monitoring. *J Med Syst*. 2018;42(7):1–7.
38. El-Miedany Y. Telehealth and telemedicine: How the digital era is changing standard health care. *Smart Homecare Technol TeleHealth*. 2017;4:43–51.
39. Lee CK. Blockchain application with health token in medical & health industrials. Atlantis Press; 2019;196(Ssphe 2018):233–6. http://doi.org/10.2991/ssphe-18.2019.55
40. Webster P. *The telemedicine referral case process key participants in the referral case process*. 2018;1–19. Available from: https://telemedicine.arizona.edu/sites/
41. Siyal AA, Junejo AZ, Zawish M, Ahmed K, Khalil A, Soursou G. Applications of blockchain technology in medicine and healthcare: Challenges and future perspectives. *Cryptography*. 2019;3(1):1–16.
42. Funk E, Riddell J, Ankel F, Cabrera D. Blockchain technology: A data framework to improve validity, trust, and accountability of information exchange in health professions education. *Acad Med*. 2018;93(12):1791–4.
43. Narayanaswami C, Nooyi R, Govindaswamy SR, Viswanathan R. Blockchain anchored supply chain automation. *IBM J Res Dev*. 2019;63(2):1.
44. Zhang P, White J, Schmidt DC, Lenz G, Rosenbloom ST. FHIRChain: Applying blockchain to securely and scalably share clinical data. *Comput Struct Biotechnol J* [Internet]. 2018;16:267–78. https://doi.org/10.1016/j.csbj.2018.07.004
45. Hang L, Choi E, Kim DH. A novel EMR integrity management based on a medical blockchain platform in hospital. *Electronics*. 2019;8(4).
46. Bhattacharya P, Tanwar S, Bodkhe U, Tyagi S, Member S. BinDaaS: Blockchain-based deep-learning as-a-service in healthcare 4.0 applications. *IEEE/ACM Trans Netw*. 2019;4697(c).
47. Fan VY, Jamison DT, Summers LH. Pandemic risk: How large are the expected losses? *Bull World Health Organ*. 2018;96(2):129–34.
48. Khan SU, Islam N, Jan Z, Din IU, Khan A, Faheem Y. An e-Health care services framework for the detection and classification of breast cancer in breast cytology images as an IoMT application. *Futur Gener Comput Syst* [Internet]. 2019;98:286–96. https://doi.org/10.1016/j.future.2019.01.033
49. Chattu VK, Nanda A, Chattu SK, Kadri SM, Knight AW. The emerging role of blockchain technology applications in routine disease surveillance systems to strengthen global health security. *Big Data Cogn Comput*. 2019;3(2):1–10.

50. Katuwal GJ, Pandey S, Hennessey M, Lamichhane B. Applications of blockchain in healthcare: Current landscape & challenges. 2018;1–17. http://arxiv.org/abs/1812.02776
51. Jervelund SS. How social media is transforming the spreading of knowledge: Implications for our perceptions concerning vaccinations and migrant health. *Scand J Public Health*. 2018;46(2):167–9.
52. Huckle S, White M. Fake news: A technological approach to proving the origins of content, using blockchains. *Big Data*. 2017;5(4):356–71.
53. Mamoshina P, Ojomoko L, Yanovich Y, Ostrovski A, Botezatu A, Prikhodko P, et al. Converging blockchain and next-generation artificial intelligence technologies to decentralize and accelerate biomedical research and healthcare. *Oncotarget*. 2018;9(5):5665–90.
54. Kostova D, Husain MJ, Sugerman D, Hong Y, Saraiya M, Keltz J, et al. Synergies between communicable and noncommunicable disease programs to enhance global health security. *Emerg Infect Dis*. 2017;23(December):S40–6.
55. Bhattacharya S, Singh A, Hossain MM. Strengthening public health surveillance through blockchain technology. *AIMS Public Heal*. 2019;6(3):326–33.
56. Dwivedi AD, Srivastava G, Dhar S, Singh R. A decentralized privacy-preserving healthcare blockchain for IoT. *Sensors* (Switzerland). 2019;19(2):1–17.
57. Lupton D, Maslen S. Telemedicine and the senses: A review. *Sociol Heal Illn*. 2017;39(8):1557–71.
58. Jamil F, Hang L, Kim KH, Kim DH. A novel medical blockchain model for drug supply chain integrity management in a smart hospital. *Electron*. 2019;8(5):1–32.
59. Underwood S. Blockchain beyond bitcoin. *Commun ACM*. 2016;59(11):15–17.
60. Du X, Chen B, Ma M, Zhang Y. Research on the application of blockchain in educational resources. *ACM Int Conf Proceeding Ser*. 2021;1–5. Available from: https://doi.org/10.1145/3503047.3503092
61. Chen H, Pendleton M, Njilla L, Xu S. A survey on ethereum systems security: Vulnerabilities, attacks, and defenses. *ACM Comput Surv*. 2020;53(3):1–29.
62. Kamel Boulos MN, Wilson JT, Clauson KA. Geospatial blockchain: Promises, challenges, and scenarios in health and healthcare. *Int J Health Geogr* [Internet]. 2018;17(1):1–10. https://doi.org/10.1186/s12942-018-0144-x
63. Azzi R, Chamoun RK, Sokhn M. The power of a blockchain-based supply chain. *Comput Ind Eng* [Internet]. 2019;135(August 2018):582–92. https://doi.org/10.1016/j.cie.2019.06.042
64. Wachter RM. Making IT work: Harnessing the power of health IT to improve care in England. *Natl Advis Gr Heal Inf Technol* [Internet]. 2016:1–69. Available from: www.gov.uk/government/uploads/system/uploads/attachment_data/file/550866/Wachter_Review_Accessible.pdf%0Ahttps://assets.publishing.service.gov.uk/government/uploads/system/uploads/attachment_data/file/550866/Wachter_Review_Accessible.pdf
65. Herlihy M. Atomic cross-chain swaps. *Proc Annu ACM Symp Princ Distrib Comput*. 2018:245–54.
66. Bennett B. Blockchain HIE overview: A framework for healthcare interoperability. *Telehealth Med Today*. 2018;2(3):1–6.
67. Mense A, Flatscher M. Security vulnerabilities in ethereum smart contracts. *ACM Int Conf Proceeding Ser*. 2018:375–80.
68. Chen HS, Jarrell JT, Carpenter KA, Cohen DS HX. Blockchain in healthcare: A patient-centered model. *Biomed J Sci Tech Res*. 2019;10(3):1–10.
69. Powles J, Hodson H. Google DeepMind and healthcare in an age of algorithms. *Health Technol* (Berl). 2017;7(4):351–67.
70. Mandl KD, Szolovits P, Kohane IS. Public standards and patients' control: How to keep electronic medical records accessible but private. *Br Med J*. 2001;322(7281):283–7.
71. Dinh-Le C, Chuang R, Chokshi S, Mann D. Wearable health technology and electronic health record integration: Scoping review and future directions. *JMIR mHealth uHealth*. 2019;7(9).
72. Roehrs A, da Costa CA, da Rosa Righi R. OmniPHR: A distributed architecture model to integrate personal health records. *J Biomed Inform* [Internet]. 2017;71:70–81. http://doi.org/10.1016/j.jbi.2017.05.012
73. Flach JM, Schanely P, Kuenneke L, Chidoro B, Mubaslat J, Howard B. Electronic health records and evidence-based practice: Solving the little-data problem. *Proc Int Symp Hum Factors Ergon Heal Care*. 2018;7(1):30–5.

4

Application of Blockchain in Tracking Diseases and Outbreaks

Phool Chandra, Zeeshan Ali, Neetu Sachan,
Vaibhav Rastogi, Mayur Porwal, and Anurag Verma

4.1 Introduction

In 2008, blockchain technology was initially used by Satoshi Nakamoto to create the Bitcoin cryptocurrency system. Since that time, numerous industries, including business and banking, as well as the healthcare industry, have implemented blockchain technology [1]. A blockchain is a decentralized information and dispersed logbook that is accessible from all nodes in a system. Since a blockchain stores data online, it can be compared to an electronic database. Blockchain technology may one day be used to safeguard individual patients' health records in the healthcare sector. Blockchain technology allows for the direct exchange of digital assets between users, removing the requirement for a third person during the procedure. Blockchain is a distributed ledger that maintains information in a series of blocks secured by cryptographic hashes [2]. The decentralized character of blockchain and its immutability, visibility, and audibility all promote increased safety as well as reliability of transactions and other operations. A blockchain is a type of dispersed document that includes an ever-expanding data, which is referred to as blocks [3]. Blockchain technology has uses outside of the sphere of cryptocurrencies, covering the financial as well as social sectors, risk managing systems, and healthcare delivery networks, among others [4,5]. On a blockchain network, a block consists of four components—details about the hash (identification number) of the current block, the hash of the preceding block, and the date and time—that connect every new block to its antecedent. Blockchain technology comes in three basic architectural flavors: public (permissionless), private (permission), and hybrid blockchains. Everyone can join public blockchains because they are created to be open-sourced. Furthermore, all transactions carried out on a public blockchain are fully viewable to all participants; therefore, there is no control via any one user or entity, because evidence of work has become the most well-known method applied for public blockchains [6]. Contrarily, users of private blockchains must first obtain permission to join the network, and all transactions can only be accessed by those users who have been granted access. In contrast, because hybrid blockchains are adaptable, users can choose which information should be kept accessible to the public and which should be kept private [7]. In the industry, the health system is an essential sector. In addition to a standard physical examination, numerous medical traceability devices can be used to diagnose patients' body states, such as heart rate, blood sugar levels, electroencephalograms, and other crucial biomedical signals [8], or increased healthfulness [9]. Sharing a quite-large amount of information among institutions might hasten scientific work, clinical problem-solving, and the development of policy. For example, when deciding on the best method of action, a doctor may need accessibility to a patient's medical data stored at numerous sites. Also, this market will have a significant impression on the economy [10]. User trust is essential for the achievement of health records exchange. Any flaw may result in the patient feeling insecure of the online healthcare industry. Blockchain allows marketers to retain a perspective of the items applied in medicine. Blockchain technologies will help the drugs and health sectors get rid of fake medications and make it possible to trace all these products [11,12]. It aids in identifying the root of falsity. Blockchain can guarantee the confidentiality of patient documents and, once created, may preserve medical history in a permanent manner. The hospital uses these decentralized networks with all common hardware. With the energy conserved by these gadgets, researchers may calculate estimates for treatments, medications, and remedies for various ailments and conditions [13]. Healthcare suppliers and clients can both benefit from studies on healthcare content exchange. Several cloud-based options for transferring healthcare information have been put forth, but the reliability of a third-party cloud system is in doubt. Still, blockchain has been offered for healthcare document sharing which does not depend on accepting a third party. Nevertheless, current methods primarily concentrate on the data gathered from physician exams. They are useless at sharing continuous data streams produced by sensors and other surveillance equipment [14]. Blockchain is a decentralized database that continuously includes new items and never modifies them without broad consensus. The worth of a blockchain hash is determined by the cryptographic hash that connects each database block with recently revised information block records [15]. Data is processed decentralized, and visible, and responds to all network participants because of the distributed blockchain database design. A single attack is prevented by this decentralized structure, thereby bolstering and securing it. By minimizing two times as much medical practice and monitoring, it improves patient care and allows for greater control of health data while saving time and resources for both clients and clinicians.

Maintaining medical data on a blockchain will enable the patient to monitor where their documentation is going [16]. A blockchain system uses program agreement to enable peer-to-peer value transactions without the need for an agent. It begins operating on the internet on a network of P2P computers that are all operating the program and have a precise copy of the transactions log. Public, private, hybrid, along with group blockchain technologies are just a few of the different flavors available [17]. In the field of healthcare, growth is rapid, at increasing rates. Higher-quality healthcare services that are backed by advanced technology are in great interest today. In this case, blockchain may play a significant role in revolutionizing the healthcare sector. Additionally, the framework of the medical sector is changing in support of a patient-centered approach that places special emphasis on the following two factors: readily available services and adequate healthcare supplies at all times [4]. Blockchain recovers healthcare organizations' capacity to perform proper patient attention and top-notch medical facilities. With this technique, the time-consuming and repetitious course of health information exchange, which raises expenses for the healthcare industry, can be promptly resolved [18]. Blockchain technology enables public participation in health research projects. Also, better public welfare research and information exchange will enhance treatments for several groups. A centralized database is used to administer the entire healthcare sector, along with the organizations [19].

4.2 Healthcare

Infectious illnesses like the flu or SARS have hallmarks of fast breakout, high infection levels, and possibly fatal sickness. The threats to public health posed by these infectious illnesses have become more serious [20]. The blockchain enables healthcare organizations to provide high-quality patient care more effectively. Blockchain technology offers enormous capability in the requirement for a more patient-centered strategy to healthcare organizations because of its capacity to interconnect different systems and enhance the reliability of electronic health records (EHR). Blockchain technology is continually gaining more importance in the healthcare sector due to its many applications. Only a few examples of usage fields include public healthcare management, health data, computerized health claim judgments, patient portal accessibility, individual clinical data interchange, user-centered health research, pharmaceutical forgeries, novel treatments, and targeted medicines [21,22]. The application of blockchain technologies and SCs especially can help with endpoint flipping, limited clinical trial publications, client informed consent, and data scavenging, including misplaced data findings. An EHR contains details on a patient's condition, clinical progress, medical history, records, information, forecasts, as well as any other documentation about a patient's health. A blockchain-based EHR system can be viewed as a protocol that customers use to get and maintain the security and confidentiality of their medical data. There are many advantages to using an EHR system powered by blockchain. The central as well as proprietor of information that has been destroyed or breached is recognized, and documents are maintained in a dispersed format that is simple for non-affiliated service firms to verify. A single, consistent data collection is created by combining data from several sources, which is updated and delivered regularly. A more effective and protected system is required in the healthcare sector to handle increasingly complex transactions and records, maintain medical information, pre-authorize fees, resolve insurance claims, or execute more difficult activities [23,24]. One of the essential qualities of blockchain software is transparency. Securing personal details and data about the patients receiving treatment is essential. The extent of fraudulent news on social media platforms causes worry and dread, since the information is unreliable. Due to its capacity to evaluate data and deliver real-time data improvements, blockchain technology may offer a potential means of ensuring the examination of data accuracy. It can make the transition easier from connectivity controlled by organizations to patient-centered interoperability [25,26]. Only hospital or healthcare practitioner networks now have access to electronic medical information, which is kept in data centers. This kind of information centralization can be expensive to manage and is liable to security breaches. In order to resolve this, the blockchain keeps a detailed record of every patient's medical history. This safer method includes the patient's, doctors', regulators', hospitals', and even insurers' oversight. In order to reduce insurance claims and use doctors to make correct medicine recommendations, this assures precautionary measures for keeping medical records and patients' comprehensive medical history, altering medical practices to promote a patient-centered strategy. Blockchain-based healthcare systems can improve patient data security and privacy by granting patients access to their medical records [27,28]. These platforms can also combine patient data by facilitating the sharing of patient history among various healthcare facilities. Keeping tracking of patients' healthcare records is essential in the healthcare industry. Due to its exceptional sensitivity, this information is a top target for hackers. All sensitive data must be kept secure. Data control is an additional element that will aid in providing the patient with the best possible care. As a result, obtaining

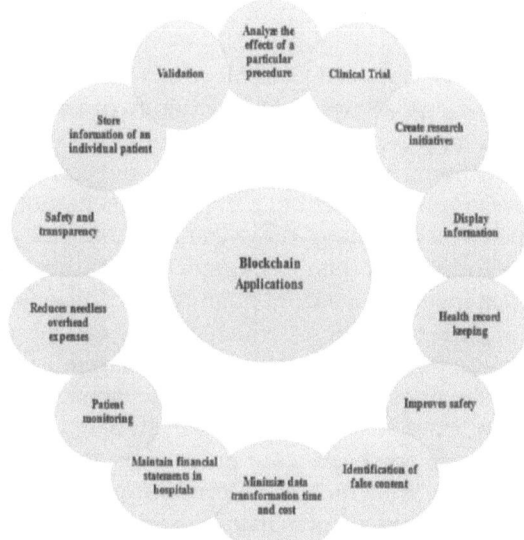

FIGURE 4.1
Blockchain technology has important uses in healthcare.

and exchanging patient health information is another application that could profit from the state-of-the-art technologies. Although blockchain technology is incredibly resilient to faults and assaults, it also offers a wide range of access control solutions. The blockchain is a great medium for healthcare data because of this [29] and the significant applications of blockchain shown in Figure 4.1.

4.3 Blockchain Technology's Capabilities in Healthcare

The entire prescription process is visible due to the blockchain, from production to store shelves. IoT and blockchain can be utilized to monitor traffic and freight direction, including speed. The quantity of healthcare information available is growing incredibly quickly as a result of the growth of medical information technology. The efficient use of medical resources, clinical decision support, medical quality control, precision medicine, or disease risk evaluation and predictions have all benefited from the exchange and utilization of medical information [30,31]. It offers the chance to strategically schedule purchases to prevent disruptions and limitations of a specific medicine in pharmacies, clinics, and various other healthcare facilities. Blockchain-based digital structures would be used to help assure that the logistical data is protected from unauthorized changes [32]. It encourages self-assurance and prevents those who are attracted in acquiring drugs from dealing data, money, or pharmaceuticals in an unauthorized way. Technology can greatly improve patients' situations while keeping expenses down. It removes all hurdles and difficulties in multi-level authentication [33–35]. Blockchain is the best technology for protection because it can keep an unchangeable, decentralized, and open record of all medical information. Blockchain, on the other hand, is both open and closed, hiding any individual's identity behind complex and protected algorithms which can keep confidentiality of medical information [36]. The technology's decentralized design enables rapid and safe information sharing between patients, doctors, and various other healthcare workers. Blockchain technology allows the transition to interoperability, led by patients allowing patients to maintain accessibility to their medical records and by allowing them to follow laws. In addition to increasing security and confidentiality, this also gives patients more power over their confidential data. Implementation, evaluation, and quality verification are difficult tasks. Any of these technical issues could be solved by usage of the blockchain in the industry. When tracking drugs, authorities will use blockchain reports to distinguish real medications from phony ones. This ensures that all authorized participants can trade digital transactions, which include patient information. By amending a single approval, patients who get doctors may share all their information [37,38]. An increasing number of businesses are embracing blockchain, including the healthcare sector. Also, early users of the health ecosystem's technology are pleased with them. In order to completely transform the healthcare industry in the arriving years, blockchain has a comprehensive strategy that includes addressing the issues influencing the current framework. Doctors, patients, or pharmacists can quickly reach all the data at any time thanks to it. Day or night, medical firms study, test, and learn regarding blockchain technologies for application in the medical field for health data [39]. It has made a name for itself as a vital instrument in healthcare by incorporating medications, improving payment options, and decentralizing patients' health-related history data. Blockchain is a crucial technology for the medical industry, besides other modern technologies, such as machine learning, as well as artificial intelligence. Undoubtedly, there are correct ways that blockchain is changing the healthcare industry. The system is designed to analyze the medical supply chain using blockchain technology [40]. The capacity of blockchain allows for the creation of a complex data storage structure that documents a person's complete medical history, including diagnoses, test results, previous regimens, or even measurements made by intelligent sensors. This strategy makes it simple for a doctor to get all the data needed to ensure accuracy diagnoses or recommendations. While all the data is maintained in a particular blockchain system, it is secured from loss and change [41]. Blockchain can be utilized to circumvent internal networks in businesses. A substantial organization with numerous autonomous participants, with different degrees of power on a blockchain database that is encrypted, can protect organizations from hazards and attacks from the outside world. These rescue attacks and other issues, like computer conflicts, as well as hardware defect, will be eradicated if a healthcare provider properly adopts a blockchain network [42]. Blockchain is a category of shared database from the standpoint of information management, where a lot of data, as well as information, is kept with the decentralization, highly available, or high trustworthiness capabilities of blockchain technology seen in Figure 4.2. Based on this, blockchain can create an efficient data analysis and collection, but also a real-time monitoring process that can encourage the extremely logical affiliation of physical "data islands" and realize evidence chunking, "turning scatter into a whole," or "turning points into the surfaces," while improving the efficiency of communication among system participants. When it comes to social governance, blockchain software provides a safe distributed computer network for establishing dependable cooperative relationships and decentralized collaborative frameworks [43]. More than 10 years old, China's public healthcare emergency response program is crucial to the country's daily control of public medical emergencies or early detection of infectious ailments. The blockchain system can be improved for the protection and management of infectious illnesses, achieving more focused and multi-party distributed

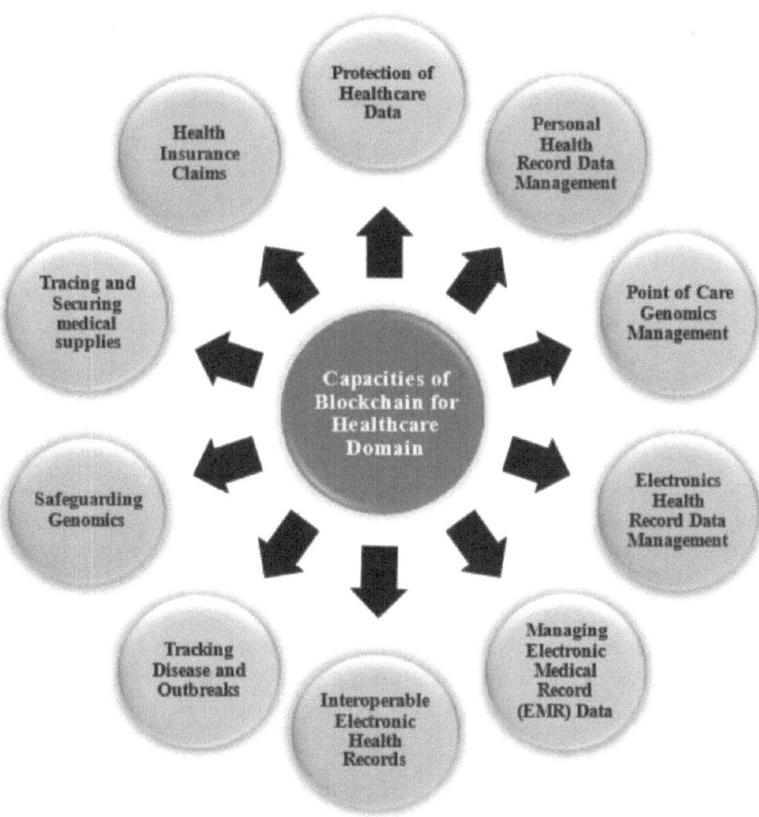

FIGURE 4.2
Potential of blockchain technology in the healthcare sector.

monitoring, as well as traceability for infectious illnesses, depending on the current real-time surveillance and early warning technology.

4.4 Functions for Storing and Tracking Information about Infectious Diseases

Utilizing blockchain technology, data storage for infectious diseases will enable data recompiling and storage throughout an epidemic. Each entity in that kind of disease-direct tracking system can upload disease-related information as well as data on an automated node basis. Utilizing blockchain technology, data storage for contagious diseases will enable data recording as well as storage throughout an epidemic. Each entity in that kind of disease direct reporting process can upload disease-related data as well as details on an autonomous node basis. The data the hospital collected about infectious diseases, like as verified cases, suspected cases, information about diseased patients, etc., are handled by hospital 1. The blockchain automatically records the upload time along with the time stamp. A fixed-length hash value of the supplied data would be kept on the blockchain in addition to a time stamp. Another node on the blockchain would have access to the disease data uploaded by hospital 1 through the blockchain agreement, allowing them to view it. The hash function converts data of any length into a fixed-length function value. A hash mechanism can hash the contents and produce a fixed-length hash result during the upload of disease-related information to the blockchain [44]. Every unit of data has an irreversible, one-of-a-kind hash value. The resultant hash value will vary dramatically once the input data even slightly differs or changes. Consequently, it simply requires computing a hash function on the actual disease evidence and comparing the results to the hash maintained on the blockchain to determine whether the record on a blockchain has been altered. If the two results match each other, the disease details can be assumed to be valid (no forgery or manipulation). In order to ensure data security, the hospital can check the preceding pieces of material through its hash when it needs to submit new disease cases (hospital 2). The updated data would still be kept as a hash even if hospital 2 also had fresh disease information to submit to the blockchain. From this tamper-proof keeping approach, the tamper-resistant illness-preserving data assures the veracity of tracing. According to the chain retention of blockchain, all the evidence for the update of communicable diseases information must be stored in chronological sequence and cannot be changed. Hence, each node of a health institution will submit an information amendment query to the contagious diseases blockchain system for consensual confirmation whenever it determines that the recorded infectious disease information has to be updated once more [45,46]. If the newly revised information regarding infectious diseases is accepted by the consensus, then it will be stored on the blockchain alongside the most recent upload time. After that, the system will send a broadcast to the national CDC as well as the managing department in order to validate and modify the information that is displayed at the terminals. In the end, the national CDC and pertinent organization agencies disseminate it to any nodes that were participating. When it comes to the function of tracking, the information gathering and keeping in the illness reporting system does not follow a hierarchical sequence. This means that the lower-level nodes do not gather data to send up to the higher-level nodes. Instead, every node in the country that can collect relevant data would participate in the uploading and storing activities, which would result in the establishment of a horizontal process for the transfer of disease information. A data transfer procedure, also known as a transaction on the blockchain, is initiated each time the preceding node completes its recording, commencing at the beginning of the illness information record and continuing until its conclusion [47]. A new block would be produced for each disease conversion transaction to keep a record of the methodology of the transaction. The move-out party's, along with the move-in party's, transactions addresses, the overall price of the transaction, the period of time it took to complete, and any linked contents are all included in this segment. (This information is unmodifiable.) The from-address is a representation of the exceptional address labelling of the node that came before this one, and the to-address is a representation of the exceptional address labelling of the node that is now being communicated with. And thus, focusing on a block of details of the conveying of disease information, we are able to unequivocally understand the process of disease storing information (for example, party inputting, information input) that took place immediately prior to the information recording with the node of the existing organization. This is because the information was transferred. Since the blockchain is linked by the hash feature value created by the earlier block, which forms the sequences planning of previous transactions, any node can trace back, relying on the transaction address of the instant last output node, and question all the transaction-relevant data that comprises this particular transaction address, till it arrives at the transaction input node. This is possible because the blockchain is linked by the hash function value produced by the previous block, which attaches the blockchain and produces the sequential procedure of preceding transactions. Once the "transaction" of illness information between the previous node and the next node has been completed successfully, the information will be saved in the blockchain, which will establish a database, called a "transaction" database [48], shown in Figure 4.3 and Figure 4.4. All transaction is stored in its block, and each block has its unique hash value to identify it. This particular block contains informational contents regarding the originator, the receivers, the period the transaction occurred, the message that was sent during the transaction, and other related information. The entity that was used as input in the preceding block will be used as output in the block that comes after it, linking the blockchain. You can identify the transaction details in the

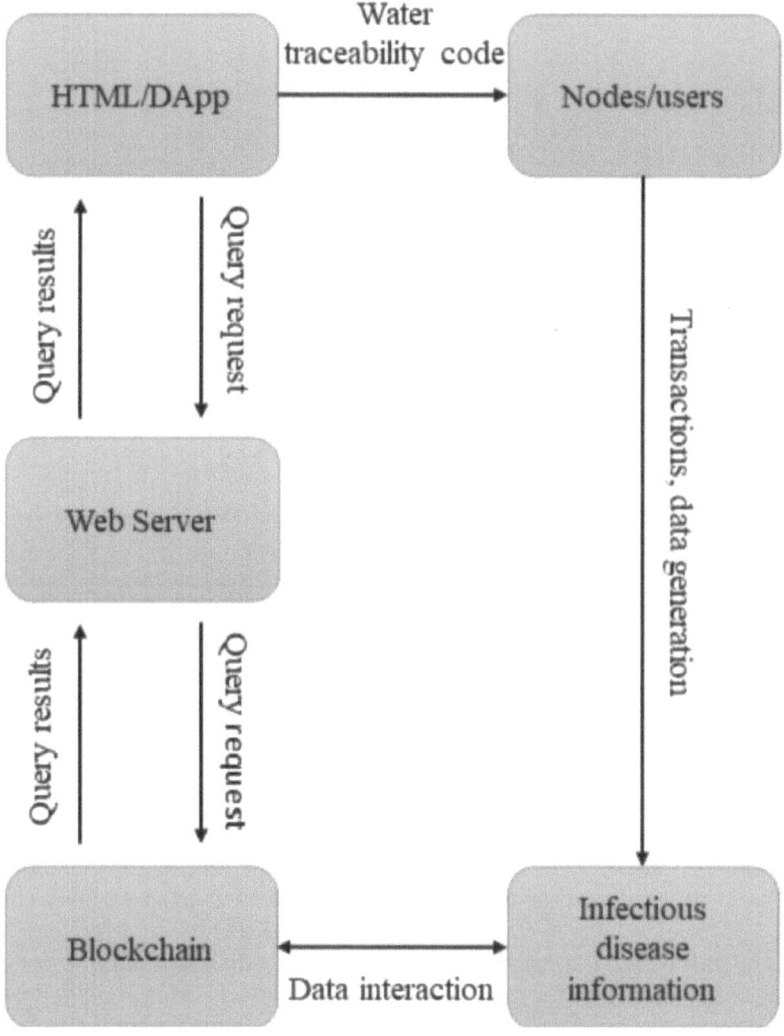

FIGURE 4.3
Interaction workflow of tracing.

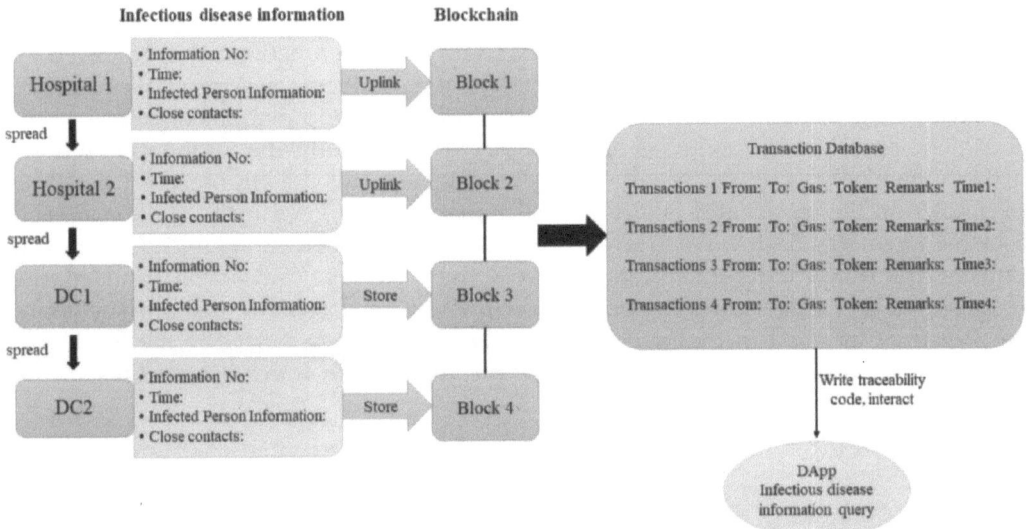

FIGURE 4.4
Storing and tracking information about infections and diseases.

blockchain, which contains the address, by entering the location of the existing transaction exporter. This allows you to query any and all communicable diseases pathogen evidence that satisfies the necessities of the situations and, ultimately, discover the primary contamination condition when the contagious disease spreads. The relevant entity that satisfies the authority can access the final result of the tracing process by using the front-end page or the DApp application (a dispersed application). When associated entities send query requests to a web server, the web server forwards such requests to the blockchain monitoring system by utilizing SDK or API techniques. Lastly, the blockchain tracking system evaluates the source based on the transaction that was validated by all parties, delivers the results of the inquiry, and shows the relevant data in the display manner on the frontend visualization platform. Take, for instance, how traceability refers to the process of locating patients who are infected. It is of the highest priority to avoid the transmission of the coronavirus. With blockchain software, one is able to record direct fighting activities, follow the travels of infected patients, and offer real-time data about afflicted locations. The usage of blockchain technology to create surveillance of a person's activities in virus-free regions is another interesting application for the technology. The blockchain is utilized to keep track of safety zone details, like population, location, as well as the status of the existing coronavirus epidemic. In order to maintain openness and honesty across the medical supply chain, it is essential that products and medical resources be regularly monitored and traced. This monitoring is made feasible by the blockchain network's ability for recording transactions and monitoring their progress [49]. The platforms that address the problem of providing great healthcare at a reasonable price were powered by blockchain technology. It has the opportunity to provide a workable approach to tracking the illness epidemic in order to safeguard a greater number of people. It permits real-time regimen checking, which enables the position of infected persons to be tracked so that they can receive the appropriate therapy at the appropriate time. Fewer errors in diagnosis may occur if hospitals and medical practitioners have access to a database of medical histories that is both safe and dependable [50,51]. Figure 4.3 shows interaction workflow of tracing. Storing and tracking information about infections and diseases are depicted in Figure 4.4.

4.4.1 At Hospital Level

The technological facilities necessary for the implementation of decentralized software is provided by a blockchain. It is made up of a connected series of blocks that are connected utilizing hash pointers; every block has transaction data for an item that can be digitized [52]. So at its foundation, blockchain software is dependent on hash-based data formats, which offer benefits, such as the elimination of collisions, the binding of data, and the concealment of data. One of the prevalent technologies utilized in electronic medical records (EMR) in contemporary hospital infrastructures in manufacturing areas is blockchain. *EMR* stands for "electronic medical information." The characteristics of decentralization, data provenance, or robustness are among those that have considered blockchain technology suited for keeping, maintaining, and exchanging confidential health information in electronic medical records (EMR) [53]. In contrast, "health chain" is an electronic medical record (EMR) system that was built on the blockchain and utilized IBM's Hyperledger Fabric. This technology contributes to the achievement of scalable data protection as well as the optimization of the EMR system's productivity. Transactions in the billing sector, insurance occurrences, and monitoring measures such as nosocomial infection observation are thought to benefit, at the very least, from the usage of blockchain technology [4,54]. The benefit of utilizing this technique is that it enables a lot of information to be saved, processed, and distributed to the relevant parties in a very timely manner, free of any link failures or delays. It can revise health database interoperability with built-in verification mechanisms, hence reducing the dangers of data theft [55].

4.4.2 Resource Management in Health Systems

The management of logistical and human factors in healthcare systems can be simplified with the help of blockchain technology. For instance, external vendors may supply healthcare systems with counterfeit pharmaceuticals and instruments that are of a lower quality than such systems require. The utilization of blockchain technology allows for the validation of quality requirements at various points along the supplier chain management and the notification of relevant authorities on potentially problematic deviations [56]. In addition, managing human resources in today's digital age necessitates storing and making use of employee data for tracking attendance and leaves, assessing productivity, and implementing security precautions that involve complex authentication procedures. The application of blockchain technology has the potential to make such procedures more effective and help the growth of more intelligent health service organizations [57,58]. This section will study the various applications of blockchain technology that can be used in the field of medicine, such as the maintenance of critical patient data and the management of healthcare records. Because its increasingly widespread application has the potential to enhance people's overall quality of life, blockchain technology has gained societal importance in the domain of medicine. Using the same line of reasoning, computation has the potential to alleviate some of the issues that exist in this sector. The field of informatics, for instance, makes a contribution to the digitized medical documents by guaranteeing a more dependable transmission of data, applicability in other areas, and log management [59,60].

4.4.3 Patient-Level Applications

Blockchain technology is progressively used to exchange health information with individuals and their carers because of the decentralized qualities it possesses that address data safety issues. Blockchain technology was developed by Bitcoin creator Satoshi Nakamoto. The patient participation initiatives also encourage the effective use of health information technology and boost patient–provider contact through digital channels [61]. Moreover, blockchain technology–based mobile health measures are allowing distant patients to observe via the usage of biosensors, which helps bridge accessible barriers in patient-level healthcare [62,63]. The creation of fresh patient data certificates for use by medical professionals in different institutions is required by blockchain technology. The freshly added information is typically repetitious and causes a waste of time, which is a significant health malfunction. This is a problem since new knowledge might cause health problems. Because of their place in the supplier chain, every individual may have a unique set of rights or choices about accessibility. Furthermore, any block that contains information about medicine will have a hash connecting it to another block, regardless of whose block it was [64]. In addition, the data transparency characteristic that is a part of the blockchain design will be able to assist in finding the full root route and putting an end to the circulation of falsified pharmaceuticals. When a patient attends a different clinic, that patient is issued a fresh medical card, which is then filed away in a certain location. These specifics are typically withheld from the general citizens and consist of records compiled from caretakers at the facilities in question. Blockchain technology offers a practical solution to a number of data processing issues. Using this technique will enable the development of transparent and comparable blockchain medical information across the world [65–67]. The monitoring and discussing of patient medical information is another use case for blockchain technology's potential applications. Patients may have trouble accessing their medical documents because these records are typically housed in several different healthcare services. The blockchain concept may make it possible for patients to have complete and protected access to all their records as well as their medical history [68]. There have been some proposals made for using blockchain technology to organize patient medical information and facilitate access to those records. By the application of disseminated blockchain principles, the information managing system MedBlock, which is dependent on blockchain technology, provides efficient EMR access and retrieval [69,70]. This program has a significantly better consensus process, which assures that the network will not get overburdened by activity. When implementing software like blockchain, which continues to increase in functionality over time, there is a risk of overloading the network. Access control and cryptographic both contribute significantly to MedBlock's high level of security [71,72].

4.4.4 Disease Surveillance at the Community Level

The term "surveillance" refers to the "systematic, continuous collection, collation, and data evaluation and the timely distribution of details to those who require to understand so that the acts can be taken" [73] regarding communicable and noncommunicable illnesses by all the general health processes based on the national priority areas as per WHO's International Health Regulations (IHR). For instance, a fatal virus such as Nipah can spread around the world in just 36 hours, and it has the potential to produce a pandemic by jeopardizing the state of health security caused by increased urbanization and globalization [74,75]. The monitoring of communicable diseases is a continuous operation that is complicated and ineffective due to the large number of self-regulating entities that send data to a centralized information system. Hence, ensuring that information continues to flow without interruption and in a timely fashion is a difficult task. In addition, there are no rewards that are provided for ordinary staff members [45,76]. The benefits of blockchain technology are beneficial to disease monitoring systems in a variety of ways, as will be addressed further on. The timely reporting done by the health workers at the district level is what makes district-level monitoring so effective. A warning sign can be produced by making use of data taken from prescriptions and the most common complaints. In the same manner, the facilities can be linked as a participatory node whenever a specific favorable check for a prioritized disease will operate as an induction so that early public health actions can be done. This will allow for the best possible outcome [77]. It is also possible to use this technique with other technologies, such as geographical data systems, in order to speed up the routine examinations of epidemics. Supply chain systems for drugs and vaccines can additionally be made more efficient by ensuring that they are delivered on time. These blockchain apps may also assess the price of different treatment approaches now accessible and disseminate the data at a quick movement, conserving time by minimizing the amount of redundancy that occurs in reporting. The second crucial feature is that the blockchain can circumvent the constraints of the district's health information systems that are previously in place, since it ensures visibility and accurate reporting, like in the instance of declaring deaths caused by a specific outbreak shown in Figure 4.5 [45].

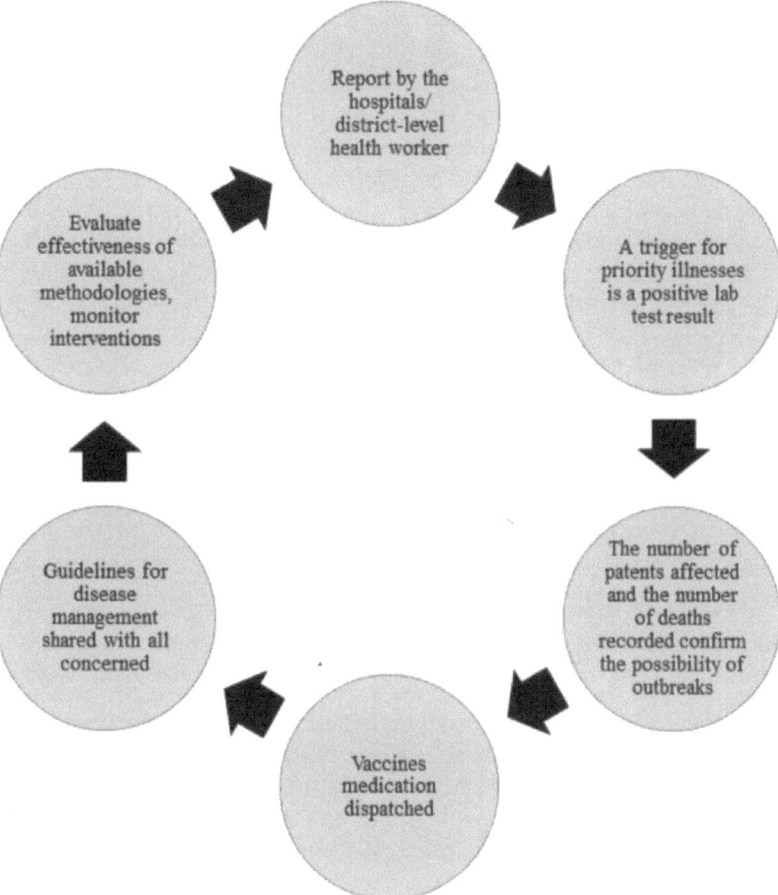

FIGURE 4.5
Sequencing of incidents in an illness surveillance system.

4.4.5 In the Early Detection and Surveillance of Infectious Diseases

The existing early alert system in China for the avoidance and management of infectious illnesses needs data to be collected and described via layer-by-layer inspections. As a result, the system is not enough for dealing with unanticipated contagious diseases and has glaring weaknesses. When used to the construction of a platform for the avoidance and management of infectious illnesses, using blockchain technology has the potential to effectively create detection and early indication of newly emerging serious illnesses [78]. Research and implementation on a local and international scale of blockchain software for contagious disease surveillance and early advising, in conjunction with other technologies, include artificial intelligence and consensus processes, as well as smart transactions [79]. Utilizing smart radio frequency electronic recognition tags to gather monitoring data of feasible and clarified Ebola virus infection into the SERIS and smart IoT to connect telephone companies, Ebola virus surveillance branches, Ebola vaccine supply agencies, as well as transport agencies to establish a national epidemic monitoring network via blockchain, the Democratic Republic of the Congo, for example, can monitor the spread of the Ebola virus throughout the country. This is accomplished by using blockchain software to form a national network for Ebola virus monitoring [80]. This serves as an excellent template for constructing a comprehensive contagious disease epidemic surveillance system in China. In the national study on applications relating to the area of communicable disease monitoring and earlier warnings under the guise of blockchain technology, to create a contagious disease initial warning methodology, the model incorporates and communicates big information resources through the use of smart contracts. This provides a contagious disease shared data platform that is necessary for the development of China's rapid acute contagious illness monitoring and earlier warning system. There is a shortage of systematic studies on early communicable diseases data gathering, geographic warning systems, and interconnection of government as well as social resources, which is found to be the primary focus of the existing domestic blockchain medical software research. However, it has been discovered that this research is primarily cantered on the giving of medical data information [81]. Using blockchain technology, a four-level pandemic preventive chain network can be built by integrating communicable disease monitoring and emergency alert networks at the district, municipal, regional, and national stages [80,82]. Primary healthcare institutes (hospitals) are incorporated in the four-level pandemic avoidance sequence to obtain encoded information sharing and a two-level automatic early detection process at the local and national levels. This is accomplished through the integration of the national CDC, the specific network documentation system, the national automatic early detection system for contagious diseases, the nationwide three-level public healthcare information exchange framework, and the national automatic early warning system for contagious diseases [78,83].

4.4.6 Utilizing Blockchain Technology to Streamline the Reporting, Establishing a Distributed Procedure for Infectious Diseases

The core component of blockchain technology is a disseminated database that is jointly managed by various parties. This database should implement a decentralized data collection and control model even though all entities can acquire an entire copy of the information and engage in the space to storing as well as the monitoring of the data. In between the base layer of the blockchain P2P system and the information-applying layers, a covering of multi-party protected computing (MPC) or data protection sharing layer is assembled. This allows for the realization of the efficient sharing of communicable disease data within the area and among various institutions under the assumption of defending privacy rights and organizational data security [84]. At the identical time, the data cipher text is kept under the security of the key interchange algorithm or MPC architecture, and smart contracts are automatically alerted. After a contagious disease pandemic, the data cipher text is released by the geographic notice smart agreement and given to medical centers in the surrounding areas for expressing health-related and personal information about the pandemic. The method of reporting infectious diseases benefits greatly from blockchain technology as well [85]. At the moment, the national infectious illness reporting system expects an excessive amount of thoroughness and precision from the data that is reported on infectious diseases. While there is the possibility of "suspected cases," the first signs and complications of new illnesses often aren't obvious and can't be diagnosed precisely. In addition, hospitals and medical professionals are under a lot of pressure to report, which can cause them to miss the early warning signs. Through the use of blockchain technology, potential incidents are initially submitted immediately to the blockchain networks by monitoring sentinel sites that are responsible for certificate maintenance. The data on the reported case is encrypted using a digital certificate by the sentinel software, and the person's public key is forwarded to every hospital node that is a part of the four-level chain that prevents epidemics. Case ciphertext information is distributed around the whole hospital node using a P2P network [86]. The regional pandemic protection chain has a leader node that is in charge of beginning verification and consensus. This node is also responsible for ensuring that the final document is automatically synced to all the nodes across the network. Earlier notification will create extensive utilization of the regional pandemic preventative measures chain smart agreement threshold judgment and the big records examination provided by the national automatic communicable diseases alert system; at the similar time, confirmation, geographic consultation, pathogen investigation, specialist discussion, and the last verification of communicable diseases will be performed concurrently. The blockchain system will allow for parallel reporting of detected and proven cases, which will reduce the amount of decision-making needed during an epidemic [13,87].

In order to ensure that the product is effective, testing must be carried out methodically, and trustworthy information regarding the total number of tests conducted must be maintained. To achieve this objective, the technology of blockchain can be used to facilitate the construction of dispersed check-in locations for evaluating patients. The organizers of each of these check-in locations are capable of performing the duties of nodes inside the identically distributed blockchain system [88]. These network sites can continuously update information about the number of tests performed and the quantity of cases with laboratory confirmation at their local check-in station. All healthcare professionals and governmental organizations can have confidence in storing knowledge in the network even though blockchain is unchangeable and makes tampering impossible. All of a person's data, involving gender, age, medical records, underlying health issues, the seriousness of the condition, the symptoms experienced, and the recommended plan of treatment, are securely uploaded to the Internet when they evaluate positive for a disease. Soon, every medical facility handling a reported case will be allowed to consult this research to forecast the kind of facilities and treatments required to handle the current problem [89].

4.5 Blockchain Technology in the Pharmaceutical Industry

Blockchain is a recent technology which is being applied to create innovative solutions across numerous sectors, particularly healthcare. Blockchain software is used in the healthcare industry to store and exchange patient data between hospitals, diagnostic laboratories, pharmaceutical companies, and physicians. Blockchain technology can accurately spot significant mistakes in the field of healthcare, even ones that could be fatal. It can also improve the effectiveness, security, or openness of exchanging medical details in the healthcare system. Medical organizations can use this technology to better understand and analyze patient records [4,19]. In healthcare companies, applications for blockchains are numerous. Security, a major concern, is addressed by the use of cryptographic methods that analyze blocks of private data. Different paradigms are used to create security elements. The security risk presented by fake drugs has been addressed using sequential. With this technique, serial numbers are authenticated throughout the whole supply chain system, thanks to confirmation checks. Pharmaceutical quality control is accomplished by utilizing electronic signatures, blockchain chain identifiers, health-related information, or data analysts distributed from the producer to the pharmacy to keep the constant quality. Medication tracking has also been improved to minimize theft [90–92].

4.5.1 Counterfeit Prevention

Pharmaceuticals are serialized and given safety determinants so that customers can validate them and differentiate between genuine and counterfeit products. By transactions that are exposed and based on chain codes, the blockchain network also improves security. The medical sector needs trust and openness, and that's why, lacking it, the counterfeiting profession flourishes and exposes the public to risks associated with poor-quality or subpar medicines. By using blockchains for quality control as well as the identification of phony medications, protection is enhanced and lives are protected [93]. Counterfeiting can be avoided using several strategies, such as the Anti-Counterfeit Medication System (ACMS). As follows, ACMS makes use of the Ethereum blockchain and InterPlanetary File System (IPFS) networks:

- To avoid cloning, implement ownership standards for both retail and non-retail medications.
- Create Ethereum smart contracts using IPFS networks as well as the Ethereum blockchain for effective ACMS administration.
- Introduce the program for small businesses.
- Assess and examine the suggested system. The ACMS successfully thwarts fraud. Upon starting a transaction, participants provide a chain code. The approvals are gathered and submitted to the purchasing services, where transactional confirmation is the final stage after the signature is validated by endorsing team members [94,95].

4.5.2 Product Distribution

The existence of various dealers and middlemen creates the potential for unethical business practices, which in turn reduce the effectiveness of the supply network. The use of blockchain technology to stop the distribution of substandard drugs has received widespread praise. Pharmaceuticals that do not meet quality standards are removed from circulation, and an inquiry is conducted into how they made their way into the supply system for pharmaceuticals. To enhance pharmaceutical distribution, accounting systems, chains code, and serialization—a process in which sequence numbers are allocated to pharmaceuticals to permit recognition and segmentation utilized. Information stored on blockchains is subject to stringent regulations to prevent illegal access, which would put the integrity of protection systems at risk. The use of the Internet of Things (IoT) in the delivery of pharmaceuticals results in increased productivity [96–98].

4.5.3 Tracking and Tracing

It is only natural that items that are in transportation should be monitored and identified from the point of shipment to their final destination. Stoppages in delivery have a negative impact on corporate processes in general, while issues in the healthcare and pharmaceutical sectors can destroy life or aggravation of the illness. The distribution of pharmaceuticals is now possible with the use of blockchain software. The monitoring and tracing of drugs is necessary for the successful running of businesses, the protection of patient's health, and also the fulfillment of regulatory requirements. It is now possible to conduct pharmaceutical trade and patient monitoring without interruption due to sophisticated and safe tracking or tracing technology. These technologies ensure that commodities in circulation are supplied on schedule to the appropriate locations. A protected international register was established in order to ease the process of medicine supply on a global scale. Even though the technology has great prospects for giant pharmaceutical companies, it is expected that smaller firms would also gain [4,99].

4.5.4 Safety and Security

Because pharmaceuticals are such high-value commodity, it is imperative that they be protected by security measures. The cryptographic capabilities offered by blockchain applications form the foundation of the pharmaceutical company's security and privacy systems. The capabilities of tracing or tracking drugs fulfill the regulatory standards, and cryptography technology improves the safety of drugs. Theft and the distribution of fake medications are both actively being combated by increased security measures. Unauthorized drug alterations are also minimized, which prohibits opportunist pharmaceutical stakeholders from modifying pharmaceuticals and lowering safety in this way. The governance of supply chain networks is based on the implementation of strong safety or security procedures, which, if compromised, trigger an alarm [90,100].

4.6 Conclusion

In the medicine sector, blockchain technology is utilized for many different uses, including protecting patient data and regulating the distribution of pharmaceuticals. The widespread adoption of supporting innovative technologies throughout the ecosystem will have a significant impact on how helpful Blockchain will be in the medical sector. It typically entails tracing networks, recording medications, running studies, and assuring healthcare. Clinical trials gain from the credibility and results that blockchain technology offers. By keeping them in a computerized fingerprint, this information can be stored on the blockchain in the manner of smart contracts. The usage of blockchain technique in healthcare has many benefits, some of which include the improvement of network services security on all stages, the confirmation and verification of the identities of all attendees, and the standardization of authorization procedures for accessing electronic medical records. A distributed ledger called a blockchain is utilized to keep the surveillance of the pharmaceutical delivery system and to keep track of who is responsible for which medications. Because this technology may be used to store the data of even a single patient, it is useful for helping to assess and confirm the consequences of a certain procedure. It helps hospitals keep their financial statements up-to-date and reduces the amount of time and money spent on record transformation. The decentralized ledger system of blockchain makes it possible to transmit patient healthcare documents in a safe manner, improves the protection of healthcare data, regulates the supply chain for medicines, and assists investigators in the medical field in decoding genetic information.

References

1. Angraal S, Krumholz HM, Schulz WL. Blockchain Technology. *Circ Cardiovasc Qual Outcomes* [Internet]. 2017 Sep;10(9). Available from: www.ahajournals.org/doi/10.1161/CIRCOUTCOMES.117.003800
2. Xu Y, Li X, Zeng X, Cao J, Jiang W. Application of Blockchain Technology in Food Safety Control: Current Trends and Future Prospects. *Crit Rev Food Sci Nutr* [Internet]. 2022 Apr 5;62(10):2800–19. Available from: www.tandfonline.com/doi/full/10.1080/10408398.2020.1858752
3. Sivasankari B, Varalakshmi P. *Blockchain and IoT Technology in Healthcare: A Review*; 2022. Available from: https://ebooks.iospress.nl/doi/10.3233/SHTI220455
4. Haleem A, Javaid M, Singh RP, Suman R, Rab S. Blockchain Technology Applications in Healthcare: An Overview. *Int J Intell Netw* [Internet]. 2021;2:130–9. Available from: https://linkinghub.elsevier.com/retrieve/pii/S266660302100021X
5. Salah K, Rehman MHU, Nizamuddin N, Al-Fuqaha A. Blockchain for AI: Review and Open Research Challenges. *IEEE Access* [Internet]. 2019;7:10127–49. Available from: https://ieeexplore.ieee.org/document/8598784/
6. Abu-elezz I, Hassan A, Nazeemudeen A, Househ M, Abd-alrazaq A. The Benefits and Threats of Blockchain Technology in Healthcare: A Scoping Review. *Int J Med Inform* [Internet]. 2020 Oct;142:104246. Available from: https://linkinghub.elsevier.com/retrieve/pii/S1386505620301544
7. Aste T, Tasca P, Di Matteo T. Blockchain Technologies: The Foreseeable Impact on Society and Industry. *Computer* (Long Beach Calif) [Internet]. 2017;50(9):18–28. Available from: http://ieeexplore.ieee.org/document/8048633/
8. Hossain M, Islam SMR, Ali F, Kwak K-S, Hasan R. An Internet of Things-based Health Prescription Assistant and Its Security System Design. *Futur Gener Comput Syst* [Internet]. 2018 May;82:422–39. Available from: https://linkinghub.elsevier.com/retrieve/pii/S0167739X17314085
9. Badawi HF, Dong H, El Saddik A. Mobile Cloud-Based Physical Activity Advisory System Using Biofeedback Sensors. *Futur Gener Comput Syst* [Internet]. 2017 Jan;66:59–70. Available from: https://linkinghub.elsevier.com/retrieve/pii/S0167739X15003428
10. Gordon WJ, Catalini C. Blockchain Technology for Healthcare: Facilitating the Transition to Patient-Driven Interoperability. *Comput Struct Biotechnol J* [Internet]. 2018;16:224–30. Available from: https://linkinghub.elsevier.com/retrieve/pii/S200103701830028X
11. Xia Q, Sifah EB, Smahi A, Amofa S, Zhang X. BBDS: Blockchain-Based Data Sharing for Electronic Medical Records in Cloud Environments. *Information*. 2017;8(2):44.
12. Kassab M, DeFranco J, Malas T, Laplante P, Destefanis G, Neto VVG. Exploring Research in Blockchain for Healthcare and a Roadmap for the Future. *IEEE Trans Emerg Top Comput* [Internet]. 2021 Oct 1;9(4):1835–52. Available from: https://ieeexplore.ieee.org/document/8809781/
13. Shen B, Guo J, Yang Y. MedChain: Efficient Healthcare Data Sharing via Blockchain. *Appl Sci* [Internet]. 2019 Mar 22;9(6):1207. Available from: www.mdpi.com/2076-3417/9/6/1207

14. Menachemi N, Rahurkar S, Harle CA, Vest JR. The Benefits of Health Information Exchange: An Updated Systematic Review. *J Am Med Informatics Assoc* [Internet]. 2018 Sep 1;25(9):1259–65. Available from: https://academic.oup.com/jamia/article/25/9/1259/4990601
15. Chelladurai U, Pandian S. A Novel Blockchain Based Electronic Health Record Automation System for Healthcare. *J Ambient Intell Humaniz Comput* [Internet]. 2022 Jan 23;13(1):693–703. Available from: https://link.springer.com/10.1007/s12652-021-03163-3
16. Zhang P, Schmidt DC, White J, Lenz G. *Blockchain Technology Use Cases in Healthcare*; 2018, pp. 1–41. Available from: https://linkinghub.elsevier.com/retrieve/pii/S0065245818300196
17. Hölbl M, Kompara M, Kamišalić A, Nemec Zlatolas L. A Systematic Review of the Use of Blockchain in Healthcare. *Symmetry* (Basel) [Internet]. 2018 Oct 10;10(10):470. Available from: www.mdpi.com/2073-8994/10/10/470
18. Mettler M. Blockchain Technology in Healthcare: The Revolution Starts Here. In: *2016 IEEE 18th International Conference on e-Health Networking, Applications and Services (Healthcom)* [Internet]. IEEE; 2016, pp. 1–3. Available from: http://ieeexplore.ieee.org/document/7749510/
19. Farouk A, Alahmadi A, Ghose S, Mashatan A. Blockchain Platform for Industrial Healthcare: Vision and Future Opportunities. *Comput Commun* [Internet]. 2020 Mar;154:223–35. Available from: https://linkinghub.elsevier.com/retrieve/pii/S014036641931953X
20. Smith RD. Responding to Global Infectious Disease Outbreaks: Lessons from SARS on the Role of Risk Perception, Communication and Management. *Soc Sci Med* [Internet]. 2006 Dec;63(12):3113–23. Available from: https://linkinghub.elsevier.com/retrieve/pii/S0277953606004060
21. Linn LA, Koo MB. *ONC/NIST Use of Blockchain for Healthcare and Research Workshop*. ONC/NIST; 2016.
22. Kombe C, Ally M, Sam A. A Review on Healthcare Information Systems and Consensus Protocols in Blockchain Technology. *Int J Adv Technol Eng Explor* [Internet]. 2018 Dec 21;5(49):473–83. Available from: http://accentsjournals.org/PaperDirectory/Journal/IJATEE/2018/12/1.pdf
23. Weiss M, Botha A, Herselman M, Loots G. Blockchain as an Enabler for Public mHealth Solutions in South Africa. In: *2017 IST-Africa Week Conference* (IST-Africa). IEEE; 2017, pp. 1–8.
24. Bryatov S, Borodinov A. Blockchain Technology in the Pharmaceutical Supply Chain: Researching a Business Model Based on Hyperledger Fabric. In: *Proceedings of the V International Conference Information Technology and Nanotechnology 2019* [Internet]. IP Zaitsev V.D.; 2019, pp. 134–40. Available from: http://ceur-ws.org/Vol-2416/paper18.pdf
25. Alhadhrami Z, Alghfeli S, Alghfeli M, Abedlla JA, Shuaib K. Introducing Blockchains for Healthcare. In: *2017 International Conference on Electrical and Computing Technologies and Applications (ICECTA)* [Internet]. IEEE; 2017, pp. 1–4. Available from: http://ieeexplore.ieee.org/document/8252043/
26. Dimitrov DV. Blockchain Applications for Healthcare Data Management. *Healthc Inform Res* [Internet]. 2019;25(1):51. Available from: http://e-hir.org/journal/view.php?id=10.4258/hir.2019.25.1.51
27. Greenspan G. Multichain Private Blockchain. *White Pap*; 2015. Available from: https://www.multichain.com/download/MultiChain-White-Paper.pdf
28. Alketbi A, Nasir Q, Talib MA. Blockchain for Government Services—Use Cases, Security Benefits and Challenges. In: *2018 15th Learning and Technology Conference (L&T)* [Internet]. IEEE; 2018, pp. 112–19. Available from: https://ieeexplore.ieee.org/document/8368494/
29. Casino F, Dasaklis TK, Patsakis C. A Systematic Literature Review of Blockchain-Based Applications: Current Status, Classification and Open Issues. *Telemat Informatics* [Internet]. 2019 Mar;36:55–81. Available from: https://linkinghub.elsevier.com/retrieve/pii/S0736585318306324
30. Mackey TK, Kuo T-T, Gummadi B, Clauson KA, Church G, Grishin D, et al. 'Fit-for-Purpose?'—Challenges and Opportunities for Applications of Blockchain Technology in the Future of Healthcare. *BMC Med* [Internet]. 2019 Dec 27;17(1):68. Available from: https://bmcmedicine.biomedcentral.com/articles/10.1186/s12916-019-1296-7
31. Justinia T. Blockchain Technologies: Opportunities for Solving Real-World Problems in Healthcare and Biomedical Sciences. *Acta Inform Medica* [Internet]. 2019;27(4):284. Available from: www.ejmanager.com/fulltextpdf.php?mno=302645059
32. Griggs KN, Ossipova O, Kohlios CP, Baccarini AN, Howson EA, Hayajneh T. Healthcare Blockchain System Using Smart Contracts for Secure Automated Remote Patient Monitoring. *J Med Syst*. 2018;42:1–7.

33. Tripathi G, Ahad MA, Paiva S. S2HS: A Blockchain Based Approach for Smart Healthcare System. *Healthcare* [Internet]. 2020 Mar;8(1):100391. Available from: https://linkinghub.elsevier.com/retrieve/pii/S2213076419302532
34. Gupta R, Tanwar S, Tyagi S, Kumar N, Obaidat MS, Sadoun B. HaBiTs: Blockchain-based Telesurgery Framework for Healthcare 4.0. In: *2019 International Conference on Computer, Information and Telecommunication Systems (CITS)* [Internet]. IEEE; 2019, pp. 1–5. Available from: https://ieeexplore.ieee.org/document/8862127/
35. Srivastava G, Parizi RM, Dehghantanha A. *The Future of Blockchain Technology in Healthcare Internet of Things Security*; 2020, pp. 161–84. Available from: http://link.springer.com/10.1007/978-3-030-38181-3_9
36. Ahmad SS, Khan S, Kamal MA. What is Blockchain Technology and its Significance in the Current Healthcare System? A Brief Insight. *Curr Pharm Des* [Internet]. 2019 Aug 9;25(12):1402–8. Available from: www.eurekaselect.com/172892/article
37. Bhavin M, Tanwar S, Sharma N, Tyagi S, Kumar N. Blockchain and Quantum Blind Signature-Based Hybrid Scheme for Healthcare 5.0 Applications. *J Inf Secur Appl* [Internet]. 2021 Feb;56:102673. Available from: https://linkinghub.elsevier.com/retrieve/pii/S2214212620308255
38. Rathee G, Sharma A, Saini H, Kumar R, Iqbal R. A Hybrid Framework for Multimedia Data Processing in IoT-Healthcare Using Blockchain Technology. *Multimed Tools Appl* [Internet]. 2020 Apr 3;79(15–16):9711–33. Available from: http://link.springer.com/10.1007/s11042-019-07835-3
39. Chukwu E, Garg L. A Systematic Review of Blockchain in Healthcare: Frameworks, Prototypes, and Implementations. *IEEE Access* [Internet]. 2020;8:21196–214. Available from: https://ieeexplore.ieee.org/document/8972918/
40. Houtan B, Hafid AS, Makrakis D. A Survey on Blockchain-Based Self-Sovereign Patient Identity in Healthcare. *IEEE Access* [Internet]. 2020;8:90478–94. Available from: https://ieeexplore.ieee.org/document/9091543/
41. Rejeb A, Bell L. Potentials of Blockchain for Healthcare: Case of Tunisia. *SSRN Electron J* [Internet]. 2019. Available from: www.ssrn.com/abstract=3475246
42. Paranjape K, Parker M, Houlding D, Car J. Implementation Considerations for Blockchain in Healthcare Institutions. *Blockchain Healthc Today* [Internet]. 2019 Jul 4;2. Available from: https://blockchainhealthcaretoday.com/index.php/journal/article/view/114
43. Hussien HM, Yasin SM, Udzir NI, Ninggal MIH, Salman S. Blockchain Technology in the Healthcare Industry: Trends and Opportunities. *J Ind Inf Integr*. 2021;22:100217.
44. Li J, Wu J, Jiang G, Srikanthan T. Blockchain-Based Public Auditing for Big Data in Cloud Storage. *Inf Process Manag* [Internet]. 2020 Nov;57(6):102382. Available from: https://linkinghub.elsevier.com/retrieve/pii/S0306457320308773
45. Chattu VK, Nanda A, Chattu SK, Kadri SM, Knight AW. The Emerging Role of Blockchain Technology Applications in Routine Disease Surveillance Systems to Strengthen Global Health Security. *Big Data Cogn Comput* [Internet]. 2019 May 8;3(2):25. Available from: www.mdpi.com/2504-2289/3/2/25
46. Queiroz MM, Fosso Wamba S. Blockchain Adoption Challenges in Supply Chain: An Empirical Investigation of the Main Drivers in India and the USA. *Int J Inf Manage* [Internet]. 2019 Jun;46:70–82. Available from: https://linkinghub.elsevier.com/retrieve/pii/S0268401218309447
47. Sultana T, Almogren A, Akbar M, Zuair M, Ullah I, Javaid N. Data Sharing System Integrating Access Control Mechanism Using Blockchain-Based Smart Contracts for IoT Devices. *Appl Sci* [Internet]. 2020 Jan 9;10(2):488. Available from: www.mdpi.com/2076-3417/10/2/488
48. Wang Y, Cai S, Lin C, Chen Z, Wang T, Gao Z, et al. Study of Blockchains's Consensus Mechanism Based on Credit. *IEEE Access* [Internet]. 2019;7:10224–31. Available from: https://ieeexplore.ieee.org/document/8605507/
49. Govindan K, Mina H, Alavi B. A Decision Support System for Demand Management in Healthcare Supply Chains Considering the Epidemic Outbreaks: A Case Study of Coronavirus Disease 2019 (COVID-19). *Transp Res Part E Logist Transp Rev* [Internet]. 2020 Jun;138:101967. Available from: https://linkinghub.elsevier.com/retrieve/pii/S1366554520306189
50. Antal C, Cioara T, Antal M, Anghel I. Blockchain Platform for COVID-19 Vaccine Supply Management. *IEEE Open J Comput Soc* [Internet]. 2021;2:164–78. Available from: https://ieeexplore.ieee.org/document/9382850/

51. Juma H, Shaalan K, Kamel I. A Survey on Using Blockchain in Trade Supply Chain Solutions. *IEEE Access* [Internet]. 2019;7:184115–32. Available from: https://ieeexplore.ieee.org/document/8936386/
52. Sriman B, Ganesh Kumar S, Shamili P. *Blockchain Technology: Consensus Protocol Proof of Work and Proof of Stake*; 2021, pp. 395–406. Available from: http://link.springer.com/10.1007/978-981-15-5566-4_34
53. Roman-Belmonte JM, De la Corte-Rodriguez H, Rodriguez-Merchan EC. How Blockchain Technology Can Change Medicine. *Postgrad Med* [Internet]. 2018 May 19;130(4):420–7. Available from: www.tandfonline.com/doi/full/10.1080/00325481.2018.1472996
54. Thomas C, Bindu V, Aby AA, Anjalikrishna UR, Kesari A, Sabu D. Blockchain-Based Medical Insurance Storage Systems. In: *Recent Trends in Blockchain for Information Systems Security and Privacy*. CRC Press; 2021, pp. 219–35.
55. Vazirani AA, O'Donoghue O, Brindley D, Meinert E. Implementing Blockchains for Efficient Health Care: Systematic Review. *J Med Internet Res* [Internet]. 2019 Feb 12;21(2):e12439. Available from: www.jmir.org/2019/2/e12439/
56. Tseng J-H, Liao Y-C, Chong B, Liao S. Governance on the Drug Supply Chain via Gcoin Blockchain. *Int J Environ Res Public Health* [Internet]. 2018 May 23;15(6):1055. Available from: www.mdpi.com/1660-4601/15/6/1055
57. Munsing E, Mather J, Moura S. Blockchains for Decentralized Optimization of Energy Resources in Microgrid Networks. In: *2017 IEEE Conference on Control Technology and Applications (CCTA)* [Internet]. IEEE; 2017, pp. 2164–71. Available from: http://ieeexplore.ieee.org/document/8062773/
58. Meinert E, Alturkistani A, Foley KA, Osama T, Car J, Majeed A, et al. Blockchain Implementation in Health Care: Protocol for a Systematic Review. *JMIR Res Protoc* [Internet]. 2019 Feb 8;8(2):e10994. Available from: www.researchprotocols.org/2019/2/e10994/
59. Pop C, Antal M, Cioara T, Anghel I, Sera D, Salomie I, et al. Blockchain-Based Scalable and Tamper-Evident Solution for Registering Energy Data. *Sensors* [Internet]. 2019 Jul 10;19(14):3033. Available from: www.mdpi.com/1424-8220/19/14/3033
60. Azaria A, Ekblaw A, Vieira T, Lippman A. MedRec: Using Blockchain for Medical Data Access and Permission Management. In: *2016 2nd International Conference on Open and Big Data (OBD)* [Internet]. IEEE; 2016, pp. 25–30. Available from: http://ieeexplore.ieee.org/document/7573685/
61. Engelhardt MA. Hitching Healthcare to the Chain: An Introduction to Blockchain Technology in the Healthcare Sector. *Technol Innov Manag Rev* [Internet]. 2017 Oct 27;7(10):22–34. Available from: http://timreview.ca/article/1111
62. Bansal A, Garg C, Padappayil RP. Optimizing the Implementation of COVID-19 "Immunity Certificates" Using Blockchain. *J Med Syst* [Internet]. 2020 Sep 19;44(9):140. Available from: https://link.springer.com/10.1007/s10916-020-01616-4
63. Saravanan M, Shubha R, Marks AM, Iyer V. SMEAD: A Secured Mobile Enabled Assisting Device for Diabetics Monitoring. In: *2017 IEEE International Conference on Advanced Networks and Telecommunications Systems (ANTS)* [Internet]. IEEE; 2017, pp. 1–6. Available from: https://ieeexplore.ieee.org/document/8384099/
64. Chen X, Xu X, Shao H, Hu D, Su Y, Mao X, et al. Blockchain-Based Emergency Information Sharing System for Public Health Security. *Chinese J Eng Sci* [Internet]. 2021;23(5):41. Available from: https://journal.hep.com.cn/sscae/EN/10.15302/J-SSCAE-2021.05.006
65. Miyachi K, Mackey TK. hOCBS: A Privacy-Preserving Blockchain Framework for Healthcare Data Leveraging an On-chain and Off-chain System Design. *Inf Process Manag* [Internet]. 2021 May;58(3):102535. Available from: https://linkinghub.elsevier.com/retrieve/pii/S0306457321000431
66. Bell L, Buchanan WJ, Cameron J, Lo O. Applications of Blockchain Within Healthcare. *Blockchain Healthc Today* [Internet]. 2018 Jul 9;1. Available from: https://blockchainhealthcaretoday.com/index.php/journal/article/view/8
67. Bhuiyan MZA, Zaman A, Wang T, Wang G, Tao H, Hassan MM. Blockchain and Big Data to Transform the Healthcare. In: *Proceedings of the International Conference on Data Processing and Applications* [Internet]. ACM; 2018, pp. 62–8. Available from: https://dl.acm.org/doi/10.1145/3224207.3224220

68. Al Omar A, Rahman MS, Basu A, Kiyomoto S. Medibchain: A Blockchain Based Privacy Preserving Platform for Healthcare Data. In: *Security, Privacy, and Anonymity in Computation, Communication, and Storage: SpaCCS 2017 International Workshops, Guangzhou, China, December 12–15, 2017, Proceedings 10*. Springer; 2017, pp. 534–43.
69. Kuo T-T, Kim H-E, Ohno-Machado L. Blockchain Distributed Ledger Technologies for Biomedical and Health Care Applications. *J Am Med Informatics Assoc* [Internet]. 2017 Nov 1;24(6):1211–20. Available from: https://academic.oup.com/jamia/article/24/6/1211/4108087
70. Fan K, Wang S, Ren Y, Li H, Yang Y. MedBlock: Efficient and Secure Medical Data Sharing Via Blockchain. *J Med Syst* [Internet]. 2018 Aug 21;42(8):136. Available from: http://link.springer.com/10.1007/s10916-018-0993-7
71. Agbo C, Mahmoud Q, Eklund J. Blockchain Technology in Healthcare: A Systematic Review. *Healthcare* [Internet]. 2019 Apr 4;7(2):56. Available from: www.mdpi.com/2227-9032/7/2/56
72. Li H, Zhu L, Shen M, Gao F, Tao X, Liu S. Blockchain-Based Data Preservation System for Medical Data. *J Med Syst* [Internet]. 2018 Aug 28;42(8):141. Available from: http://link.springer.com/10.1007/s10916-018-0997-3
73. Tandon A, Dhir A, Islam AKMN, Mäntymäki M. Blockchain in Healthcare: A Systematic Literature Review, Synthesizing Framework and Future Research Agenda. *Comput Ind* [Internet]. 2020 Nov;122:103290. Available from: https://linkinghub.elsevier.com/retrieve/pii/S0166361520305248
74. Chang MC, Park D. How Can Blockchain Help People in the Event of Pandemics Such as the COVID-19? *J Med Syst* [Internet]. 2020 May 16;44(5):102. Available from: https://link.springer.com/10.1007/s10916-020-01577-8
75. Fan VY, Jamison DT, Summers LH. Pandemic Risk: How Large Are the Expected Losses? *Bull World Health Organ* [Internet]. 2018 Feb 1;96(2):129–34. Available from: www.ncbi.nlm.nih.gov/pmc/articles/PMC5791779/pdf/BLT.17.199588.pdf/
76. Islam N, Faheem Y, Din IU, Talha M, Guizani M, Khalil M. A Blockchain-Based Fog Computing Framework for Activity Recognition as an Application to e-Healthcare Services. *Futur Gener Comput Syst* [Internet]. 2019 Nov;100:569–78. Available from: https://linkinghub.elsevier.com/retrieve/pii/S0167739X19309860
77. Sharma V, Gupta A, Hasan NU, Shabaz M, Ofori I. Blockchain in Secure Healthcare Systems: State of the Art, Limitations, and Future Directions. Soni M, editor. *Secur Commun Netw* [Internet]. 2022 May 21;2022:1–15. Available from: www.hindawi.com/journals/scn/2022/9697545/
78. Liu J, Jin C, Huang Y, Zhang K, Li W, Cui L. Research on Infectious Disease Surveillance and Traceability System Based on Blockchain Technology. In: *Proceedings of the 4th International Conference on Economic Management and Model Engineering, ICEMME 2022, November 18–20, 2022*. Nanjing, China; 2023.
79. Rifi N, Rachkidi E, Agoulmine N, Taher NC. Towards Using Blockchain Technology for eHealth Data Access Management. In: *2017 Fourth International Conference on Advances in Biomedical Engineering (ICABME)*. IEEE; 2017, pp. 1–4.
80. Liberman DF, Ducatman AM, Fink R. Biotechnology: Is There a Role for Medical Surveillance. *Bioprocess Saf Work Comm Saf Health Considerations*. 1990;1051:101.
81. Radanović I, Likić R. Opportunities for use of blockchain technology in medicine. *Appl Health Econ Health Policy*. 2018;16:583–90.
82. Panwar A, Bhatnagar V, Khari M, Salehi AW, Gupta G. A Blockchain Framework to Secure Personal Health Record (PHR) in IBM Cloud-Based Data Lake. Aler R, editor. *Comput Intell Neurosci* [Internet]. 2022 Apr 12;2022:1–19. Available from: www.hindawi.com/journals/cin/2022/3045107/
83. Bocek T, Rodrigues BB, Strasser T, Stiller B. Blockchains Everywhere—A Use-case of Blockchains in the Pharma Supply-chain. In: *2017 IFIP/IEEE Symposium on Integrated Network and Service Management (IM)* [Internet]. IEEE; 2017, pp. 772–7. Available from: http://ieeexplore.ieee.org/document/7987376/
84. Gad AG, Mosa DT, Abualigah L, Abohany AA. Emerging Trends in Blockchain Technology and Applications: A Review and Outlook. *J King Saud Univ—Comput Inf Sci* [Internet]. 2022 Oct;34(9):6719–42. Available from: https://linkinghub.elsevier.com/retrieve/pii/S1319157822000891
85. Abd-alrazaq AA, Alajlani M, Alhuwail D, Erbad A, Giannicchi A, Shah Z, et al. Blockchain Technologies to Mitigate COVID-19 Challenges: A Scoping Review. *Comput Methods Programs*

Biomed Updat [Internet]. 2021;1:100001. Available from: https://linkinghub.elsevier.com/retrieve/pii/S266699002030001X
86. Alsaed Z, Khweiled R, Hamad M, Daraghmi E, Cheikhrouhou O, Alhakami W, et al. Role of Blockchain Technology in Combating COVID-19 Crisis. *Appl Sci* [Internet]. 2021 Dec 17;11(24):12063. Available from: www.mdpi.com/2076-3417/11/24/12063
87. Krichen M, Ammi M, Mihoub A, Almutiq M. Blockchain for Modern Applications: A Survey. *Sensors* [Internet]. 2022 Jul 14;22(14):5274. Available from: www.mdpi.com/1424-8220/22/14/5274
88. Sharma A, Bahl S, Bagha AK, Javaid M, Shukla DK, Haleem A. Blockchain Technology and Its Applications to Combat COVID-19 Pandemic. *Res Biomed Eng* [Internet]. 2022 Mar 22;38(1):173–80. Available from: https://link.springer.com/10.1007/s42600-020-00106-3
89. Behnaminia F, Samet S. Blockchain Technology Applications in Patient Tracking Systems Regarding Privacy-Preserving Concerns and COVID-19 Pandemic. *Int J Inf Commun Eng*. 2023;17(2):144–156. Available from: https://publications.waset.org/10012975/blockchain-technology-applications-in-patient-tracking-systems-regarding-privacy-preserving-concerns-and-covid-19-pandemic
90. Sinclair D, Shahriar H, Zhang C. Security Requirement Prototyping with Hyperledger Composer for Drug Supply Chain. In: *Proceedings of the 3rd International Conference on Cryptography, Security and Privacy* [Internet]. ACM; 2019, pp. 158–63. Available from: https://dl.acm.org/doi/10.1145/3309074.3309104
91. Alshahrani W, Alshahrani R. Assessment of Blockchain Technology Application in the Improvement of Pharmaceutical Industry. In: *2021 International Conference of Women in Data Science at Taif University (WiDSTaif)* [Internet]. IEEE; 2021, pp. 1–5. Available from: https://ieeexplore.ieee.org/document/9430210/
92. Huang Y, Wu J, Long C. Drugledger: A Practical Blockchain System for Drug Traceability and Regulation. In: *2018 IEEE International Conference on Internet of Things (iThings) and IEEE Green Computing and Communications (GreenCom) and IEEE Cyber, Physical and Social Computing (CPSCom) and IEEE Smart Data (SmartData)* [Internet]. IEEE; 2018, pp. 1137–44. Available from: https://ieeexplore.ieee.org/document/8726740/
93. Adsul KB, Kosbatwar SP. A Novel Approach for Traceability & Detection of Counterfeit Medicines Through Blockchain. *Int J Curr Eng Technol*. 2020;(8):1025–30. Available from: http://inpressco.com/wp-content/uploads/2021/02/Paper2141025-1030.pdf
94. Kumar A, Choudhary D, Raju MS, Chaudhary DK, Sagar RK. Combating Counterfeit Drugs: A Quantitative Analysis on Cracking Down the Fake Drug Industry by Using Blockchain Technology. In: *2019 9th International Conference on Cloud Computing, Data Science & Engineering (Confluence)* [Internet]. IEEE; 2019, pp. 174–8. Available from: https://ieeexplore.ieee.org/document/8776891/
95. Saxena N, Thomas I, Gope P, Burnap P, Kumar N. PharmaCrypt: Blockchain for Critical Pharmaceutical Industry to Counterfeit Drugs. *Computer* (Long Beach Calif) [Internet]. 2020 Jul;53(7):29–44. Available from: https://ieeexplore.ieee.org/document/9130418/
96. Hulea M, Rosu O, Miron R, Astilean A. Pharmaceutical Cold Chain Management: Platform Based on a Distributed Ledger. In: *2018 IEEE International Conference on Automation, Quality and Testing, Robotics (AQTR)* [Internet]. IEEE; 2018, pp. 1–6. Available from: https://ieeexplore.ieee.org/document/8402709/
97. Dwivedi SK, Amin R, Vollala S. Blockchain Based Secured Information Sharing Protocol in Supply Chain Management System with Key Distribution Mechanism. *J Inf Secur Appl* [Internet]. 2020 Oct;54:102554. Available from: https://linkinghub.elsevier.com/retrieve/pii/S2214212620301484
98. Botcha KM, Chakravarthy VV, Anurag. Enhancing Traceability in Pharmaceutical Supply Chain using Internet of Things (IoT) and Blockchain. In: *2019 IEEE International Conference on Intelligent Systems and Green Technology (ICISGT)* [Internet]. IEEE; 2019, pp. 45–453. Available from: https://ieeexplore.ieee.org/document/8998114/
99. Mani V, Prakash M, Lai WC. Cloud-based Blockchain Technology to Identify Counterfeits. *J Cloud Comput*. 2022;11(1):1–15.
100. Plotnikov V, Kuznetsova V. The Prospects for the Use of Digital Technology "Blockchain" in the Pharmaceutical Market. Mottaeva A, Melović B, editors. *MATEC Web Conf* [Internet]. 2018 Aug 20;193:02029. Available from: www.matec-conferences.org/10.1051/matecconf/201819302029

5

Building Efficient Smart Contract for Healthcare 4.0

Kanika Agrawal and Mayank Aggarwal

5.1 Introduction

With technological advancements, the demand for usage of safe and secure online communication system is growing. As the flow of data and use of Internet are growing, the threats to security of data have tremendously increased [1]. Hackers attack the channel of communication to steal information and disrupt the connection. Thus, it has become important to consider security concerns along with concerns related to data integrity, redundancy, and heterogeneity. Security is the most important issue to be considered in any institution [2,3]. The unauthorized data breaching and information leakage lead to wastage of resources and huge financial losses. The lack of a robust and secure model makes the system suffer from different attacks. These attacks usually affect security and privacy. With the huge number of cyber hacking and cyberattacks, confidentiality, authorization, integrity, and access control are to be taken care of. With time, many centralized and client–server architectures were introduced to lessen the aforementioned issues. But the problem was, these were central servers, which when failed led to the crashing down of the system. Many security mechanisms such as advanced encryption standard (AES) were also used to protect data and the system, but they faced significant computation power and communication overhead. Thus, to mitigate the effect of the aforementioned issues on the communication channel, the blockchain and Bitcoin concepts were introduced [4]. The decentralized blockchain technique enabled digital assets transference without any support of a third party [5]. It helped in the development of a system and supporting the Bitcoin cryptocurrency. In 2008, for the first time, the blockchain concept was proposed and executed by Satoshi Nakamoto in 2009. The distributed blockchain concept consists of connected nodes that are chained together to store in a public ledger all the committed transactions [6]. As more transactions are created, new blocks are added in the chain. This technology has several cores, such as cryptographic hash, distributed consensus algorithms, and digital signatures. The blockchain's decentralization helped removed intermediate party interference that helped in validating and verifying the transactions [7]. Because of its safe and secure societal impact, it is applied to many domains, such as aircraft, e-voting, supply chain, academics, etc., worldwide.

There are many blockchain-based applications, out of which the healthcare domain uses blockchain to help hospital management systems as well as save the lives of patients [8]. However, with time, the healthcare industry has faced drastic changes and transformation, from healthcare 1.0 version to healthcare 4.0.

Healthcare 1.0 allowed patients' medical history to be maintained manually by the doctors and thus was more doctor-centric. But healthcare 2.0 came into existence and replaced these manual records with electronic records. However, the usage of wearable devices (WDs) came in healthcare 3.0, which helped in patients' history real-time tracking [9]. After some time, the electronic health record (EHR) system was developed, which helped in the electronic storage of patient records in databases. To ensure patients' data security, healthcare 4.0 was developed to deliver uninterrupted services in real time and also to store in the centralized EHR system patients' details [10]. Patient's health was monitored through implantable medical devices (MDs) and WDs. WDs have healthcare sensors [11] that help in blood pressure, glucose level, heart rate, and temperature analysis of the patient remotely and help store them in a centralized EHR. Telehealthcare with Internet of Things (IoT) helped coordinate disease management [12]. Healthcare Internet of Things put tremendous effect on the healthcare domain. It usually generates a lot of data that help hackers make various security attacks, such as data confidentiality and integrity attacks at regular intervals of time. The traditional systems were not able to handle the real-time data, so this led to the evolution of cloud technology that helps process and store massive amounts of data securely. Moreover, to secure health information and to improve the national healthcare system, the healthcare industries have paved the path for different health-related acts.

5.1.1 Blockchain Overview

Initially, centralized and decentralized systems were developed with the need to store data and have network access. However, the centralized system provided the facility of storing data only on a single node or server, large network access, on-demand self-service, processing, big data management, and availability. Due to the central server storage, it faced a disadvantage of full data loss if storing node got corrupted [13]. Thus, decentralized system came into existence to overcome the limitations of the centralized system. The features provided by this system were better security, transparency, immutability, and after-settlements. However, this system lacks a secure distributed system for efficient working in different locations. Thus, this led to the evolution of blockchain technology much after the development of centralized and decentralized systems.

5.1.2 Blockchain

Blockchain technology is an immutable and distributed system that consists of blocks connected together through hash in the form of chain. The data saved on blockchain is safe and secure and cannot be altered or tampered. This helps in making transactions traceable and helps synchronize the environment along with invalidation of transactions [14]. It creates a non-centralized environment that helps network users interact safely. In blockchain, using previous nodes, the history of transactions occurred can easily be traced, which makes it trustworthy for usage. Each node has the previous block's hash and a unique identification [15]. It also uses a consensus mechanism that makes blockchain secure, transparent, and trusted. Also, these algorithms help non-central blockchain system to add a new node in the chain [16]. In blockchain, all transactions are arranged in a sequence to the previous node and are time-stamped.

5.1.3 Blockchain Architecture

Blockchain architecture consists of five modules [16,17]. These are:

- *Data module.* Data module creates the blockchain system in distributed and shared databases.
- *Transaction module.* It manages the transactions of the blockchain system.
- *Block creation module.* This module helps miners develop blocks that contain the details over network nodes.
- *Consensus module.* This module uses consensus algorithms, such as proof-of-stake and proof-of-work, which help in maintaining the consistency of the transactions.
- *Connection and interface module.* The module helps in tracking transactions and real-time data.

5.1.4 Blockchain Characteristics

The important blockchain characteristics [18] that make it unique, secure, and safe to be used for future applications are shown here:

1. *Transparent.* The data stored on network is traceable, visible, and transparent throughout the network lifetime.
2. *Decentralized.* The data present on the system is efficiently monitored, updated, accessed, and stored on various systems.
3. *Autonomy.* Without any interference from a third party, the node on the blockchain system can easily secure data safely.
4. *Immutable.* Due to the provision of time stamps, the data doesn't change with time in a blockchain network.
5. *Irreversible.* For each transaction ever made in a blockchain system, a fix and verifiable record is kept in a network which cannot be reversed.
6. *Open-source.* The blockchain system network usually provides an open-source access with the sense of hierarchy to everyone.
7. *Anonymity.* Blockchain helps in hiding the identity of an individual during the data transfer between nodes.
8. *Contract automation or smart contracting.* Smart contracts are the computerized programs that are usually coded and have functions that provide better security and lower transaction costs. These include the conditions for penalties, rules, and actions for all involved parties in a transaction.
9. *Ownership and uniqueness.* For each and every document exchanged, the uniqueness and ownership are recorded on blockchain using a unique hash code.

5.1.5 Blockchain Consensus Mechanisms

In the blockchain system, consensus mechanisms [19] are the procedures or mechanisms that are used by different participating nodes so as to solve a problem for a definite conclusion. The important consensus algorithms in blockchain are:

1. *Proof-of-work*. In the year 2008, Satoshi Nakamoto suggested the proof-of-work (PoW) consensus mechanism. In this, the participating blocks need to solve a complex mathematical problem. The node that helps in solving the given problem gets an opportunity to generate the required block. However, during this process, a big loss of resources and energy is encountered.
2. *Proof-of-stake (PoS)*. The decentralization of a blockchain system is preserved by this mechanism. The node in this process gets $n\%$ time for $n\%$ resources so as to create a new block. It also helps save time and resources for blockchain network.
3. *Proof-of-authority (PoA)*. PoA is an algorithm that helps few nodes to be designated as authority and thus validates the transactions to create new nodes.
4. *Proof-of-space (PoS)*. PoS or proof-of-capacity is a mechanism that makes the need to prove capacity and storage for a node to help solve complex problems. This helps in the next block generation and validation in blockchain.
5. *Practical Byzantine fault tolerance (PBFT)*. PBFT uses three phases to reach consensus. It usually tolerates big message complexities and also uses less of resources. Thus, it is mostly used in blockchain system of small networks.

5.2 Applications of Blockchain System in the Healthcare Domain

Today, the safety of patients' data is of huge importance. To have a safe facility for the patient and his data, the need for blockchain technology is required. The technology has immutable data with peer-to-peer (P2P) node, where blocks are used to store transactions in a connected form of chain with a digital ledger [20]. Blockchain is used in various sectors, like finance, banking, supply chain, etc., and helps protect data from attackers. One such application is in healthcare, which also uses blockchain for safety and security of hospital management systems.

Blockchain has various applications in healthcare domain, such as EHR medical, pharmaceuticals, biomedical, disease prediction, and genomics [21]. These are described in the following.

5.2.1 Biomedical

One of the main tasks for future researches in the biomedical field is the storage of biological samples in a high-quality and better condition. However, today, there exist web-based applications for different tasks, such as informed consent, respect for quality, confidentiality, safety standards, non-profit, and traceability of samples. The research [22] described smart contracts based on blockchain for traceability of the processes in a biobank. The concept helped in providing security and integrity of the processes.

In blockchain-based medical applications, alteration of data are not allowed. It only helps in safe and secure transactions. One of the most important concerns while handling data related to biomedicine is that of data privacy on the Internet of Medical Things. To overcome such issues, the authors in [23] proposed a blockchain-based safe and secure k-medoids to ensure authenticity, which is implemented with the help of partial homomorphic cryptosystem (Paillier). They used the Hyperledger tool to implement the concept to help eliminate dependency on third parties and thus ensure data security and privacy. However, the work is less reliable, thus has a future scope for the development of lightweight privacy-preserving and securing machine learning methods.

The chapter [24] presented a deep literature review on current research deployed using blockchain technology in the biomedical domain. The results showed that the area still needs improvement as it is in early stages. The biomedical sector is the application where the products related to the sector should be secure and can easily be traced. If this doesn't happen, then the chances for modification of initial data increase, thus leading to the potential risk for patients. Hence, the work [25] proposed a new way that helped lessen the control and operational issues of using blockchain-based Hyperledger chains. The novelty of the approach is that it controls and helps eliminate the possibility of changing the blockchain system. Since the technology helps improve accessibility, it is used in various healthcare subdomains also.

The research [26] proposed a blockchain-based consensus or federated private network along with AADHAAR infrastructure and the health information exchange model to resolve the concerns related to transparency, full ownership, and privacy of users. The research [27] designed a model based on blockchain to eliminate the issue of privacy and disease overlapping of patients' related medical data. However, the work lacks in-depth analysis and thus needs to improve the difficulty level used for the outcome. Table 5.1 depicts the different blockchain applications in the field of biomedicine in the healthcare domain.

5.2.2 Prediction of Diseases

One of the most important applications of blockchain in healthcare is that for disease prediction. It helps predict various kinds of diseases that help in proper analysis of the patients. The research [28] proposed a learning situation to learn from heterogeneous respiratory and multi-class medical data. The system leverages blockchain technology and ensures privacy to aggregate the local model. This work introduced the technique that involves weight manipulation and used local model as the important parameter to test privacy. The resulting metric scores showed that the performance is analogous to a model that is single-sourced. The novel aggregation technique was used to achieve for five classes the highest accuracy test of 88.10%, compared to the other single-source model that has accuracy of 88.60%.

The work [29] proposed a blockchain-aided improved system that helped detect different diseases of COVID-19 patients past their recovery period. The disease kind is organized and trained based on post-symptoms of patients for disease prediction. However, the work lacks in-depth analysis and needs to utilize prevention techniques for disease prediction.

The research [30] proposed a detection scheme based on blockchain for diabetes that has three phases of registration, second is user authentication, and finally, Internet of Things (IoT) data upload for evaluation. In this research, the first step included registration during its first phase, and then the user verification of identity using electronic health records with the manager. The tool used for the research was the InterPlanetary File System (IPFS) but still needs further investigation of machine learning techniques.

The research [31] analyzed and detected the heart risk using blockchain with machine learning concept. Using AI methods and IoT, they anticipated the dangers of a coronary episode. Using AI model, an android application was used that helped get the forecast and, furthermore, helped get the client's pulse information using the brilliant band.

For disease prediction, the work [32] used fog computing and proposed safe, secure, and efficient blockchain-based medical care services. For the work, the authors used diabetic and cardio diseases data. Also, for future work, the security of the model can be enhanced and the hybrid classification models can also be added.

TABLE 5.1
Blockchain Application in the Biomedical Domain

Authors	Year	Tools Used	Objective	Key Contribution	Limitation	Future Scope
Lizcano et al. [22]	2023	Hyperledger Fabric	Described blockchain-based smart contract to ensure the traceability and storage of biological samples in a biobank in a safe manner.	To overcome the problem of storing biological samples in better condition, the authors described blockchain-based smart contract to ensure the traceability and storage of biological samples in a biobank.	Less-reliable	Usage of smart contract developed in different software.
Akter et al. [23]	2022	Hyperledger	Proposed secure k- medoids with partial homomorphic cryptosystem (Paillier) and blockchain for data privacy.	To overcome data privacy issues, the authors proposed a secure k-medoids with blockchain and partial homomorphic cryptosystem (Paillier) to eliminate dependency on third parties and ensure data privacy.	Less-efficient	Development of lightweight privacy-preserving machine learning methods.
Soni et al. [24]	2021	—	Addressed the impact of blockchain on healthcare and the biomedical industry.	The authors presented the findings in the biomedical sector using exhaustive literature review of blockchain technology deployment.	Lacks in-depth analysis	Improve security and efficiency.
Amin et al. [25]	2021	Hyperledger Fabric, Hyperledger Caliper	Proposed blockchain-based biomedical engineering supply chain (BESC).	The authors proposed a data-dealing approach to alleviate security issues using Hyperledger Fabric blockchain-based BESC. It is a novel approach that eliminates the possibility of tampering the blockchain system.	Less-secure	Improve efficiency.
Jeet et al. [27]	2020	RStudio	To design a novel approach to overcome the problem of disease overlapping.	The authors designed a novel approach using blockchain technology so as to manage patients' details.	Lacks in-depth analysis	Improve the difficulty level.

With the increased coronary heart disease (CHD) diagnosis medical-related data, it became important to help doctors make accurate clinical diagnosis of the patients. Hence, the research [33] proposed a novel contextual online learning model based on blockchain in mobile edge computing for CHD diagnosis under local differential privacy. The work helped guarantee the diagnosis of patients in a real-time, personalized environment and also considered the patient's heterogeneity. Table 5.2 shows the various blockchain applications in the field of disease prediction in the healthcare domain.

5.2.3 Electronic Health Record (EHR)

Earlier, the systems failed to share health records with security and privacy. But with the electronic health record (EHR) systems, it has become possible, and they also have reduced healthcare costs with fewer medical errors. The research [34] involved an experimental analysis to examine blockchain with patients and EHR systems. The confirmatory factor analysis was used to test reliability. Moreover, using regression analysis, the endogeneity problems were addressed in the research. Results were based on structural equation modeling and regression analysis.

In EHR, the decentralized ledger helps protect data from any hacker. In the blockchain network, each block stores data and ledgers updated copy and thus help validate and protect the copy [35] from hacking. Different stakeholders are involved in permissioned blockchain system, such as hospital, labs, and doctors that access patients' details after taking patients' permission. With strong security and sharing facility for data on blockchain, the security solutions of blockchain are significantly in usage.

For securing and maintaining medical data, the work [36] presented an enhanced study with or without cloud computing for modern blockchain-based solutions. The authors evaluated the different methods using blockchain technology and presented the future roadmap, research gaps, and challenges that boost the healthcare 4.0 technology. However, work lacks efficiency and scalability and suggests quantum-aware blockchain for the future.

To safeguard patients' data in terms of immutability, transparency, traceability, decentralization, and trustworthiness, the research [37] proposed patient-controlled blockchain-enabled EHRs as a way to help patients maintain their records. Also, to evaluate the suggested solutions, different performance criteria, such as accuracy and cost, were used.

The research [38] proposed a cloud computing blockchain-based sharing scheme for patient-controlled EHRs.

The research [39] introduced the blockchain-based electronic health records (BEHR) that helped in transmission between healthcare stakeholders. The authors also proposed an integrated approach that used Internet of Things–based cloud environment with blockchain to reduce the latency in transmission of healthcare records.

The research [40] implemented and designed the blockchain-based e-health system with the facility of patient-centric EHR storage. The research [41] presented systematic literature review that elaborated the different standards for electronic health records so as to achieve semantic interoperability and maturity in blockchain. The work helped in building privacy-preserving solutions for data record storage, sharing, and the state-of-the-art for EHR sharing with cross-chain interoperability.

The research [42] proposed a blockchain-based secure EHR system. With the evolution of wireless and wearable technology, the telemedicine turned into the telecare medicine information system (TMIS). The research [43] proposed a security-preserving electronic health record that helps share the protocol for improved diagnosis in TMIS. Table 5.3 shows the various blockchain applications in the field of electric health records in the healthcare domain.

TABLE 5.2
Blockchain Application in Disease Prediction

Authors	Year	Tools Used	Objective	Key Contribution	Limitation	Future Scope
Noman et al. [28]	2023	Python	Proposed a mechanism of federated learning mechanism from heterogeneous respiratory and multi-class medical data.	The authors introduced the weight manipulation technique that used local model as the important parameter to test privacy. The resulting metric scores showed that the performance is analogous to a single-source model.	Less-efficient	Can be extended to non-medical use cases.
Sivaparthipan et al. [29]	2022	—	Proposed an improved dragonfly algorithm–based deep neural network (IDADNN) algorithm to detect different diseases for COVID-19 patients.	The authors designed deep learning algorithm for COVID-19 patients to detect different diseases.	Lacks efficiency	For disease prediction, use prevention techniques.
Chen et al. [30]	2021	InterPlanetary File System (IPFS)	Presented blockchain-based diabetes disease detection framework.	The authors proposed diabetes disease detection framework using blockchain that detects disease with various machine learning classification algorithms and securely maintains EHRs of the patients.	Less-reliable	Investigate more machine learning algorithms.
Anand et al. [31]	2021	Google Fit API	Analyzed heart risk detection using machine learning and blockchain.	The authors anticipated the danger of coronary episode using AI and IoT methods. An android application helped made a brilliant band to get clients' pulse information and also helped get the forecast by using the AI model.	Lacks reliability	Improve reliability.
Liu et al. [33]	2020	—	Proposed a BC-enabled contextual online learning model for coronary heart disease (CHD) diagnosis under local differential privacy in mobile edge computing.	To guarantee the real-time personalized diagnosis for patients, a novel context-aware online learning algorithm for CHD diagnosis was proposed and considered the heterogeneity of patients.	Less accurate	Improve accuracy and consider more elements.

TABLE 5.3
Blockchain Application in Electronic Health Records

Authors	Year	Tools Used	Objective	Key Contribution	Limitation	Future Scope
Hajian et al. [34]	2023	R	Conducted an experimental analysis to examine blockchain with patients and EHR. The confirmatory factor analysis was used for the model's reliability and validity tests.	The authors conducted an experimental analysis to examine blockchain with patients and EHR systems.	Less-reliable	Improve reliability.
Mahajan et al. [36]	2022	NetBeans IDE Hyperledger	Study of modern blockchain-based solutions for medical data security.	The authors presented the systematic study for safeguarding medical data using blockchain and cloud computing. The outcomes presented the research gaps, future roadmap, and to boost healthcare 4.0 technology.	Lacks efficiency	Quantum-aware blockchain.
Rai et al. [37]	2022	Ethereum Ganache Remix IDE	Proposed patient-controlled electronic health records using blockchain.	The author's proposed work provided with secure storage and access rules for medical data.	Lacks in-depth analysis	Improve efficiency.
Pang et al. [38]	2022	—	Proposed cloud computing and blockchain-based patient-controlled electronic health records sharing scheme.	The authors proposed the encryption-and-encryption scheme based on multi-keyword based on attribute to encrypt electronic health records.	Lacks reliability	Improvise the proposed consensus algorithm.
Mallikarjuna et al. [39]	2021	Node.js Apache JMeter	Developed an efficient e-health records using Internet of Things.	The authors proposed an approach that integrated blockchain 4.0 and IoT-based cloud environment.	Lacks complete implementation of technologies with blockchain 4.0	To apply data science and AI in COVID-19 data.

5.2.4 Genomics

Blockchain has created data revolution in the field of genomics. To protect patient's privacy, collaborative privacy-preserving modeling allowed the construction of more predictive models in general. The work [44] designed a quorum mechanism that helped hierarchical network address the site availability issue. The work combined a hierarchical learning algorithm design of blockchain smart contracts. During the initialization and iteration phases, the QuorumChain was constructed and evaluated the site-unavailability scenarios in modeling process on genomic datasets. The results showed that HierarchicalChain wouldn't function if one or more sites would become unavailable; however, QuorumChain significantly improved the predictive correctness.

By genomic data ownership, by enabling the transparent genomic data sharing, and by reducing the individual genome sequencing costs [45], blockchain is used significantly in the genomics domain. Using nested database indexing method, the work [46] developed a novel blockchain private network so as to store personal genomic variants.

The research [47] proposed a framework based on blockchain for PGx data sharing. Using private Ethereum blockchain, the proof-of-concept implementation on PGxChain was stimulated. PGxChain helped in sharing of PGx and medical data. However, it has its existence only in limited number of browsers. With implementation, the need to secure the data and preserve its efficiency was required. Thus, the research [48] proposed gene data management. The model included two semi-private storage and private storage. However, its efficiency and security, needed to develop real gene data storage server.

The work [49] proposed dynamic consent architecture based on blockchain and implemented proof-of-concept to support genomic data sharing for the proposed architecture. To support genomic data sharing, the work [50] focused on benchmarking blockchain strategies. Using three methods of Index Everything, Dual-Scenario Indexing, and Query Index, the researchers developed a feasible solution for patient records sharing on gene–drug interactions using blockchain.

For safe and secure sharing of de-identified patient data and with a focus on late-stage cancer, authors in [51] piloted a blockchain-authenticated system derived from standard of genomic testing, electronic health records (EHRs), and care imaging called the Cancer Gene Trust (CGT). The work [52] proposed a layered architecture of blockchain in genomics and healthcare. To improve privacy and security, and with encouraged genetic research, the designed architecture showed how communication between researchers, medical professionals, and users was improved. Table 5.4 shows the various blockchain applications in the field of genomics in the healthcare domain.

5.2.5 Pharmaceuticals

The counterfeit drugs have been a source of major concern. Thus, for solution, the research [53] conducted a review. The authors used an automated content analysis in blockchain-based pharmaceuticals and helped identify various points of pharmaceuticals, avenues for future studies, and the usage of smart contracts to lessen counterfeit drugs. Also, managerial and theoretical implications were also discussed.

The pharmaceuticals involve supply chain at each and every phase, and thus, blockchain helps trace every minute detail of the medicine and its components so as to regularly detect the defects caused in supply chain at each and every step [54]. Thus, many researches were carried out that helped in doing so. The work [55] presented an integrated system for data integrity and analytics in the pharmaceutical industry. The monitoring

TABLE 5.4
Blockchain Application in Genomics

Authors	Year	Tools Used	Objective	Key Contribution	Limitation	Future Scope
Kuo et al. [44]	2023	—	Designed a source-verifiable quorum mechanism that helped hierarchical network to address the site-availability issue.	The authors designed an immutable and source-verifiable quorum mechanism that helped hierarchical network address the site-availability issue.	Recovery of site yet to be explored	Improve efficiency.
Gursoy et al. [46]	2022	SAMchain VCFtools	Developed a private blockchain system to store reference-aligned genomic variants and reads on-chain.	The authors used nested database indexing to rapidly analyze the data.	Lacks efficiency	Improve scalability.
Albalwy et al. [47]	2022	Ethereum Hyperledger Caliper	Proposed a framework using blockchain so as to support sharing of pharmacogenetic data.	The authors proposed a methodology that used blockchain-based PGxChain framework and used smart contracts implemented so as to address the issue for identifiable genomic data and its storage and movement.	Available only on some Internet browsers	Aggregate the system with an identity management service of NHS Identity or GOV.UK Verify.
Park et al. [48]	2021	Ethereum	Using local differential privacy (LDP), proposed a secure genomic data management system.	The authors provided a model with semi-private and private storage, where only the irreversibly modified gene data was dealt with the external users and original gene data reside in the internal system.	Less-secure	To construct real gene data storage server.
Kuo et al. [50]	2021	iDASH2.0 Amazon Web Services (AWS)	Focused on using blockchain for sharing records of gene-drug interactions.	The authors developed a feasible solution using three methods of Index Everything, Dual-Scenario Indexing, and Query Index to share patient records using blockchain on gene-drug interactions.	Less-efficient	Improve efficiency.

techniques helped identify the production yield discrepancies, conducted predictive analytics for business process to estimate important parameters, and also identified sources of data errors. The work in [56] elaborated the potential usage of blockchain technology in the healthcare domain. The work explored the standard data processing problems and drug tracing approaches.

The research [57] elaborated about the factors that encouraged and hindered the application of blockchain technology in pharmaceutical domain. Some of the common factors were illiterate stakeholders, limited network, and individuals that restricted the application of blockchain technology in pharmaceutical industries. For secure record transactions, and to enhance trust between parties, the research [58] proposed the blockchain in the supply chain model assessment of pharmaceutical.

The research [59] investigated the incentive alignment opportunities of supply chain members and considered a two-stage supply chain. It was comprised of a common retailer and two medicine manufacturers that had more accurate demand information than the manufacturers. To verify the authenticity of transactions in ledger, blockchain network was used to help healthcare supply chain stakeholders. The authors in [60] investigated different applications of blockchain technology and their benefit in healthcare supply machine management. Table 5.5 shows the various blockchain applications in the field of pharmaceuticals in the healthcare domain.

5.3 Tools for Blockchain Systems

Different frameworks are used to develop blockchain systems. For example, the authors in [61] built the healthcare system using Wireshark framework, which helped measure the blockchain's performance and round-trip time. Also, Spyder IDE was used for statistical data evaluation. Thus, this section deals with various tools that are used in healthcare applications.

5.3.1 Hyperledger Fabric

Hyperledger Fabric is a tool that uses modular architecture [62] for developing applications. It uses plug-and-play components of membership services and consensus for deployment. From Linux Foundation, the tool is found to be an open-source project. It is written in chaincode and uses smart contract model–based permissioned architecture. It supports a wide variety of languages, such as Java, JavaScript, and Go. It uses channel technology for confidential transactions and thus helps in easy initialization. However, Hyperledger Fabric has minimum APIs and SDKs with complex architecture. Also, it lacks skilled programmers [63] and is not network fault-tolerant.

5.3.2 Hyperledger Sawtooth

Hyperledger Sawtooth is a framework that builds distributed ledgers scalable. It helps deploy and execute the ledgers [64]. It is an open-source platform and a blockchain-as-a-service that deploys smart contracts without main and core system knowledge. Various organizations such as Linux Project, IBM, SAP, and Intel sponsor Sawtooth. It supports two main consensus algorithms also.

TABLE 5.5
Blockchain Application in Pharmaceuticals

Authors	Year	Tools Used	Objective	Key Contribution	Limitation	Future Scope
Kordestani et al. [53]	2023	—	Conducted a systematic literature review to find a proper solution for counterfeiting drugs.	The authors used an automated content analysis in blockchain-based pharmaceuticals and helped identify various points of pharmaceuticals, avenues for future studies, and the usage of smart contracts to lessen counterfeit drugs.	Lacks in-depth analysis	Consider more paper for analysis.
Sahana et al. [56]	2022	IPFS	Explored the problems related with drug tracing approaches and standard data processing.	The authors showed the importance of blockchain-based new digital platforms as an emergence for seamless and fast interaction between data providers.	Less-efficient	Improve efficiency.
Alshahrani et al. [57]	2021	—	Explored the importance of improving pharmaceutical industries using blockchain in Saudi Arabia.	The authors discussed various factors that encouraged as well as hindered the pharmaceutical industries blockchain applications.	Lacks in-depth analysis	Improve reliability.
Badhotiya et al. [58]	2021	—	Proposed investigation in the pharmaceutical supply chain model using blockchain and to securely record transactions and enhance trust between parties.	The authors discussed the blockchain adaptation to address the supply chain challenges.	Fewer number of papers are taken into account	Add recent papers for evaluation.

5.3.3 Ethereum

Ethereum [65] is a decentralized and an open-source blockchain that utilizes the functionality of smart contract. The cryptocurrency used for this platform is Ether (ETH). It works in a public network [66] and uses distributed ledger. It uses consensus mechanisms, but when PoW mechanism is used, it creates blocks in chain in blockchain. Also, it faces dependability issues and hard forks.

5.3.4 InterPlanetary File System (IPFS)

The IPFS [67] uses a distributed file system to share and store data. To identify each and every file in a global namespace, it uses content-addressing that helps connect each and every computing device. For static webpage delivery, the gateways replace the protocols used. The tool also helps in communication for local network users, provides higher bandwidth, and helps the creators in distribution of work. But sometimes IPFS consumes a high bandwidth, which makes it delimited for usage.

5.3.5 Postman

Postman is a standalone software testing application programming interface (API). It helps build up, design, test, document, and modify APIs. It streamlines each and every step of the API cycle that helps create better APIs. By leveraging security warnings, alerts, and reports, the platform advanced intelligence about API operations. Personal workspaces, team workspaces, and public workspaces are the three types of workspaces for Postman. With Postman API and open-source technologies, it is extensible easily. It is available for free and also offers different paid plans for better usage [68].

5.3.6 Ganache

Ganache is a personal blockchain for development of Ethereum and rapid Corda-distributed application. It helps in developing, deploying, and testing DApps in a safer environment. It has command line interface and user interface as two flavors to be used. It helps in testing Solidity contracts using personal Ethereum blockchain. It shows benefits and features more than Remix [69].

5.3.7 Blockchain Testnet

Blockchain testnet is an instance of blockchain network that helps in experimentation and testing without any risk to real funds and main chain. The testnet coins are from faucets for free and are usually different from the mainnet coins. While in use, they are used for analyzing BC data on a smaller scale and can easily be reset at any time.

5.3.8 Iroha

Iroha is BC framework that is embedded inside infrastructure projects using distributed ledger technology [70]. The distributed feature in BC ledger allows data to be publicly shared. Architecture, consensus mechanism, and functional/logical flow are the three major roles of the tool Iroha. It is hosted by the Linux Foundation and was launched in May 2019. It is used to help merchants buy goods, build national identities, and allow financial services access. It also provides the facility of plugin modular design for blockchain running and multiple signatures for transactions.

5.3.9 Geth

The original implementation of protocol of Ethereum is Go Ethereum. It is written in Go [71] and is an open-source framework provided. It can easily be used as a library by embedding in Go, android project, or iOS. Geth mines Ether and serves as a node that helps create software for users of Ethereum virtual machine (EVM).

5.3.10 Hyperledger Composer

Hyperledger Composer is a framework for open development for easy making of blockchain applications. It helps in solving business-related problems and aims at improving operational efficiencies. With corporate members, the Linux Foundation hosts it and provides an example of BaaS. It uses JavaScript and is part of the Hyperledger Fabric platform. For more scalability and reusability, to make the utilities, it uses built-in libraries. It supports scalability, sharing for business implementation, and reusability across organizations of different components and helps in generating the required APIs [72].

5.3.11 MATLAB

MATLAB is developed by MathWorks [73] and is a numeric computing environment and multi-paradigm proprietary programming language. It provides various features for the plotting of data, matrix manipulations, and helps in proper interfacing with that of programs written in other languages and implementation of algorithms. It helps in iterative analysis with programming language and usually expresses the results in an array in mathematics or matrix directly. The interpreter is written in Java language for MATLAB. However, besides these advantages, it takes more time for execution, requires large amount of memory, and is expensive too.

5.3.12 Truffle

Truffle uses the Ethereum virtual machine (EVM) and is a development environment, testing framework, and asset pipeline for blockchain [74]. It has more than 1.5 million downloads and is the most used popular tool for BC applications.

5.3.13 Wireshark

Wireshark is a free packet analyzer and an open-source that is used for network analysis, education, troubleshooting, and communications protocol development. It stores the traffic on the local network and stores data for offline analysis. It is legal for usage but becomes illegal if handled without authorization. It identifies wireless network attacks, such as disassociation, authentication denial of service attacks, de-authentication, and beacon flooding using filters. The tool is safe to use and is freely available for many platforms. It can deeply analyze the information floating in the network easily. The healthcare department uses this tool for working. However, the tool is unable to detect the intruders in the network as well as cannot send data, etc. [75].

5.3.14 Spyder IDE

Spyder IDE is a cross-platform open-source IDE that is used mainly for scientific programming using Python language. It helps in writing scripts but doesn't support complex Python programs. It helps support machine learning, data science, but doesn't support web development. It helps generate figures quickly and debug the existing codes that help users understand the results easily. Different software layouts are also available that can be selected and used according to the requirement by the users. However, the result tab is not so effective to be used, and also, the tutorials provided for Spyder usage should be developed and uploaded more [76].

5.3.15 SPSS

SPSS is a statistical suite that is used for data management, business intelligence, advanced analytics, criminal investigation, and multivariate analysis. It is also used for statistical, batched, and interactive analysis and was developed by IBM. The software is available commercially with copyright and is not free. Students access SPSS for free via institution or in free trial version. It is used mainly by market researchers, companies of survey, health researchers, government entities, marketing organizations, education researchers, data miners, etc. that analyze survey data for results. Java language is used to write graphical user interface (GUI) of SPSS. It is easy to use, provides good user interface, and handles large data easily. However, it is very expensive and has limited functionalities [77].

5.4 Analysis Tools for Blockchain Ethereum Smart Contracts

There are various tools present that are used to analyze the Ethereum blockchain-based smart contracts.

5.4.1 Echidna

Echidna [78] was invented in 2020 and is a static analysis tool that is open-source and publicly available that takes input in the form of viper or Solidity code. It is developed in Haskell and a smart contract fuzzer of Ethereum that supports three properties of assertion checking, user-defined properties, and gas use estimation. It has two steps involved: (1) Pre-processing: to analyze smart contracts, it leverages Slither. (2) Fuzzing campaign: in this property, violations are detected and random transactions are generated. Thus, Echidna helps in easy usage and helps support the development of contract frameworks. Also, it has fast execution that produces results very fast.

5.4.2 Eth2Vec

Eth2Vec [79] is a tool based on command line and was developed in the year 2021. It analyzes smart contracts and uses machine learning approach to get the knowledge of EVM features of byte code. Finally, it matches the similarity in the target EVM and code of EVM to detect the vulnerabilities.

5.4.3 Gastap

Gastap [80] was developed in 2018 and is basically a statical analysis tool. This tool analyzes the EVM byte code or Solidity code or disassembled byte code of EVM. For its functions, it deduces the requirements of gas bounds and then compares the gas limit paid and deduced gas requirement.

5.4.4 Remix IDE

Remix IDE [81] is an open-access tool that analyzes smart contracts in Solidity code and provides an easy way to write the code. It was invented in 2016 and is a JavaScript implementation of EVM. It is based on browser and is a user's interface. The source code is present in the GitHub Repository. It has the Solidity static analysis plugin that has 21 analysis modules under four different categories: gas and economy, security, ERC, and miscellaneous, in Remix IDE v0.10.1.

5.4.5 Slither

Slither [82] was invented in 2018 and is an open-source tool which is developed in the Python language. It inputs Solidity code for analysis and also uses an intermediate representation of SlithIR. To detect vulnerabilities, Slither analyzes data flow of the tracking approaches. The open version predicts almost 20 bugs too.

5.4.6 SmartAnvil

SmartAnvil [83], invented in 2018, is an open-source platform which was developed in Smalltalk. For smart contract analysis, it is constructed using various modules. This platform has three component tools, such as SmaCC-Solidity, which is a parser used to support static code of Solidity smart contract. Second is SmartInspect, which is a component usually used to detect the Solidity smart contract internal state, and third is Ukulele, which helps fetch required data using this query language from the blockchain.

5.4.7 SmartBugs

SmartBugs [84] was invented in 2020 and is a publicly available static analysis framework that is executed in the Python language. For analyzing the smart contracts, it supports ten tools. It has five components: tools dockers image, command-line interpreter, SmartBugs runner, tools configuration, and dataset.

5.4.8 SmartCheck

SmartCheck [85] was developed in Java and invented in 2017. It is an open-source, publicly available static analysis tool. To analyze the smart contract, SmartCheck employs syntactical analysis and lexical analysis approaches. Using custom Solidity grammar and ANTLR (a parser generator) for an intermediate representation, the generation of an XML parse tree is done. For detecting vulnerabilities, usage of XPath queries is done so as to process the intermediate representation. It detects almost 20 bugs, like style guide violation, implicit visibility level, etc.

5.4.9 DefectChecker

DefectChecker [86] was deployed in 2021 and was developed in the Java language. It has four sections for processing: inputter, defect identifier, feature detector, and CFG builder. It takes byte code as an input and then extracts the opcodes as output. For symbolic execution, all the opcodes are clustered and categorized accordingly into different categories. Finally, for detection of defects in the smart contract, control flow graph is constructed.

5.4.10 GasChecker

GasChecker [87] was invented in 2020. The tool does analyses on the basis of ten programming patterns or gas inefficient codes.

5.4.11 Gasper

Gasper [88] is written in the Python language. It was invented in 2017. It helps in gas cost analysis of patterns in smart contracts that are based on the EVM byte code. It identifies seven gas cost patterns as costly loop-related patterns and unnecessary code-related patterns. Thus, it can be concluded that the Gasper tool is based on the execution on symbolics and is a pattern checker based on gas cost that works on byte code.

5.4.12 HoneyBadger

HoneyBadger [89] is an open-source, publicly available tool which was developed using the Python language. For honeypot smart contracts, it performs systematic analysis. It has a structure consisting of analysis pipeline of three different types, named honeypot analysis, symbolic analysis, and cash flow analysis. The satisfiability of constraints is checked by each and every type of analysis using Z3 SMT solver.

5.4.13 MadMax

MadMax [90] is an openly available public source of static analysis tool which came into existence in 2018. For static analysis performance, it uses Gigahose IR. The first one includes a control-flow-analysis decompiler, and the last is queries. Thus, it helps identify the concepts related to specific high-level area.

5.4.14 Mythril

Mythril [91] is an open-source analysis, publicly available tool which was deployed and executed by ConsenSys using Python programming language in 2017. For input, EVM byte code is provided for analysis in the tool. Mythril helps in the analyses of the important Ethereum smart contracts that are basically based on blockchain and also helps improve performance on platforms of blockchain.

5.4.15 Oyente

Oyente [92] is a static analysis and open-source, publicly available tool which came into existence in 2016 and is deployed and executed in Python. For analyses of smart contracts, it employs symbolic execution and also helps in statistical and path-by-path analyses of the program code. From consideration to eliminate provably the infeasible traces, the Validator and Explorer uses Z3 bit-vector solver.

5.4.16 Securify

Securify [93] is a static analysis and open-source, publicly available tool which is executed and deployed in the Java language and was invented in the year 2018. To check whether it is safe or not, it helps checks smart contract behavior associated to a particular feature or parameter and also helps in a fully automated security analysis. The input is byte code of EVM and security patterns set for the tool.

5.4.17 Vandal

Vandal [94] is a static analysis open-source, publicly available tool which is implemented in the Python language and was invented in 2018. Its analysis pipeline helps in the transformation of the EVM byte code into semantic logics relation. It shows vulnerability analysis into declarative language of soufflé. Vandal's analysis pipeline has several stages: extractor, scrapper, decompiler, and disassembler, to produce the logic relations.

5.4.18 Manticore

Manticore [95] is a dynamic analysis open-source, publicly available tool which is executed in Python in the year 2017. It is a symbolic-type execution analysis tool that is dynamic in nature that allows user customization for analysis purposes in Manticore. Its architecture has components which are the core engine and Ethereum execution modules.

5.5 Building Smart Contracts

Smart contracts are the simple programs that are usually stored on a blockchain and execute when required conditions are met. They include participants and don't involve any third-party intermediary or time loss. [96]

Smart contract uses simple "if–else" statements to write codes on blockchain. A specified computer network gets involved and helps in executing the code. This helps in releasing funds to the actual parties involved, sending notifications, registering a vehicle, or issuing a ticket. The blockchain is regularly updated after transaction is completed. Thus, this helps in saving of transaction without any fear of alteration on blockchain.

Some of the benefits of smart contracts are discussed in what follows.

5.5.1 Speed and Accuracy

The contract executes immediately, soon after the conditions are met. Since the smart contracts are automated and digital, there's no need for any manual paperwork and filling-in documents.

5.5.2 Transparency and Trust

Due to the non-involvement of any third party and the usage of encrypted records of transactions, there's no chance of any alteration of information. Thus, this helps in building trust and transparency among users.

Building Efficient Smart Contract for Healthcare 4.0

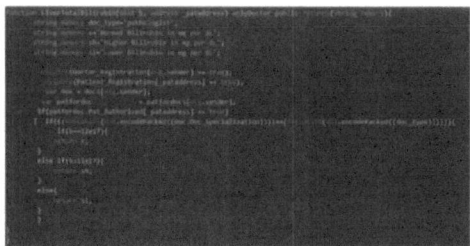

FIGURE 5.1
Healthcare smart contract with LiverTotalBilirubinfunction().

5.5.3 Security

The transaction stored on blockchain is encrypted and is hard to hack. Since each record is well connected to the subsequent and previous records on a ledger, it makes it difficult for hackers to alter a single record.

5.5.4 Savings

Smart contracts don't involve any intermediary and helps handle transactions without any time delays and fees.

Figure 5.1 shows the working of a healthcare smart contract that includes the LiverTotalBilirubinfunction() in Remix IDE [97]. This function helps in easy analysis of the patient's amount of total bilirubin in liver. When doctor checks his patient, he enters the amount of bilirubin in the form of ethers along with the patient's address. The function then checks various parameters. Such as:

1. If the doctor is already registered in the hospital.
2. If the patient is already registered in the hospital.
3. If the particular patient is authorized to this particular doctor.
4. If the doctor specialization, for example, "pathologist," is same as the doctor the patient wants to concern.
5. After all these conditions are met, the function checks the amount of bilirubin. If the amount is equal to 12 mg per deciliter, then the patient has "Normal Bilirubin in mg per dL." If the amount is greater than 12 mg per deciliter, then the patient has "Higher Bilirubin in mg per dL." Else, if both the conditions turn false, then the patient has "Lower Bilirubin in mg per dL."

5.6 Solidity Static Analysis

After the writing of smart contracts in Remix IDE, the vulnerabilities are usually generated. Thus, it becomes important to reduce these vulnerabilities and debug the code. To do so, various tools are provided, and one such tool is Solidity static analysis [98].

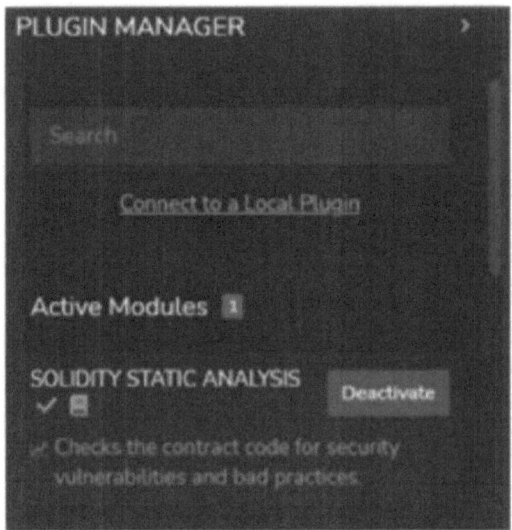

FIGURE 5.2
Activated Solidity static analysis plugin in Remix IDE.

Solidity static analysis is a plugin that helps perform static analysis on smart contracts after compilation. It is usually activated from the Remix Plugin Manager.

Figure 5.2 shows the activated Solidity static analysis plugin in the Solidity environment of Remix IDE that helps check all the bad practices and security vulnerabilities of the code. This plugin provides us with different modules that help in debugging a code. These include security, gas and economy, ERC, and miscellaneous. One has to select/deselect these modules for analysis.

Figure 5.3 shows all four modules of Solidity static analysis and shows the detailed sub-modules of a security module. By default, all modules are selected during analysis of smart contract.

After the deployment of our smart contract with LiverTotalBilirubin function, the need to check for vulnerabilities arose. Thus, to reduce the gas cost incurred, it becomes necessary to check vulnerabilities.

Figure 5.4 shows certain changes in the LiverTotalBilirubin() function to reduce gas cost and vulnerabilities. These are:

1. Similar variable names.
2. This includes "Variables have very similar names," "patfordoc" and "patfordocs." Thus, "patfordoc" is replaced with "pfordoc." Also, "doc" and "docs" show similar error. Thus, "doc" is replaced with variable "d."
3. Also, local variables to display return statements are removed, and simple one-return string-type variable is used to return the statement.
4. The use of "var" keyword is deprecated. Instead, use *storage* keyword for storage.
5. Make functions "external" so as to reduce the gas cost.
6. Since bytes consumes less gas than string, use bytes keywords and variables wherever possible in code.

Building Efficient Smart Contract for Healthcare 4.0

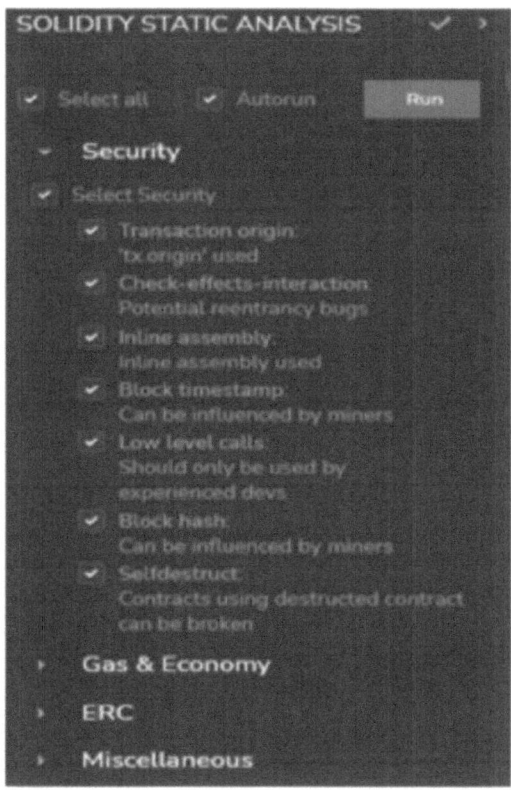

FIGURE 5.3
All four modules of Solidity static analysis.

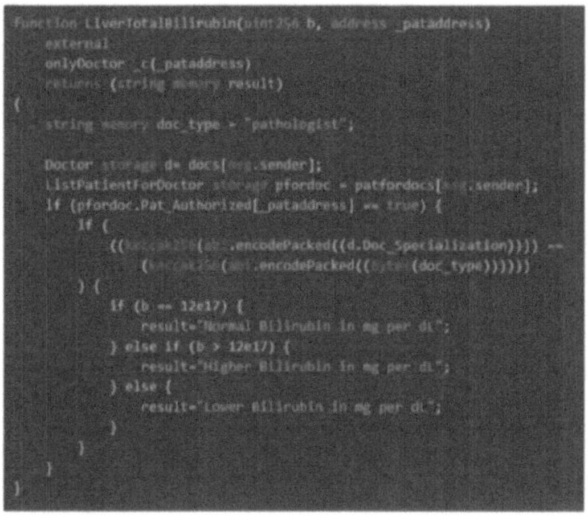

FIGURE 5.4
Final healthcare smart contract with reduced vulnerabilities.

5.7 Research Challenges in Healthcare

The traditional healthcare sector faced various challenges [99]. However, with advancement in blockchain technology, these limitations were solved, and possible solutions were suggested using blockchain. Some of the research challenges and their possible solutions for healthcare sector are discussed next.

5.7.1 Patient Data Management

In the healthcare domain, with the registration of new patient and doctor in the hospital, the database is being maintained to store the data securely. Patients are checked by the doctors, and the prescriptions are provided. Thus, to get correct future prescription, the previous data of the patient has to be provided to the authorized doctor. This stimulates the need to transfer medical information of the patient to the doctor or pharmacists. This increases a sense of insecurity toward medical data exposure. To solve this issue, blockchain technology helps in generating hash for each and every patient's private information. The medical data is evaluated using blockchain API for an affected patient without revealing his identity. Also, the patient gets the power to decide accessibility of data [100]. Thus, this helps in proper management of patient data in hospital healthcare system.

5.7.2 Clinical Trials

Patients are always eager for their personal and confidential information safe storage. One never wants their data to be exposed and provided to an unauthorized party. Thus, with the usage of hashing algorithms and blockchain, it becomes almost impossible to modify the stored and private data of the patients. The healthcare industry has always needed a safe and secure data sharing method so as to safely share data with authorized parties. With blockchain, it becomes easy to manage data within multiple sites, systems, and protocols. Also, patients, with certain permissions, can access their health information [101].

5.7.3 Drug Traceability

Today, the main problem is drug counterfeiting in the pharmacology sector. The recent survey on drugs shows that about 10 to 30 percentages of the drugs are duplicate and fake. This results in severe patient's health damage and drug's improper usage by different stakeholders. Thus, all this problem is solved using blockchain technology, which helps store the whole route of drugs operation and detect frauds carried from manufacturer till supply.

5.7.4 Latency

In the validation process, many traditional systems allowed all the participants to participate, due to which the patient's real-time data becomes unpredictable and unreliable. This also made the process very time-consuming and a little cumbersome. Thus, to solve this problem, blockchain follows proper consensus mechanism in the validation process that allows an easy working of the healthcare system so as to increase processing speed and performance of the whole system [102].

5.7.5 Scalability

One of the main concerns regarding scalability in traditional systems included the block's limited size and its frequency. But with blockchain, it helps provide the facility for execution of millions of transactions per second. Various other solutions have also been provided by blockchain, such as soft fork (SegWit), lighting network, hard fork (Bitcoin Cash), and plasma cash, so as to remove the scalability issues.

5.7.6 Interoperability

Earlier healthcare systems faced issues related to secure access and sharing of patient information. Privacy and security are the most important elements to be considered for the healthcare management sector. Thus, to rectify the issue, developers tested the features of different prototypes of blockchain. This resulted in blockchain's deployment and adoption in an operational healthcare system. Blockchain provides an open standard for interoperability in healthcare and enables data access using APIs between various products [102].

5.7.7 Security and Privacy

In a network, hackers are always there to attack and steal information. To solve this issue and to preserve the privacy and the security of the patient's data, the usage of permissioned blockchain like private and consortium are implemented. This technology uses smart contracts for the execution of transactions in blocks without any third-party interference. These transactions are usually irreversible and traceable in nature [102,103].

5.8 Conclusion

This chapter provides an in-depth analysis about blockchain importance in the healthcare domain. The chapter discusses the basics of blockchain, its characteristics, its architecture, the consensus mechanisms used in blockchain, as well as provides a literature survey on blockchain's role in different healthcare applications, such as genomics, electronic health records, pharmaceuticals, biomedicine, and prediction of diseases. Further, it provides details of 15 frameworks, such as Ganache, Hyperledger Fabric, Truffle, Ethereum, etc., that help in building blockchain system. Also discussed are 18 different tools, such as Solidity static analysis, Oyente, Securify, SmartCheck, etc., that help in the analysis of different bugs and vulnerabilities of the blockchain systems. Apart from this, the details regarding the building of smart contracts on Remix IDE using Solidity and detection of vulnerabilities using Solidity static analysis plugin are also explained. Thus, this chapter helps readers have an easy understanding of the concept of blockchain and effective smart contract execution in the healthcare 4.0 industry, along with in-depth knowledge of different performance analysis tools.

References

[1] Gambhire G, Gujar T, Pathak S. Business potential and impact of industry 4.0 in manufacturing organizations. In: *Fourth International Conference on Computing Communication Control and Automation (ICCUBEA)*. Vol. 2018; 2018. pp. 1–6. https://doi.org/10.1109/ICCUBEA.2018.8697552.

[2] Fraga-Lamas P, Fernández-Caramés TM. A review on blockchain technologies for an advanced and cyber-resilient automotive industry. *IEEE Access*. 2019;7:17578–98. https://doi.org/10.1109/ACCESS.2019.2895302.

[3] Makhdoom I, Abolhasan M, Abbas H, Ni W. Blockchain's adoption in IoT: The challenges, and a way forward. *J NetwComput Appl*. 2019;125:251–79. https://doi.org/10.1016/j.jnca.2018.10.019.

[4] Nakamoto S. Bitcoin: A peer-to-peer electronic cash system. *Decentralized Bus Rev*. 2008:21260.

[5] Aste T, Tasca P, Di Matteo T. Blockchain technologies: The foreseeable impact on society and industry. *Computer*. 2017;50(9):18–28. https://doi.org/10.1109/MC.2017.3571064.

[6] Salah K, Rehman MHU, Nizamuddin N, Al-Fuqaha A. Blockchain for AI: Review and open research challenges. *IEEE Access*. 2019;7:10127–49. https://doi.org/10.1109/ACCESS.2018.2890507.

[7] Litke A, Anagnostopoulos D, Varvarigou T. Blockchains for supply chain management: Architectural elements and challenges towards a global scale deployment. *Logistics*. 2019;3(1):5. https://doi.org/10.3390/logistics3010005.

[8] Aloini D, Benevento E, Stefanini A, Zerbino P. Transforming healthcare ecosystems through blockchain: Opportunities and capabilities for business process innovation. *Technovation*. 2023;119:102557. https://doi.org/10.1016/j.technovation.2022.102557.

[9] Hathaliya JJ, Tanwar S, Tyagi S, Kumar N. Securing electronics healthcare records in healthcare 4.0: A biometric-based approach. *ComputElectr Eng*. 2019;76:398–410. https://doi.org/10.1016/j.compeleceng.2019.04.017.

[10] Coventry L, Branley D. Cybersecurity in healthcare: A narrative review of trends, threats and ways forward. *Maturitas*. 2018;113:48–52. https://doi.org/10.1016/j.maturitas.2018.04.008.

[11] Al-rawashdeh M, Keikhosrokiani P, Belaton B, Alawida M, Zwiri A. IoT adoption and application for smart healthcare: A systematic review. *Sensors* (Basel). 2022;22(14). https://doi.org/10.3390/s22145377.

[12] Hamil H, Zidelmal Z, Azzaz MS, Sakhi S, Kaibou R, Djilali S, et al. Design of a secured telehealth system based on multiple biosignals diagnosis and classification for IoT application. *Expert Syst*. 2022;39(4):e12765. https://doi.org/10.1111/exsy.12765.

[13] Hathaliya JJ, Tanwar S. An exhaustive survey on security and privacy issues in healthcare 4.0. *ComputCommun*. 2020;153:311–35. https://doi.org/10.1016/j.comcom.2020.02.018.

[14] Gupta R, Kumari A, Tanwar S. Fusion of blockchain and artificial intelligence for secure drone networking underlying 5-g communications. *Trans EmergTelecommun Technol*. 2021;32(1):1–20. https://doi.org/10.1002/ett.4176.

[15] Gupta R, Kumari A, Tanwar S. A taxonomy of blockchain envisioned edge-as-a-connected autonomous vehicles. *Trans EmergTelecommun Technol*. 2021;32(6):1–24. https://doi.org/10.1002/ett.4009.

[16] Dutta P, Choi TM, Somani S, Butala R. Blockchain technology in supply chain operations: Applications, challenges and research opportunities. *Transp Res E LogistTransp Rev*. 2020;142:102067. https://doi.org/10.1016/j.tre.2020.102067.

[17] Chen M, Malook T, Rehman AU, Muhammad Y, Alshehri MD, Akbar A, et al. Blockchain-enabled healthcare system for detection of diabetes. *J Inf Sec Appl*. 2021;58:1–12. https://doi.org/10.1016/j.jisa.2021.102771.

[18] Dutta P, Choi TM, Somani S, Butala R. Blockchain technology in supply chain operations: Applications, challenges and research opportunities. *Transp Res E LogistTransp Rev*. 2020;142:102067. https://doi.org/10.1016/j.tre.2020.102067.

[19] Gupta S, Sadoghi M. Blockchain transaction processing. *arXiv:2107.11592*. 2018;5.

[20] Bodkhe U, Bhattacharya P, Tanwar S, Tyagi S, Kumar N, Obaidat MS. Blohost: Blockchain enabled smart tourism and hospitality management. In: *International Conference on Computer, Information and Telecommunication Systems (CITS)*. Vol. 2019; 2019. pp. 1–5. https://doi.org/10.1109/CITS.2019.8862001.

[21] Hathaliya J, Sharma P, Tanwar S, Gupta R. Blockchain-based remote patient monitoring in healthcare 4.0. In: *9th International Conference on Advanced Computing (IACC)*. IEEE Publications; 2019. pp. 87–91. https://doi.org/10.1109/IACC48062.2019.8971593.

[22] Ortiz-Lizcano MI, Arias-Antunez E, Hernandez Bravo A, Caminero MB, Rojo Guillen T, Nam Cha SH. Increasing the security and traceability of biological samples in biobanks by blockchain technology. *Comput Methods Programs Biomed*. 2023;231:107379.

[23] Akter S, Reza F, Ahmed M. Convergence of blockchain, kmedoids and homomorphic encryption for privacy preserving biomedical data classification. *Internet Things Cyber-Phys Syst*. 2022;2:99–110. https://doi.org/10.1016/j.iotcps.2022.05.006.

[24] Soni M, Singh DK. Blockchain-based security & privacy for biomedical and healthcare information exchange systems. *Mater Today Proc*. 2021. Available from: https://doi.org/10.1016/j.matpr.2021.02.094.

[25] Amin MR, Zuhairi MF, Saadat MN. Transparent data dealing: Hyperledger fabric based biomedical engineering supply chain. In: *15th International Conference on Ubiquitous Information Management and Communication (IMCOM)*. Vol. 2021; 2021. pp. 1–5. https://doi.org/10.1109/IMCOM51814.2021.9377418.

[26] Haidar M, Kumar S. Smart healthcare system for biomedical and health care applications using aadhaar and blockchain. In: *5th International Conference on Information Systems and Computer Networks (ISCON)*. Vol. 2021; 2021. pp. 1–5. https://doi.org/10.1109/ISCON52037.2021.9702306.

[27] Jeet R, Kang SS. E-biomedical: A positive prospect to monitor human healthcare system using blockchain technology. *World J Eng*. 2022;19(1):13–20. https://doi.org/10.1108/WJE-10-2020-0475.

[28] Noman AA, Rahaman M, Pranto TH, Rahman RM. Blockchain for medical collaboration: A federated learning-based approach for multi-class respiratory disease classification. *Healthc Anal*. 2023;3:100135. https://doi.org/10.1016/j.health.2023.100135.

[29] Sivaparthipan CB, Muthu BA, Fathima G, Kumar PM, Alazab M, Díaz VG. Blockchain assisted disease identification of Covid-19 patients with the help of ida-dnn classifier. *Wirel Personal Commun*. 2022;126(3):2597–620. https://doi.org/10.1007/s11277-022-09831-7.

[30] Chen M, Malook T, Rehman AU, Muhammad Y, Alshehri MD, Akbar A, et al. Blockchain-enabled healthcare system for detection of diabetes. *J Inf Sec Appl*. 2021;58:102771. https://doi.org/10.1016/j.jisa.2021.102771.

[31] Anand R, Fazlul Kareem S, Mohamed Arshad Mubeen RM, Ramesh S, Vignesh B. Analysis of heart risk detection in machine learning using blockchain. In: *6th International Conference on Signal Processing, Computing and Control (ISPCC)*. Vol. 2021; 2021. pp. 685–9. https://doi.org/10.1109/ISPCC53510.2021.9609353.

[32] Shynu PG, Menon VG, Kumar RL, Kadry S, Nam Y. Blockchain-based secure healthcare application for diabetic-cardio disease prediction in fog computing. *IEEE Access*. 2021;9:45706–20. https://doi.org/10.1109/ACCESS.2021.3065440.

[33] Liu X, Zhou P, Qiu T, Wu DO. Blockchain-enabled contextual online learning under local differential privacy for coronary heart disease diagnosis in mobile edge computing. *IEEE J Biomed Health Inform*. 2020;8:2177–88. https://doi.org/10.1109/JBHI.2020.2999497.

[34] Hajian A, Prybutok VR, Chang H-C. An empirical study for blockchain-based information sharing systems in electronic health records: A mediation perspective. *Comput Hum Behav*. 2023;138:107471. https://doi.org/10.1016/j.chb.2022.107471.

[35] Tanwar S, Parekh K, Evans R. Blockchain-based electronic healthcare record system for healthcare 4.0 applications. *J Inf Sec Appl*. 2020;50:102407. https://doi.org/10.1016/j.jisa.2019.102407.

[36] Mahajan HB, Rashid AS, Junnarkar AA, Uke N, Deshpande SD, Futane PR, et al. Integration of healthcare 4.0 and blockchain into secure cloud-based electronic health records systems. *Appl Nanosci*. 2022:1–14. https://doi.org/10.1007/s13204-021-02164-0.

[37] Rai BK. Pcbehr: Patient-controlled blockchain enabled electronic health records for healthcare 4.0. *Health Serv Outcomes Res Methodol*. 2022:1–23. https://doi.org/10.1007/s10742-022-00279-7.

[38] Pang Z, Yao Y, Li Q, Zhang X, Zhang J. Electronic health records sharing model based on blockchain with checkable state PBFT consensus algorithm. *IEEE Access*. 2022;10:87803–15. https://doi.org/10.1109/ACCESS.2022.3186682.

[39] Mallikarjuna B, Kiranmayee D, Saritha V, Krishna PV. Development of efficient e-health records using iot and blockchain technology. In: *ICC—IEEE International Conference on Communications*. Vol. 2021; 2021. pp. 1–7. https://doi.org/10.1109/ICC42927.2021.9500390.

[40] Chelladurai MU, Pandian DS, Ramasamy DK. A blockchain based patient centric electronic health record storage and integrity management for e-health systems. *Health Policy Technol.* 2021;10(4):100513. https://doi.org/10.1016/j.hlpt.2021.100513.

[41] Sonkamble RG, Phansalkar SP, Potdar VM, Bongale AM. Survey of interoperability in electronic health records management and proposed blockchain based framework: Myblockehr. *IEEE Access.* 2021;9:158367–401. https://doi.org/10.1109/ACCESS.2021.3129284.

[42] Sharma Y, Balamurugan B. Preserving the privacy of electronic health records using blockchain. *Procedia Comput Sci.* International Conference on Smart Sustainable Intelligent Computing and Applications under ICITETM2020. 2020;173:171–80. https://doi.org/10.1016/j.procs.2020.06.021.

[43] Shamshad S, Minahil, Mahmood K, Kumari S, Chen C. A secure blockchain-based e-health records storage and sharing scheme. *J Inf Sec Appl.* 2020;55:102590. https://doi.org/10.1016/j.jisa.2020.102590.

[44] Kuo TT, Pham A. Quorum-based model learning on a blockchain hierarchical clinical research network using smart contracts. *Int J Med Inform.* 2023;169:104924. https://doi.org/10.1016/j.ijmedinf.2022.104924.

[45] Mackey TK, Kuo TT, Gummadi B, Clauson KA, Church G, Grishin D, et al. 'Fitforpurpose?'-challenges and opportunities for applications of blockchain technology in the future of healthcare. *BMC Med.* 2019;17(1):68. https://doi.org/10.1186/s12916-019-1296-7.

[46] Gursoy G, Brannon CM, Ni E, Wagner S, Khanna A, Gerstein M. Storing and analyzing a genome on a blockchain. *Genome Biol.* 2022;23(1):1. https://doi.org/10.1186/s13059-021-02568-9.

[47] Albalwy F, McDermott JH, Newman WG, Brass A, Davies A. A blockchain-based framework to support pharmacogenetic data sharing. *Pharmacogenomics J.* 2022;22(5–6):264–75. https://doi.org/10.1038/s41397-022-00285-5.

[48] Park Y-H, Kim Y, Shim J. Blockchain-based privacy-preserving system for genomic data management using local differential privacy. *Electronics.* 2021;10(23). https://doi.org/10.3390/electronics10233019.

[49] Albalwy F, Brass A, Davies A. A blockchain-based dynamic consent architecture to support clinical genomic data sharing (consentchain): Proof-of-concept study. *JMIR Med Inform.* 2021;9(11):e27816. https://doi.org/10.2196/27816, PMID 34730538.

[50] Kuo TT, Bath T, Ma S, Pattengale N, Yang M, Cao Y et al. Benchmarking blockchain-based gene-drug interaction data sharing methods: A case study from the idash 2019 secure genome analysis competition blockchain track. *Int J Med Inform.* 2021;154:104559. https://doi.org/10.1016/j.ijmedinf.2021.104559.

[51] Glicksberg BS, Burns S, Currie R, Griffin A, Wang ZJ, Haussler D et al. Blockchain-authenticated sharing of genomic and clinical outcomes data of patients with cancer: A prospective cohort study. *J Med Internet Res.* 2020;22(3):e16810. https://doi.org/10.2196/16810.

[52] Shuaib K, Saleous H, Zaki N, Dankar F. A layered blockchain framework for healthcare and genomics. In: *IEEE International Conference on Smart Computing (SMARTCOMP)*. Vol. 2020; 2020. pp. 156–63. https://doi.org/10.1109/SMARTCOMP50058.2020.00040.

[53] Kordestani A, Oghazi P, Mostaghel R. Smart contract diffusion in the pharmaceutical blockchain: The battle of counterfeit drugs. *J Bus Res.* 2023;158:113646. https://doi.org/10.1016/j.jbusres.2023.113646.

[54] Siyal AA, Junejo AZ, Zawish M, Ahmed K, Khalil A, Soursou G. Applications of blockchain technology in medicine and healthcare: Challenges and future perspectives. *Cryptography.* 2019;3(1). https://doi.org/10.3390/cryptography3010003.

[55] Kavasidis I, Lallas E, Gerogiannis VC, Karageorgos A. Analytics and blockchain for data integrity in the pharmaceuticals industry. In: *4th International Conference on Advances in Computer Technology, Information Science and Communications (CTISC)*. Vol. 2022; 2022. pp. 1–5. https://doi.org/10.1109/CTISC54888.2022.9849776.

[56] Sahana, Thejashwini, Kamath V, Lahari Y, Mohanchandra K. Blockchain based framework for secure data sharing of medicine supply chain in health care system. *Int J ArtifIntell*. 2022;9(1):32–28. https://doi.org/10.36079/lamintang.ijai-0901.358.

[57] Alshahrani W, Alshahrani R. Assessment of blockchain technology application in the improvement of pharmaceutical industry. In: *International Conference of Women in Data Science at Taif University (WiDSTaif)*. Vol. 2021; 2021. pp. 1–5. https://doi.org/10.1109/WiDSTaif 52235.2021.9430210.

[58] Badhotiya GK, Sharma VP, Prakash S, Kalluri V, Singh R. Investigation and assessment of blockchain technology adoption in the pharmaceutical supply chain. *Mater Today Proc*. International Conference on Technological Advancements in Materials Science and Manufacturing. 2021;46:10776–80. https://doi.org/10.1016/j.matpr.2021.01.673.

[59] Niu B, Dong J, Liu Y. Incentive alignment for blockchain adoption in medicine supply chains. *Transp Res E*. 2021;152:102276. https://doi.org/10.1016/j.tre.2021.102276.

[60] Reda M, Kanga DB, Fatima T, Azouazi M. Blockchain in health supply chain management: State of art challenges and opportunities. *Procedia Comput Sci*. The 17th International Conference on Mobile Systems and Pervasive Computing (MobiSPC), The 15th International Conference on Future Networks and Communications (FNC), The 10th International Conference on Sustainable Energy Information Technology. 2020;175:706–9. https://doi.org/10.1016/j.procs.2020.07.104.

[61] Tanwar S, Parekh K, Evans R. Blockchain-based electronic healthcare record system for healthcare 4.0 applications. *J Inf Sec Appl*. 2020;50:102407. https://doi.org/10.1016/j.jisa.2019.102407.

[62] Cachin C. *Architecture of the Hyperledger Blockchain Fabric*; 2016. Available from: https://www.zurich.ibm.com/dccl/papers/cachin_dccl.pdf.

[63] IBM. *What is Hyperledgerfabric?*; 2023. Available from: www.ibm.com/topics/hyperledger.

[64] T.L.F. Projects. *Hyperledger Sawtooth- Hyperledger Foundation*; 2023. Available from: www.hyperledger.org/use/sawtooth.

[65] Buterin V et al. Ethereum white paper. *GIThub Repos*. 2013;1:22–3.

[66] Patel MM, Tanwar S, Gupta R, Kumar N. A deep learning-based cryptocurrency price prediction scheme for financial institutions. *J Inf Sec Appl*. 2020;55:1–12. https://doi.org/10.1016/j.jisa.2020.102583.

[67] Benet J. IPFS-content addressed, versioned, p2p file system. *arXiv preprint arXiv:1407.3561*; 2014.

[68] Blockchain. *Postman API Network*; 2023. Available from: www.postman.com/api-evangelist/workspace/blockchain/request/35240-cca6f24a-3855-49ef-8f39-89dc95ab8e59.

[69] Suite T. *Ganache Overview*. Available from: https://trufflesuite.com/docs/ganache/,february2023.

[70] H. Foundation. *Hyperledger Iroha*; 2023. Available from: www.hyperledger.org/use/iroha.

[71] Ethereum G. *Geth Documentation*. Available from: https://geth.ethereum.org/docs/,february 2023.

[72] H. Composer. *Hyperledger Composer*; 2023. Available from: https://hyperledger.github.io/composer/v0.19/introduction/introduction.html.

[73] MathWorks. *MATLAB and Simulink*; 2023. Available from: https://in.mathworks.com/products/matlab.html.

[74] Suite T. *Truffle Smart Contracts Made Sweeter*; 2023. Available from: https://trufflesuite.com/truffle/.

[75] WIRESHARK. *About wireshark*; 2023. Available from: www.wireshark.org/about.html.

[76] Spyder. *Spyder Ide*; 2023. Available from: www.spyder-ide.org/.

[77] IS. *Statistics*. SPSS Statistics; 2023. Available from: www.ibm.com/in-en/products/spss-statistics.

[78] Grieco G, Song W, Cygan A, Feist J, Groce A. Echidna: Effective, usable, and fast fuzzing for smart contracts. In: *Proceedings of the 29th ACM SIGSOFT International Symposium on Software Testing (ISSTA)*; 2020. pp. 557–60. https://doi.org/10.1145/3395363.3404366.

[79] Ashizawa N, Yanai N, Cruz JP, Okamura S. Eth2Vec: Learning contract-wide code representations for vulnerability detection on Ethereum smart contracts. In: *Proceedings of the 3rd ACM International Symposium on Blockchain and Secure Critical Infrastructure*; 2021. pp. 47–59. https://doi.org/10.1145/3457337.3457841.

[80] Albert E, Gordillo P, Rubio A, Sergey I. Running on fumes: Preventing out-of-gas vulnerabilities in Ethereum smart contracts using static resource analysis. In: *Proceedings of the International Conference on Verification and Evaluation of Computer and Communication Systems*. Vol. 11847; 2019. pp. 63–78. https://doi.org/10.1007/978-3-030-35092-5_5.

[81] Remix-IDE [online]; 2023. Available from: https://github.com/ethereum/remix-ide.

[82] Feist J, Grieco G, Groce A. Slither: A static analysis framework for smart contracts. In: *Proceedings of the IEEE/ACM 2nd International Workshop on Emerging Trends in Software Engineering for Blockchain (WETSEB)*. Vol. 2019; 2019. pp. 8–15. https://doi.org/10.1109/WETSEB.2019.00008.

[83] Denker M. *Blockchain and Web 3.0*. Evanston, IL: Routledge; 2019. https://doi.org/10.4324/9780429029530.

[84] Ferreira JF, Cruz P, Durieux T, Abreu R. SmartBugs: A framework to analyze solidity smart contracts. In: *Proceedings of the 35th IEEE/ACM International Conference on Automated Software Engineering*; 2020. pp. 1349–52. https://doi.org/10.1145/3324884.3415298.

[85] Tikhomirov S, Voskresenskaya E, Ivanitskiy I, Takhaviev R, Marchenko E, Alexandrov Y. SmartCheck: Static analysis of Ethereum smart contracts. In: *Proceedings of the 1st International Workshop on Emerging Trends in Software Engineering for Blockchain*; 2018. pp. 9–16. https://doi.org/10.1145/3194113.3194115.

[86] Chen J, Xia X, Lo D, Grundy J, Luo X, Chen T. Defectchecker: Automated smart contract defect detection by analyzing EVM bytecode. *IEEE Trans Softw Eng*. 2021;48(7):2189–207. https://doi.org/10.1109/TSE.2021.3054928.

[87] Chen T, Feng Y, Li Z, Zhou H, Luo X, Li X, et al. GasChecker: Scalable analysis for discovering gas-inefficient smart contracts. *Comput. IEEE, Transl Emerg Topics*. 2021;9(3):1433–48. https://doi.org/10.1109/TETC.2020.2979019.

[88] Chen T, Li X, Luo X, Zhang X. Under-optimized smart contracts devour your money. In: *Proceedings of the IEEE 24th International Conference on Software Analysis*; 2017. pp. 442–6. https://doi.org/10.1109/SANER.2017.7884650.

[89] Torres CF, Steichen M. The art of the scam: Demystifying honeypots in Ethereum smart contracts. In: *Proceedings of the 28th USENIX Secursymp*; 2019. pp. 1591–607. Available from: https://dl.acm.org/doi/10.5555/3361338.3361449.

[90] Grech N, Kong M, Jurisevic A, Brent L, Scholz B, Smaragdakis Y. MadMax: Surviving out-of-gas conditions in Ethereum smart contracts. *Proc ACM Program Lang Proc ACM Program*. 2018;2(OOPSLA):1–27. https://doi.org/10.1145/3276486.

[91] Mythril [online]; 2023. Available from: https://github.com/ConsenSys/mythril.

[92] Luu L, Chu D-H, Olickel H, Saxena P, Hobor A. Making smart contracts smarter. In: *Proceedings of the ACM Conference on Computer and Communications Security*. Vols. 24–28; 2016. pp. 254–69. https://doi.org/10.1145/2976749.2978309.

[93] Tsankov P, Dan A, Drachsler-Cohen D, Gervais A, Bünzli F, Vechev M. Securify: Practical security analysis of smart contracts. In: *Proceedings of the ACM Conference on Computer and Communications Security*; 2018. pp. 67–82. https://doi.org/10.1145/3243734.3243780.

[94] Brent L, Jurisevic A, Kong M, Liu E, Gauthier F, Gramoli V, et al. Vandal: A scalable security analysis framework for smart contracts. *arXiv:1809.03981*; 2018.

[95] Mossberg M, Manzano F, Hennenfent E, Groce A, Grieco G, Feist J, et al. Manticore: A user-friendly symbolic execution framework for binaries and smart contracts. In: *Proceedings of the 34th IEEE/ACM International Conference on Automated Software Engineering (ASE)*; 2019. pp. 1186–9. https://doi.org/10.1109/ASE.2019.00133.

[96] IBM. *What Are Smart Contracts on Blockchain?*; 2023. Available from: www.ibm.com/in-en/topics/smart-contracts/.

[97] Remix-Ethereum IDE. *Remix IDE*; 2023. Available from: https://remix.ethereum.org/.

[98] SS. Analysis. *Solidity Static Analysisemix Ethereum Ide1 Documentation*; 2023. Available from: https://remix-ide.readthedocs.io/en/latest/static_analysis.html.

[99] Hathaliya J, Sharma P, Tanwar S, Gupta R. Blockchain-based remote patient monitoring in healthcare 4.0. In: *9th International Conference on Advanced Computing (IACC)*. IEEE Publications; 2019. pp. 87–91. https://doi.org/10.1109/IACC48062.2019.8971593.

[100] Iqbal N, Jamil F, Ahmad S, Kim D. A novel blockchain-based integrity and reliable veterinary clinic information management system using predictive analytics for provisioning of quality health services. *IEEE Access*. 2021;9:8069–98. https://doi.org/10.1109/ACCESS.2021.3049325.

[100] Omar I, Jayaraman R, Salah K, Yaqoob I, Ellahham S. Applications of blockchain technology in clinical trials: Review and open challenges. *Arab J Sci Eng*. 2020;46(7).
[102] Agbo CC, Mahmoud QH, Eklund JM. Blockchain technology in healthcare: A systematic review. *Healthcare* (Basel). 2019;7(2). https://doi.org/10.3390/healthcare7020056.
[103] Agrawal K, Aggarwal M, Tanwar S, Sharma G, Bokoro PN, Sharma R. An extensive blockchain based applications survey: Tools, frameworks, opportunities, challenges and solutions. *IEEE Access*. 2022;10:116858–906. https://doi.org/10.1109/ACCESS.2022.3219160.

6
Blockchain Technology: Reinventing the Management of Information Infrastructure

Shashimala Tiwari

6.1 Introduction

The welfare of society and the pleasure of individuals depend on better health. It is essential to the nation's economic development. Every day, accidents and crises involving poor health happen, and diseases are anticipated to be identified and managed [1].

A health record is a compilation of medical information on a patient's physical and mental health that has been acquired from various sources. The contents of a patient's health record include their medical history, examination findings, diagnosis, and treatment, as well as any alerts they may have, such as allergies. Both manual and electronic supervision of these medical records is possible [1].

The manual method, which uses paper and books, is a long-standing process used in the mainstream of hospitals to preserve records. This approach has significant drawbacks, including requirement for enormous storage spaces and challenge of record retrieval. Clinical records are increasingly being computerized [2] because it is convenient to store and retrieve them.

However, the possibility of manipulation without detection has grown to be a major worry. The keeping of patient records confidential is another key issue, because the patient may hold the doctor and the hospital negligent if they violate the privacy of medical records [3]. Figure 6.1 illustrates existing healthcare models.

Additionally, insufficient paper-based data can result in unnecessary repeat tests and medication. Time is wasted since this method requires extra manual labor to transfer records by mail or fax because they are scattered everywhere and not centralized [4]. Even doctors have restricted access to patient records.

By incorporating digital technologies into the healthcare system, medical institutions may swiftly and easily share patient records [5]. There are numerous concerns regarding the loading of patient data, granting access approval, security, and immutability of the data [6]. The development of a decentralized digital health infrastructure, or the incorporation of blockchain technology into the healthcare system, can address these issues [7]. By maintaining and updating records, blockchain technology has potential to recreate a new economy [8].

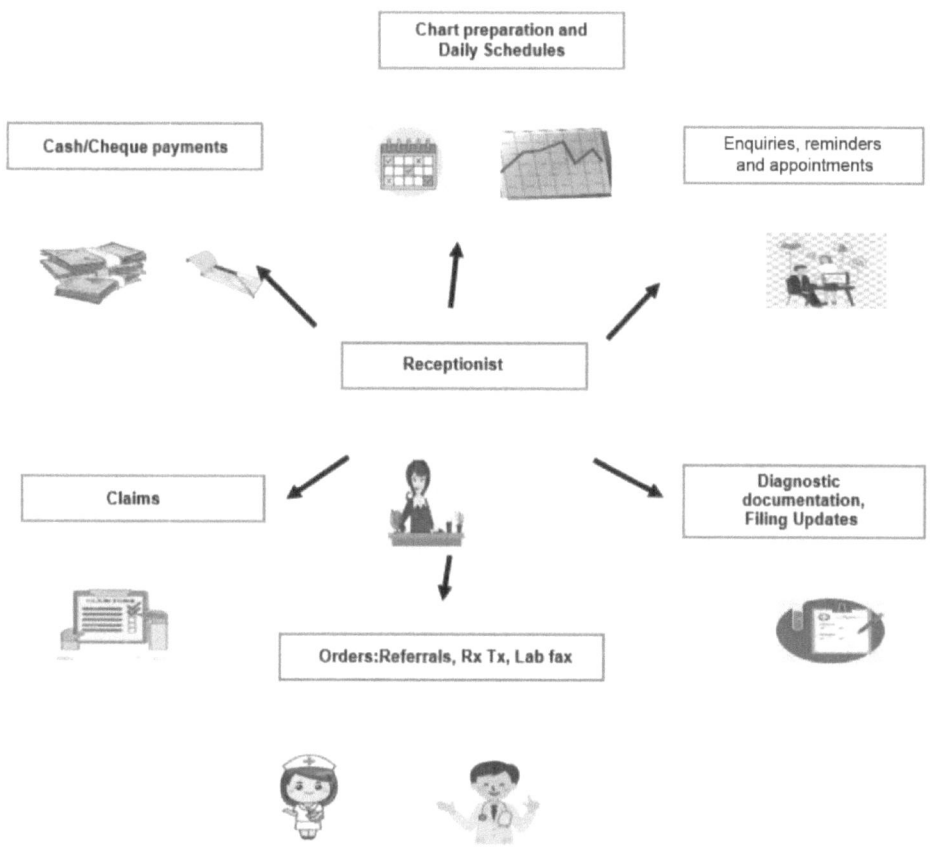

FIGURE 6.1
Existing cauterized healthcare models.

6.2 Background

6.2.1 Blockchain Technology

A *blockchain* is a constantly expanding list of transactions that is decentralized, distributed, immutable, shareable, and tamper-proof [9]. Think of blockchain as a registry with transaction data organized into time stamp blocks. Cryptographic hashes, which identify each block uniquely, are used [10]. The confusion value of a block before it is given for each block. Thus, a link is built between blocks, resulting in the formation of a series of blocks. Only when we investigate how a blockchain network functions can we obtain a clear idea of how it operates. Every node in the peer-to-peer network keeps a record of every transaction that has ever taken place on it.

Every node has its own wallet that it uses to conduct transactions. Through the use of a set of private and public keys (also known as cryptographic keys), the user and the network communicate [11]. While a public key is available to every node in the network, a private key is only used to sign one's specific transactions [12]. To complete a transaction, the sender must sign the message with their private key, which, when paired with their public key, creates a digital sign [13].

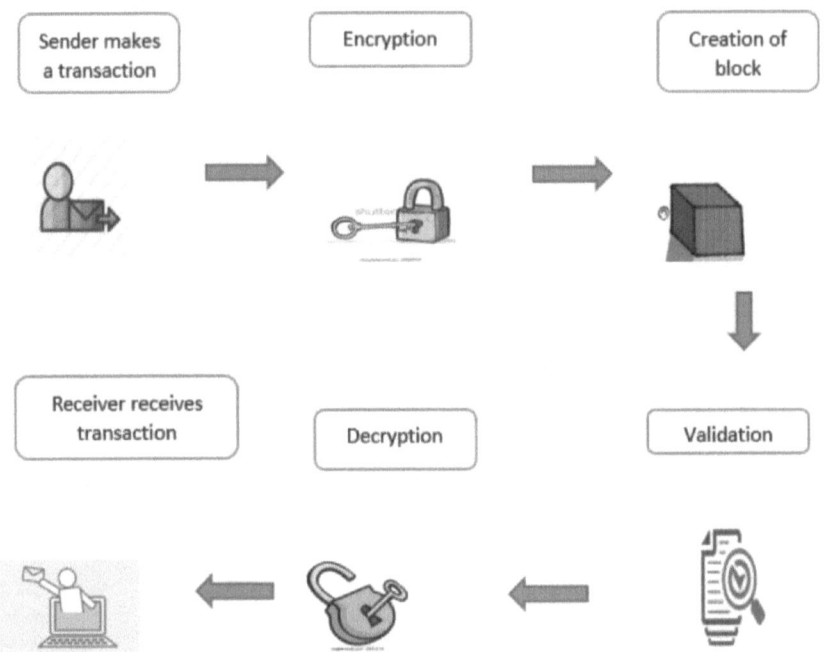

FIGURE 6.2
Working of the blockchain technology.

This transaction is published on the blockchain network, where the miners confirm it. Blockchain's high-performance nodes are known as miners [14]. Using a consensus mechanism also known as proof of work, miners make the transaction unmodifiable and irrevocable. The generation of a legitimate block is a contest between the miners, and the winner is paid [15]. Figure 6.2 describes the working of the blockchain technology.

Only when a transaction has been validated by every miner on the network is a block containing that transaction considered to be genuine and added to the longest blockchain, if more than 50% of the miners confirm the transaction [16].

6.2.2 Literature Survey

This section describes several initiatives attempted to protect health records, as well as the difficulties and potential explanations.

Towards using blockchain technology for e-health data access management. Writers highlight advantages of Blockchain and specific issues related to it for protected deployment of the health record. It offers an ascendable explanation in order to achieve the greatest presentation. They have also put out a design to address the problems with health application, in which hospitals and doctors are viewed as nodes associated to the e-health blockchain via smart contracts, and a separate database is also kept off-chain [17].

Through the data gateway, patients can communicate with blockchain and medical sensors. This study also demonstrates how completely functional systems can be developed to revolutionize future applications with usage of appropriate tools, prototypes, protocols, and blockchain technology.

Decentralized e-health architecture for enhancing healthcare analytics. In the chapter titled "Decentralized e-Health Architecture for Enhancing Healthcare Analytics," the writers discuss the difficulty connected to the analysis and safety of medical data. Additionally, they have made an attempt to deliver an explanation that elevates the bar for medical care. Based on the Exonum framework, which consists of nodes associated by peer-to-peer connections—and all nodes are validated by utilizing a public key—they have built a blockchain solution for state scale in healthcare [18]. They've also suggested that blockchain would be used to manage enormous volumes of healthcare data and sustain patient privacy.

Is blockchain technology a potential solution to security and interoperability problems affecting EMR in developing nations? The implementation of blockchain in EMR ensures uninterrupted readiness and access to real-time data, according to the chapter "Is This Solution to EMR Interoperability and Safety Challenges in Developing Countries?" Blockchain enables patients to fully access their data and have control over how it is united. Further, blockchain relies on cryptographic methods to communicate in a network without prior mutual belief. The privacy of patients is protected when their information is shared among stakeholders due to information encryption [18].

Introducing blockchain for healthcare. Authors of this chapter focused on various blockchain topologies, present blockchain problems, and provide prospective blockchain results. Even while blockchain is used to generate smart contracts between healthcare providers [19] and to grant access to specific data or patient records, it is impossible to determine who is accessing information and whether the person is authorized to do so or not. The Sybil attack is another security vulnerability that can be fixed by demanding that every miner node take part in the solution of a mathematical puzzle before attackers add a new block to blockchain [19]. Because of these issues, the author has suggested that researchers construct a new blockchain architecture that does not rely on an existing cryptographic method.

6.3 Medical Data Supervision on Blockchain

The current healthcare structure keeps track of patient health information digitally. Currently, healthcare organizations save patient data, diagnostic results, and doctor's prescriptions in a consolidated manner. Patients don't have resistor over their data, and updating documented data is a time-consuming and difficult process; thus, there is a potential that it will be leaked or used for other purposes because it is a centralized system. We are putting out the notion of converting a centralized system to a decentralized system consuming blockchain technology in an effort to address these issues. In order to integrate blockchain in healthcare, it is first necessary to comprehend the extent of the data as well as where and how it is being produced [20].

At each stage of medical therapy, such as a discussion, diagnosis, and surgery, healthcare organizations produce sensitive and important medical data. The medical information includes prescriptions written by doctors, MRI scans, X-rays, angiography, ultrasound reports, endoscopy, radiography, as well as a few other types of sensitive health information, including cancer, HIV, or psychological problems. Figure 6.3 shows medical data supervision on blockchain [20].

To advance the quality of data before placing it on the blockchain, some value must be added. Medical records for patients should be precise, clear, and organized, since unstructured data causes errors and delays in the delivery of care. Digital health records can

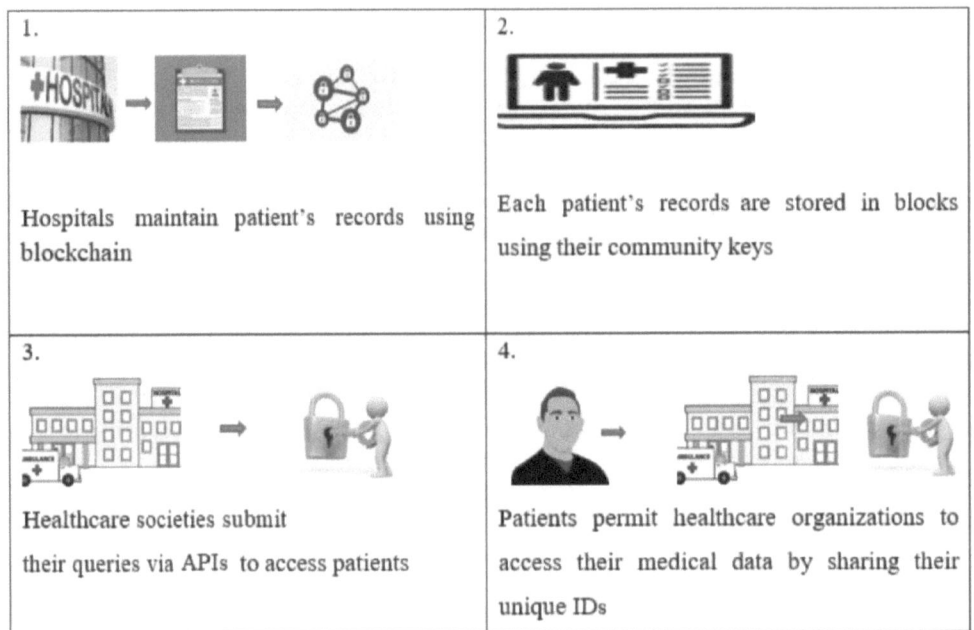

FIGURE 6.3
Medical data supervision on blockchain.

be stored across numerous nodes within a blockchain network, removing concerns connected to data centralization [20].

Patients' medical records may be saved on the blockchain network using their public keys, and transactions containing patients' medical records may be preserved using both the patients' individual IDs and public keys. Only when unique IDs match may healthcare institutions access a patient's non-identifiable data using smart contracts. Patients can, if necessary, share their public key with healthcare organizations, but data would never be identifiable without their private key.

Smart contracts are required to make sure users will share or recover the data. Smart contracts are self-executing contracts between two parties in which terms are directly written in code without the assistance of a third party. It is a procedure that supports, upholds, and authenticates contract negotiations and execution digitally [20].

The suggested notion is built as a contract with the name *healthcare* that has two nodes, each of which can be assumed to represent a hospital administrator or a lab administrator. A structure that includes the patient's address, test name, hospital name, unique ID, date, price, and signature count is formed and given the name "record."

6.3.1 Invoking the Transaction

We utilized a function Object () { [native code] } that is run automatically when a DApp is deployed and is public in nature. Only hospital administrators should start transactions on the blockchain network, as it is only he who chooses the lab admin and gives him a specific address [20].

6.3.2 Creation of New Records

To add new data to an existing record, we've built a function called "new record" that works by giving values to the corresponding arguments. Records is an array that stores the current patient records.

6.3.3 Record Validation

To be utilized for record validation, a function called "sign record" was created. If the new record is in the array of records that already exist, the hospital administrator will sign the transaction; otherwise, if the record already exists, the signature count value will be 1. In this function, the presence or absence of the new record in the existing record array is determined using the signature count. The transaction will not be signed. When the signature count equals 2, a record that has been signed is released [20].

6.4 Why Is Blockchain Technology Needed in the Healthcare Industry?

According to CNBC, human error is the third foremost cause of death in the United States.

- The safety of patient health records.
- Lack of transparency in the drug supply chain.
- The dispersion of healthcare-related data, such as patient medical histories or the qualifications of medical staff.

According to the 2020 Breach Barometer research, nearly 41 million patient records were exposed. The World Health Organization estimates that one in ten medical gadgets sold in developing countries is defective [20].

These are a few of the typical difficulties. The current situation makes it impossible to share and obtain health data on time.

The potential for blockchain technology to address these healthcare trials is great. The way patients and professionals handle and use health data will be significantly improved and transformed. Each healthcare company is attempting to integrate technologies that would simplify their procedures in the wake of the digital revolution in the healthcare sector.

However, because this sector deals with sensitive medical information, professionals must make sure that any technology they employ does not jeopardize the security of patient data. Blockchain technology is useful in this situation. There are several ways that blockchain technology might help the healthcare sector [20].

6.5 Top 10 Blockchain Use Cases in the Healthcare Area

Blockchain technology has a lot of potential to help close gaps in the current healthcare sector. Ten frequently utilized blockchain applications in healthcare are listed next.

6.5.1 Increasing Access to Medical Records

Patient record management is one of the most popular blockchain applications in healthcare. It is impossible to ascertain a patient's medical record without seeing their former care provider, because health authorities frequently isolate medical data. This process can take a while and frequently leads to mistakes brought on by human miscalculation.

The blockchain directory concept offers potential to significantly expand and change over the course of the blockchain. Its approach is very helpful for monitoring the constant and ongoing growth of medical records. By keeping a constantly expanding linked list of medical records, every block in chain arrangement of blockchain helps support the ever-increasing amount of medical information. Every block also comprises a time stamp and a link to the block before it [21].

6.5.2 Preventing Counterfeit Drug

The counterfeiting of medications is a serious problem in the healthcare industry. The lack of transparency in the medicine supply chain leads to significant tampering and counterfeiting.

Blockchain technology is a useful tool for preventing drug fraud since it offers system transparency and immutability. It provides complete end-to-end supply chain transparency [21]. Providers can gain from the usage of blockchain in pharmaceutical supply chain by being able to:

- Control inventory
- Reduce counterfeiting problems
- Reduce the chance of theft

It can also help agencies like Global Fund, USAID, and Red Cross track the distribution of contributed medicines throughout nations while ensuring products' origin, veracity, and reliability.

The unchangeable and decentralized nature of blockchain technologies allows for the tracking of drugs from their creation to the patient's consumption. This avoids the production of fake and fraudulent goods by enabling customers, healthcare professionals, and businesses to determine the origin and originality of the pharmaceuticals. As a result, the financial losses associated with fake medications and pharmaceuticals decline, while also avoiding the detrimental effects that using fake medications may have [22].

6.5.3 Tracking Medical Staff Credentials

The same way that blockchain technology helps monitor the validity of medical products, it also assists in tracking the experience of medical experts. The employment process can be made simpler by logging the credentials of employees for healthcare businesses and medical institutions.

The principal benefits of incorporating blockchain are as follows:

1. It is a chance for healthcare organizations, insurers, and medical institutions to make money off their current credentials information on former and present staff.
2. Patients are informed about the experience of medical professionals through transparency and declaration for partners [21].

6.5.4 Patient-Centric Electronic Health Record

Data fragmentation is a problem that affects every nation, which implies that patients' medical histories are incomplete for both them and their healthcare providers.

A blockchain-based medical record system that interfaces with current electronic medical record software and provides single, full view of a patient's record is one potential solution to this problem [21].

It's crucial to understand that patient data won't be stored on the blockchain. Any data that is added to blockchain, including prescriptions, test results, and doctor's notes, will be transformed into a special hash function. Each hash function is distinct, and they can only be decoded with the permission of the owner of the data. In this scenario, all modifications to patient record and the patient's consent are documented as blockchain transactions [21].

6.5.5 Smart Contracts for Insurance

Smart contracts can save costs by getting rid of middlemen from the payment process. A *smart contract* is a section of computer code that is kept on a blockchain and executed spontaneously when specific criteria are met. Transaction processing is started by smart contracts without the requirement for a third party. By eliminating all unnecessary middlemen, smart contracts can significantly improve the current insurance system. A patient can safely acquire the specifics of a medical insurance coverage on a blockchain using smart contracts. This information is less-susceptible to hacking than data kept in a conventional database [21].

Additionally, filing time-consuming insurance claims won't be necessary. The smart contract is immediately activated when a patient has an insurance-covered procedure, and money is sent from payer to the hospital.

6.5.6 Remote Monitoring by IoT Security

One of the major trends in the digital health sector is remote monitoring, in which various sensors that monitor patients' vital signs can give medical professionals a greater understanding of their patients' health and enable more active and protective care. Security is a major worry in health IoT, though, both in terms of protecting patient data privacy and security and guarding against its manipulation to provide false data [21].

Blockchain technology improves the security of medical data storage and lowers the possibility of data fraud. A blockchain-based solution to store data that cannot be altered or tampered with and that bad hackers cannot threaten to erase has been developed thanks to the decentralized and immutable properties of blockchain technology, smart contracts, and unique transactions [22].

6.5.7 Reducing Costs

According to a BIS research, healthcare blockchain can help the sector avoid spending up to $100 billion a year on IT, operations, support services, labor, and health data breaches by 2025. The research claims that using blockchain to track pharmaceuticals can help pharmaceutical corporations and lessen the $200 billion in losses from phony drugs each year.

By reducing operational and IT costs associated with the insurance process as well as health insurance fraud, blockchain will help health insurance organizations [21].

Via healthcare, the exchange of health data, by 2025, blockchain is anticipated to hold the greatest market share, with a market cap of $1.89 billion. Blockchain technology can be used to address the most pervasive problems in healthcare IT systems, including interoperability and non-standardization, which have caused data silos in industry. According to a study by Bisresearch [22], blockchain technology can help cut costs in a number of areas of the healthcare sector and is projected to provide savings of up to $100 billion per year by 2025. Through greater accessibility, blockchain technology can avoid data breaches, lessen the use of unnecessary medications, and eliminate medical errors. Additionally, blockchain provides the opportunity for more effective medical data storage, automates payments and transactions, and can lower losses brought on by prescription fraud [22].

Clinician credentialing, which frequently requires a month-long procedure, is a more concrete example of how blockchain might lower expenses. Clinician credentialing can be made quicker and more effective by facilitating this process on a blockchain, as credentials can be verified instantly rather than needing to be confirmed by numerous parties. JP Morgan estimates that blockchain technology can cut the costs and time associated with this process by 80% [23].

6.5.8 Tracking Clinical Trials

The management and tracking of samples are difficult and time-consuming. A potent fusion of technological change management and human change administration is the answer. You will require not simply technology explanation to link all the parts but also support from numerous parties with competing agendas and business interests. Technology must work to make life easier for lab personnel in the bioanalytical labs and research employees at the sites while also giving the sponsor real-time data [21].

While some solutions have addressed the technological part, the human element has been largely overlooked. The sponsor should ideally receive the necessary sample-level data in real time [21]. Clinical trial and sample management processes are becoming more reliable, transparent, and effective as a result of digitization. New technologies are accelerating transition to digital clinical trials through their capacity for digital health record collection and improved insight into data and analytics [21]. In the upcoming years, the digitalization of clinical trials will propel market expansion, and blockchain technology's applications in the medical field are virtually endless.

Blockchain technology improves the flow of information between medical researchers and can give governments and healthcare providers more precise information on the health of their constituents [23].

6.5.9 Enhancing Data Security and Management

Data security is now a major concern for patients everywhere, as data gaps rise year after year. Fortunately, ensuring data safety is a feature of modern blockchain healthcare apps. The high-security features of the technology make it nearly hard to hack or alter any data kept on blockchain. Due to the openness it offers, any modifications to data are immediately apparent, and data tampering is unmanageable [21].

Blockchain technology thus makes it possible for doctors and patients to send crucial healthcare data quickly and securely while simultaneously maintaining confidentiality and transparency, thanks to encryptions and challenging security codes.

Blockchain technology is very beneficial for efficiently and securely handling patient data because it also lowers the dangers related to data centralization. The majority of patient data is now kept in a central location, making it vulnerable to hackers, theft, and data breaches. Blockchain technology is a great solution to this problem because it dispenses data among several nodes [21].

By creating a safe way of data sharing across healthcare providers, blockchain technology can increase the accessibility and interoperability of healthcare information systems. All necessary healthcare practitioners can access patient records that are securely kept on a permissioned blockchain [22].

6.5.10 Providing Supply Chain Transparency

Declaration of authenticity of medical items is crucial for establishing their validity in the healthcare sector. With use of a blockchain-based system, customers can track products, providing them with complete visibility and transparency from the manufacturing facility to every step of the supply chain. This is serious problem for business, especially in underdeveloped nations, where tens of thousands of people die every year from using fake prescription drugs [21].

Supply chain management and transparency are some of the most cutting-edge use cases for blockchain outside of financial markets, as proven by IBM and Walmart's high-profile partnership to secure food safety in the supply chain. Because the technology and ROI have already been established, we think that this is the short-term impression of blockchain on the healthcare industry that is most important.

As previously mentioned, patients would have complete control over their data on a medical data blockchain. A patient's records can be updated and expanded by healthcare professionals, but the patient has control over who has access to their information. People being in charge of their own health data would be a significant and novel move, as accessing one's own data is currently highly challenging [23].

6.6 Blockchain Prevents Medical Errors

Blockchain technology can help prevent medical errors brought on by missing information by giving practitioners simple access to patients' records via medical data blockchain. Practitioners have immediate access to all personally identifiable information, allergies, and previously treated conditions in crucial situations, which helps them prescribe the best course of action [22].

6.7 Challenges Faced by Blockchain Technology

Scalability and storage capacity. Scalability and secrecy are the two fundamental issues with data storage on blockchain. Data on blockchain is insecure since it can be seen by everyone connected to the chain, which is not what a decentralized platform wants. The patient medical history, X-ray reports, MRI results, lab results, and many more reports would be saved in the blockchain as data, which would have a significant effect on storage ability of blockchain [24].

TABLE 6.1

Benefits and Blockades of Blockchain Technology

Benefits and Blockades of Blockchain Technology		
Benefits	Decentralized	Information kept on blockchain is dispersed across network.
	Data transparency	Data stored on blockchain is tamper-proof.
	Safety and privacy	Blockchain uses cryptographic algorithms to secure any information being kept on it.
Barriers	Scalability, storage capacity	Storing huge volumes of data on blockchain would cause storage and scalability problems.
	Lack of social skills	As blockchain is an evolving technology, and it is not a well-understood technology, so it is quite challenging to shift previously used systems on this technology.
	Lack of universally defined principles	There are no defined principles for blockchain technology that are universally applied, which makes it difficult to enforce it throughout precise domain.

Absence of social skills. Few people can comprehend how blockchain technology operates. This technology is still developing and is still in its early stages. In addition, converting from reliable EHR systems to blockchain technology will take some time since hospitals and supplementary healthcare institutions would need to convert all their systems [24].

There are no established standards for this technology because it is still in its early stages and is continually changing. As a result, implementing this technology in the healthcare industry would require additional time and effort. Because it would call for standards that have been certified by international organizations that go over standardization processes of every technology [16], the size, format, and type of data that might be kept on blockchain would be determined by these global standards. The established standards would also make it simpler to adapt to this technology, because they could be easily enforced within the businesses. Table 6.1 describes the benefits as well as blockades of blockchain technology.

6.8 Associated Work

The fundamental goal behind Satoshi Nakamoto's blockchain technology [25] was to create a decentralized currency that was cryptographically safe and useful for financial transactions. In the end, the blockchain concept was applied to many other spheres of life; the healthcare industry is one of them and plans to employ it. Numerous researchers have conducted research in this field, with their studies focusing on the viability of the idea of integrating blockchain technology in the healthcare industry. They also describe the benefits, risks, issues, and difficulties that come with using this technology. Some researchers have talked about the difficulties of really putting this into practice on a bigger scale.

6.8.1 Theoretical/Analytical Blockchain-Based Research

A study by Gordon and Catalini [26] examined how blockchain technology could benefit the healthcare industry. They concluded that hospitals, pharmaceutical firms, and other relevant parties control the healthcare industry. They cited data exchange as a primary justification for implementing blockchains in the healthcare industry. This study also suggested four techniques or elements that healthcare industry must change in order to use blockchain technology. These methods for handling digital access privileges, the availability of data, and quicker access to clinical records and patient individuality are a few examples. Additionally, it covers both on-chain and off-chain data storage. The study also covered difficulties or obstacles to using blockchain technology, such as abundance of clinical records, patient engagement, and security and confidentiality concerns [26].

In order to explore potential solutions for blockchain's scalability issue and to find projects that aim to address it, Eberhardt et al. [27] performed a study. *Blockchain* is described as a collection of different computational and economic principles built on a peer-to-peer network. Finding out which data should be saved on-chain and what can be kept off-chain was the goal of this investigation. This study included the fundamental concepts and implementation architecture for five patterns for off-chain data storage. According to authors, on-chain data is any information that has transactions made on it and is recorded on a blockchain. Off-chain data storage, however, involves placing data somewhere else on any other storage medium and excludes any transactions.

Blockchain technology, Bitcoin, and Ethereum were provided by Vujii et al. [28]. According to the authors, the environment of information technology is continually evolving, and blockchain technology is advantageous to information systems. They described Bitcoin as a decentralized peer-to-peer network utilized for Bitcoin transactions. Along with defining the notion of blockchain mining, they also established proof-of-work consensus algorithm. Authors stress that blockchain scalability is a serious issue, and that several solutions, including SegWit and Lightning, Bitcoin Cash, and Bitcoin Gold, have been proposed to address this issue [28].

A study on smart contracts and their applicability in blockchain technology was carried out by Wang et al. [29]. It begins with an introduction of smart contracts, their operating systems, and another important concept related to them. Authors also discuss how the unique concept of parallel blockchains might be applied to smart contracts. They make the point that the basis for their use is the decentralization offered by the programming language code used to generate smart contracts on blockchain.

The author went over the fundamentals of smart contracts before explaining how the multiple blockchain layers work together to maintain system functionality. Data, incentive consensus, network, contract, and application layer are these layers. The study not only describes structure and architecture used by smart contracts but also provides information on its uses and difficulties. The study also highlights a crucial future development known as parallel blockchain, which aims to build a blockchain capable of optimizing two distinct but crucial modules [29].

A review by Kuo et al. [30] examined many blockchain applications in the biomedical and healthcare industries. Perseverance of clinical records, decentralization, data pedigree, ongoing access to data, and finally, safe information being accessible to biomedical stakeholders are some of the benefits that writers observed when using blockchains for this sector. Confidentiality and the potential for malicious attack, namely, a 51% attack, were found to be the limitations of blockchain technology. Because they are used to hold private medical records, authors recognized these restrictions as being crucial for the biomedical industry. The authors' proposed solutions to these issues include storing sensitive medical data off-chain, encrypting data to preserve secrecy, and using VPNs (virtual private networks) to protect against hostile assaults [30].

6.8.2 Prototype/Implementation Blockchain-Based Research

Using the Hadoop database, Sahoo and Baruah [31] suggested a scalable foundation for blockchain technology. They suggested using scalability offered by the fundamental Hadoop database coupled with decentralization offered by blockchain technology to overcome the scalability challenge of blockchain. In instruction to increase the scalability of blockchain technology, they used a way to collect blocks on the Hadoop database.

This study suggests using the Hadoop database system, together with SHA3–256 for hashing utilized for transactions, to address scalability issue of the blockchain platform. Java was the programming language used for this architecture. This study makes easier to understand how blockchain can be used with added scalable platforms [31].

Zhang et al. [32] presented an ascendable solution for using blockchain for clinical data. The primary goal of this study was to develop a health information technology architecture that complies with guidelines established by the Office of the National Coordinator for Health Information Technology (ONC). The main issues that this technology faces were identified in this study, including concerns about secrecy, blockchain safety, scalability problems related to the enormous volume of datasets being transmitted on this platform, and lastly, lack of a globally enforceable standard for data exchange on blockchain. This study also demonstrates a decentralized application (DApp) built on the previously mentioned ONC requirements. They also talked about how to recover the FHIR chain and the lessons they had learned [32].

A method for managing medical questionnaires that aims to share data using blockchain technology was proposed by Kim et al. [33]. The aim of choosing where to store and how to share medical questionnaire data, according to the authors, is to use it for future clinical and medical research. The authors chose blockchain technology for their suggested framework because, as they underlined, it would be useful for establishing analysis systems, deciding terminologies used in EHR systems, and addressing safety challenges related with these systems [32].

The two primary purposes of this study are to create, store, and distribute data that was acquired using questionnaires. The system's validation of the questionnaire given to it is another advantage it suggests. The questions that are added to this system are evaluated to ensure that they are in the correct format, and then they are processed to separate personal records from specific data relating to the results of the questionnaire. Data sharing for upcoming research objectives would be made possible as a result. The authors address situation in which a third party asks access to questionnaire data; in that case, the doctor would need to ask the patient for permission before allowing the third party to view the data [33].

6.9 System Implementation

The system was constructed utilizing Ethereum and its dependencies, as previously stated in the earlier parts. To get insight into the system's many functions, this section goes into further detail on system implementation [33].

6.10 Advanced Contracts

Smart contracts are a critical component of DApps because they are developed to carry out fundamental tasks. The contracts listed are:

- Patient information
- Roles

These agreements are used to grant users access to DApp and carry out CRUD operations on patient data. The functionality of the provided design is the only aim of the patient records smart contract. It performs CRUD operations and creates roles for access to these features [34].

The Open Zeppelin smart contract library offers a predefined smart contract called "roles."

It is the second contract described earlier. You might utilize the smart contracts in this library, which execute a variety of functions, to build your own smart contracts. Usage of this library was motivated by the advantages it offers, namely, tested and community-approved code. Asset library, a division of OpenZeppelin library, houses the Roles smart contract. An asset library provides a number of alternative contracts for specifying access rules, but the roles library offers a detailed mechanism for character description, which was the primary factor in choosing smart contract [34].

Following is the algorithm for creating patient records smart contract. It outlines all actions taken within it, as well as the many circumstances that surround them. Additionally, it illustrates how the roles are kept up-to-date in order to allow access to a specific functionality.

6.11 Convention Scenario for Algorithm 1

The operation of smart contract for patient proceedings is described in algorithm 1. The four tasks performed by this algorithm are viewing, updating, adding, and deleting records. The system administrator and another user use these features. The administrator is responsible for performing algorithm 1's initial function, "define roles," which includes the two variables "new role" and "new account." These two variables will be used to add "new role" and "new account" to the list of "role mappings." Later on, this list would be utilized to access the system users' roles. The second function, "add patient data," is carried out by the doctor when the administrator assigns them this task in the "define roles" function [35].

Additionally, this function confirms that the work is being done at the doctor's certified public address and not by any other outside entity. In order to do this, they employ the "msg.sender" keyword, which in Solidity programming language for Ethereum is used to specify the user's address. After doing this validity check, the doctor can add the patient's records and, after doing so, would conclude the purpose by storing that record [35].

The third function, viewing patient data, calls for patient ID to be provided as an adjustable. Using this ID, the system would search for the patient's records and then return those data to the account that had originally demanded them. As a part of this function, the assigned roles of patient and doctor are also validated. Because only the patient and the doctor would have access to records, any changes to the patient's saved records are made using the fourth function, "update patient records" [35].

To make sure that only users who have been authenticated can use this function, the validation procedure is repeated. The final operation of algorithm 1 is to delete patient records, which, as its name suggests, is used to do so for the records of particular patient. After verifying that the doctor is the one doing this action, this function accepts the unique ID of the patient as input and deletes those entries. Only the system's authenticated users would have access to these functionalities, thanks to this role-based access, which would prevent unauthorized users from using them [35].

6.12 Conclusion and Future Work

Health is wealth, as the saying goes, but in the present day, we can also say that wealth contains health records. Therefore, safeguarding our medical records is more important than ever. Around the world, patient-driven interoperability—in which patients consent to on-demand access to their medical records—is starting to catch on. This paradigm holds that the patient is the exclusive owner of his medical records and determines if and with whom information should be shared. In contrast to the conventional method of data administration, blockchain efficiently addresses the issues associated with this shift from an institute-driven to patient-driven model by decentralizing the entire mechanism.

IBM's Institute for Business Value Blockchain surveyed 200 health executives, of whom 16% are prepared to use commercial blockchain. As was already mentioned, blockchain not only assists in decentralizing data but also offers real-time data access, sustains data privacy, efficiently develops large volumes of data, and authenticates and authorizes data.

Our strategy also uses smart contracts, which are fragments of code that run on their own when both parties accept a set of protocols. Here, the patient and hospital administration are seen as two different parties. The smart contract can be executed in three steps: invoking, creating records, and validation.

In this research, we propose blockchain technology as one of the potential remedies for effective upkeep of medical records. Health record management is just one application of blockchain technology; it can also be used in banking, e-voting, transportation, supply chain management, and other areas. Additional study may aid in the adoption of blockchain technology across all industries, making life easier.

References

1. Asaph Azaria, Ariel Ekblaw, Thiago Vieira, and Andrew Lippman, "Medrec: Using Blockchain for Medical Data Access and Permission Management." In *2016 2nd International Conference on Open and Big Data (OBD)*, pp. 25–30. IEEE, 2016.
2. P. Pramod, Pratyush Kumar Tripathy, Harshit Bajpai, and Manjunath R. Kounte, "Role of Natural Language Processing and Deep Learning in Intelligent Machines." In *IEEE International Conference on Electrical, Communication, Electronics, Instrumentation and Computing (ICECEIC)*, pp. 30–31. 2019.

3. Gabriel Kamau, Caroline Boore, Elizaphan Maina, and Stephen Njenga, "Blockchain Technology: Is This the Solution to EMR Interoperability and Security Issues in Developing Countries?" In *2018 IST-Africa Week Conference (IST-Africa)*, p. 1. IEEE, 2018.
4. C. Y. Simha, V. M. Harshini, L. V. S. Raghuvamsi, and M. R. Kounte, "Enabling Technologies for Internet of Things & It's Security Issues." In *2018 Second International Conference on Intelligent Computing and Control Systems (ICICCS)*, pp. 1849–1852. 2018.
5. Alexander Kuzmin, "Blockchain-Based Structures for a Secure and Operate IoT." In *Internet of Things Business Models, Users, and Networks*, pp. 1–7. IEEE, 2017.
6. Shi, Shuyun et al. "Applications of Blockchain in Ensuring the Security and Privacy of Electronic Health Record Systems: A survey." *Comput. Secur.*, vol. 97, p. 101966, 2020. https://doi.org/10.1016/j.cose.2020.101966.
7. Ujan Mukhopadhyay, Anthony Skjellum, Oluwakemi Hambolu, Jon Oakley, Lu Yu, and Richard Brooks, "A Brief Survey of Cryptocurrency Systems." In *Privacy, Security and Trust (PST), 2016 14th Annual Conference on*, pp. 745–52. IEEE, 2016.
8. Naveen Soumyalatha and Manjunath R. Kounte, "Machine Learning Based Fog Computing as an Enabler of IoT." In *International Conference on New Trends in Engineering and Technology (ICNTET)*, IEEE, 7–8 Sep 2018.
9. Chintarlapallireddy Yaswanth Simha, V. M. Harshini, L. V. S. Raghuvamsi, Manjunath R. Kounte, "Enabling Technologies for Internet of Things Its Security Issues." In *Second International Conference on Intelligent Computing and Control Systems (ICICCS 2018)*, pp 1849–52. IEEE, 14–15 June 2018.
10. Youssef Wehbe, Mohamed Al Zaabi, and Davor Svetinovic, "Blockchain AI Framework for Healthcare Records Management: Constrained Goal Model." In *2018 26th Telecommunications Forum (TELFOR)*, pp. 420–5. IEEE, 2018.
11. Akanksha Kaushik, Archana Choudhary, Chinmay Ektare, Deepti Thomas, and Syed Akram, "BlockchainLiterature Survey." In *2017 2nd IEEE International Conference on Recent Trends in Electronics, Information Communication Technology (RTEICT)*, pp. 2145–8. IEEE, 2017.
12. G. Solomon, P. Zhang, R. Brooks, and Y. Liu, "A Secure and Cost-Efficient Blockchain Facilitated IoT Software Update Framework." pp. 44879–44894. IEEE. https://doi.org/10.1109/ACCESS.2023.3272899. 11.
13. F. Fang, C. Ventre, M. Basios, et al. "Cryptocurrency Trading: A Comprehensive Survey." *Financ. Innov.*, vol. 8, p. 13, 2022. https://doi.org/10.1186/s40854-021-00321-6.
14. Nikola Bozic, Guy Pujolle, and Stefano Secci, "A Tutorial on Blockchain and Applications to Secure Network Control-Planes." In *Smart Cloud Networks Systems (SCNS)*, pp. 1–8. IEEE, 2016.
15. K. Teja, H. R. Usha, Shreevani Danai, Chintarlapallireddy Yashwanth Simha, and Manjunath R. Kounte, "Recent Trends and Working of Cryptocurrency—A New Age Digital Economy." In *International Conference on New Trends in Engineering and Technology (ICNTET)*, 7–8 Sep 2018. Available from: https://www.researchgate.net/publication/336486964_Recent_trends_and_working_of_Cryptocurrency_-A_new_age_digital_economy.
16. Tomaso Aste, Paolo Tasca, and Tiziana Di Matteo, "Blockchain Technologies: The Foreseeable Impact on Society and Industry." *Computer*, vol. 50, no. 9, pp. 18–28, 2017.
17. Nabil Rifi, Elie Rachkidi, Nazim Agoulmine, and Nada Chendeb Taher, "Towards Using Blockchain Technology for eHealth Data Access Management." In *2017 Fourth International Conference on Advances in Biomedical Engineering (ICABME)*, pp. 1–4. IEEE, 2017.
18. Igor Kotsiuba, Artem Velvkzhanin, Yury Yanovich, Iuna Skarga Ban Durova, Yuriy Dyachenko, and Viacheslav Zhygulin, "Decentralized e-Health Architecture for Boosting Healthcare Analytics." In *2018 Second World Conference on Smart Trends in Systems, Security and Sustainability (WorldS4)*, pp. 113–18. IEEE, 2018.
19. Han, Yujin et al. "Blockchain Technology for Electronic Health Records." *Int. J. Environ. Res. Public Health*, vol. 19, no. 23, p. 15577, 2022. https://doi.org/10.3390/ijerph192315577.
20. Shan Jiang, Jiannong Cao, Hanqing Wu, Yanni Yang, Mingyu Ma, and Jianfei He, "Blochie: A Blockchain-Based Platform for Healthcare Information Exchange." In *2018 IEEE International Conference on Smart Computing (SMARTCOMP)*, pp. 49–56. IEEE, 2018.
21. Sahil Gupta, *The Role of Blockchain in Healthcare*, 15 Mar 2022. Available from: https://www.parangat.com/blog/the-role-of-blockchain-in-healthcare/.

22. Global Blockchain in Healthcare Market, *Focus on Industry Analysis and Opportunity Matrix—Analysis and Forecast*, 2018–2025. Available from: https://bisresearch.com/industry-report/global-blockchain-in-healthcare-market-2025.html.
23. J. P. Morgan. Healthcare Industry Outlook. https://www.jpmorgan.com/content/dam/jpm/commercial-banking/insights/healthcare/ccbsi-healthcare-industry-outlook.pdf. (Accessed on March 2023).
24. C. Pirtle and J. Ehrenfeld, "Blockchain for Healthcare: The Next Generation of Medical Records?" *J. Med. Syst.*, vol. 42, no. 9, p. 172, 2018.
25. S. Nakamoto, *Bitcoin: A Peer-to-Peer Electrnic Cash System*, pp. 1–9, 2008. Available from: https://bitcoin.org/bitcoin.pdf.
26. W. J. Gordon and C. Catalini, "Blockchain Technology for Healthcare: Facilitating the Transition to Patient-Driven Interoperability." *Comput. Struct. Biotechnol. J.*, vol. 16, pp. 224–30, 2018.
27. J. Eberhardt and S. Tai, "On or Off the Blockchain? Insights on Off-Chaining Computation and Data." *Smart SOA Platforms Cloud Comput. Archit.*, no. October, pp. 11–45, 2014.
28. D. Vujičić, D. Jagodić, and S. Randić, "Blockchain Technology, Bitcoin, and Ethereum: A Brief Overview." In *2018 17th 2018 17th International Symposium INFOTEH-JAHORINA, Infoteh 2018—Processing*, vol. 2018-Jan, no. March, pp. 1–6, 2018. https://doi.org/10.1109/INFOTEH.2018.8345547.
29. S. Wang, Y. Yuan, X. Wang, J. Li, R. Qin, and F. Y. Wang, "An Overview of Smart Contract: Architecture, Applications, and Future Trends." *IEEE Intell. Veh. Symp. Proc.*, vol. 2018-June, no. IV, pp. 108–13, 2018.
30. T. T. Kuo, H. E. Kim, and L. Ohno-Machado, "Blockchain Distributed Ledger Technologies for Biomedical and Health Care Applications." *J. Am. Med. Informatics Assoc.*, vol. 24, no. 6, pp. 1211–20, 2017.
31. M. S. Sahoo and P. K. Baruah, "HBasechainDB-A Scalable Blockchain Framework on Hadoop Ecosystem." In *Supercomputing Frontiers*, 2018, pp. 18–29. https://doi.org/10.1007/978-3-319-69953-0_2.
32. P. Zhang, J. White, D. C. Schmidt, G. Lenz, and S.T. Rosenbloom, "FHIRChain: Applying Blockchain to Securely and Scalably Share Clinical Data." *Comput. Struct. Biotechnol. J.*, vol. 16, pp. 267–78, 2018.
33. M. G. Kim, A. R. Lee, H. J. Kwon, J. W. Kim, and I. K. Kim, "Sharing Medical Questionnaries Based on Blockchain." In *Processing—2018 IEEE International Conference on Bioinformatics and Biomedicine, BIBM 2018*, pp. 2767–9, 2019. https://doi.org/10.1109/BIBM.2018.8621154.
34. I. Grishchenko, M. Maffei, and C. Schneidewind, "A Semantic Framework for the Security Analysis of Ethereum Smart Contracts." In *Principles of Security and Trust*, 2018, pp. 243–69. https://doi.org/10.48550/arXiv.1802.08660.
35. T. Dey, S. Jaiswal, S. Sunderkrishnan, and N. Katre, "A Medical Use Case of Internet of Things and Blockchain," *2017 Int. Conf. Intell. Sustain. Syst.*, no. ICISS, pp. 486–91, 2017.

7
Potential of Blockchain in Disease Surveillance

Mohamed Yousuff, Jayashree J., Vijayashree J., and Anusha R.

7.1 Introduction

The emergence of the COVID-19 (coronavirus disease 2019) pandemic has necessitated the expeditious development of efficacious measures for managing and mitigating the disease. The potential of blockchain technology and GeoAI has been demonstrated in recent developments, as they facilitate the secure and efficient management and sharing of data to control epidemics. An obscured blockchain-based system for infection tracking [1], whereas GeoAI is used to prevent epidemics and data sharing on blockchain, is elaborated in-depth [2]. The concepts mentioned earlier underscore nascent technologies' potential in disease control and prevention while also indicating auspicious directions for future investigation. A blockchain network can record and monitor various activities, such as demands, buys, accounting, operations, and other related functions. The utilization of blockchain technology for the storage of medical data is a viable option due to its high level of security, speed, and efficiency. Utilizing blockchain technology enables tracking individuals' travel itineraries and potential contact points, thereby mitigating the transmission of the coronavirus. Efforts are underway to develop a social application and a geospatial artificial intelligence system that utilizes blockchain technology to accurately detect illnesses while simultaneously ensuring the privacy of its users [3,4].

The employment of nascent technologies such as blockchain and AI can enhance healthcare services, as evidenced by the reaction to the COVID-19 pandemic. An evidence-based analysis of blockchain's potential healthcare use cases has demonstrated that it can facilitate secure data exchange and improve healthcare outcomes for COVID-19 and other related situations [5]. Emphasized is the potential of blockchain technology in improving global health security through its ability to strengthen routine disease monitoring systems [6].

Despite their potential benefits, incorporating these technologies into healthcare systems poses a significant challenge. As mentioned earlier, the technologies' efficacy and durability necessitate meticulous contemplation of the confidentiality of data, interoperability, and regulatory compliance. In addition, the swift development of COVID-19 and other emerging infectious diseases necessitates healthcare systems that are versatile and responsive, utilizing emerging technologies to address novel challenges effectively. Utilizing the findings of the systematic review conducted [5,6], as well as the research conducted [7], numerous scholarly investigations have examined the viability of utilizing

DOI: 10.1201/9781003408246-7

blockchain-based solutions to establish a secure and decentralized platform to track infections, manage patient data, and facilitate information sharing among healthcare providers [8]. Some researchers conducted a study that evaluates several blockchain-based approaches to combat pandemics, such as contact tracing, secure data sharing, and supply chain management. Furthermore, the integration of blockchain technology with mHealth systems has been defined; it is a secure and decentralized patient data storage [9]. The investigated data reports the potential of utilizing blockchain technology and artificial intelligence in addressing pandemics such as COVID-19 [10]. As mentioned earlier, the studies underscore blockchain technology's potential utility as a valuable instrument in combating pandemics, such as the ongoing COVID-19 crisis. Implementing these technologies for epidemic management is confronted with several obstacles, such as compatibility among diverse data sources, guaranteeing the confidentiality and protection of data, and tackling concerns regarding the dependability and accuracy of data [11].

During the COVID-19 pandemic, the globe faced a massive problem as it became difficult to track down sufferers and their relationships. As a result, developing a platform to manage the COVID-19 epidemic effectively will rely heavily on blockchain technology. Using a blockchain-based platform to combat the epidemic is discussed in the study. The research has identified and discussed nine effective methods for using blockchain technology to deal with the COVID-19 epidemic. To correctly manage the COVID-19 epidemic, a platform built on blockchain technology is essential. The WHO proclaimed the global spread of COVID-19 to be an epidemic less than a month after the first cases emerged. Finding patients' contact information was the most challenging issue for most administrations. There was no reliable method for tracking new cases or calculating the prevalence of coronaviruses. Patients' records may be obtained from public hospitals and clinics, but an increased level of trust may be required, owing to the need for careful monitoring and archiving. High-risk patients may be easily identified via blockchain technology, which can be used to monitor the spread of the coronavirus. Industry 4.0, biosensors, 3D scanning, and multi-agent systems are some technologies that may be utilized to spot infections. Blockchain technology is about creating a digital record that is distributed, decentralized, and accessible to the public. Blockchain technology relies primarily on blocks, miners, and servers. Users from many walks of life, including patients, testing and clinical labs, hospitals, and government websites, use the distributed ledger's nodes. Records, samples, test findings, treatment status, discharge summaries, and histories are all in a computerized ledger. Blockchain technology provides a variety of practical answers for the COVID-19 pandemic, including the monitoring of outbreaks, the monitoring of donations, and the management of medical supply chains [3].

7.1.1 The Three Fundamental Tenants of Blockchain Technology

The three are stability, transparency, and independence. Knowledge is dispersed across a network through decentralization, eliminating the need for a centralized authority and decreasing the chance of systematic failure. Accountability is ensured since everything can be seen and followed on a public blockchain. Data entered into the blockchain cannot be changed after it has been entered, making immutability a game changer for many industries, thanks to the cryptography hash function. Each component can be uniquely identified using this technique. The immutability of blockchain ensures the integrity of stored information [12,13].

Blockchain technology allows for the decentralized, encrypted, and secure recording of digital transactions. Industries like computers, where anonymity is essential yet

Potential of Blockchain in Disease Surveillance

centralization is unnatural, stand to benefit significantly from the introduction of blockchain technology. One of the most complex parts of dealing with a pandemic is gathering reliable data on the outbreak's progression. Providing data that can be independently verified is a significant benefit of this technology. The patient's location may be monitored in real time, and the latest updates on the impacted regions can be provided, all thanks to blockchain technology. Patients, clinical and diagnostic laboratories, hospitals, and government websites utilize blockchain nodes. In the following examples, blockchain addresses the H1N1 flu epidemic [3,14].

1. *Hashlog.* Log of hashes. To combat the spread of the COVID-19 virus in the United States, a blockchain solution based on distributed ledger technology might be used [15].
2. *VeChain* is a blockchain-based infrastructure built to monitor China's vaccine manufacturing process. Distributed ledgers keep track of everything that goes into making vaccines, from raw ingredients and batch numbers to finished product packaging. Vaccine information is likewise protected against the possibility of being altered by this technique [15].
3. *PHBC.* This blockchain-based technology helps communities and businesses maintain a disease-free environment by continually and anonymously verifying that they are free of coronavirus (COVID-19) and other high-risk viruses. One of the essential functions of this blockchain-based network is its capacity to monitor the whereabouts of healthy individuals and prevent them from re-entering diseased zones [15].
4. To facilitate donations to Chinese patients with infectious diseases, *Hyperchain* was developed as a donation platform. Hyperchain's capacity to link millions of nodes means that during this epidemic, many people will be able to get the donated commodities and medical equipment they need from industries [15].

7.2 Cryptographically Secure Blockchain-Based Disease Surveillance

Over the past two years, the novel coronavirus and its highly transmissible mutant strains have caused infection in over 233 million individuals. The viral pathogen has resulted in the demise of approximately 4.8 million individuals. The United States has recorded more than 44 million confirmed cases of the illness, resulting in over 500,000 fatalities. The World Health Organization (WHO) declared COVID-19, a highly lethal virus, a worldwide pandemic on March 11, 2020. Epidemiologists suggest that contact tracing can effectively mitigate the spread of communicable diseases, particularly those that are highly contagious, by identifying individuals and their connections and collaborating with them to minimize infection rates. A potential strategy for preventing the transmission of an infectious disease is to enforce home confinement for the infected individual. Identifying individuals who may have had contact with the virus has emerged as an integral approach to mitigating the spread of COVID-19. The process of contact tracing poses significant challenges. However, it is an essential measure in mitigating the transmission of illnesses by isolating individuals exposed to the pathogen from those who have not. The utilization of patient movement tracking enables public health officials to furnish contemporaneous data on prevailing cases and classify locations according to their level of infection susceptibility. Moreover, this data is crucial for local, regional, or national governance as it can be utilized to identify areas with high incidences of illness and alert individuals to avoid specific locations [1].

The WHO strongly recommends the implementation of contact tracing as a means of mitigating the spread of COVID-19. This approach involves both forward and reverse tracing capabilities. In order to mitigate the occurrence of future epidemics, healthcare professionals must prioritize the reduction of information falsification and the enhancement of the credibility of trustworthy sources. The implementation of contact tracing measures guarantees that individuals who are not infected with a particular disease can obtain accurate and current information. The current pandemic situation requires the creation of innovative contact tracing methods that are automated, efficient, precise, and that safeguard users' privacy. The primary aim was to create a contact tracing system utilizing blockchain technology for disease management to mitigate the challenges previously outlined. The utilization of sophisticated cryptographic methods by blockchain renders its data immutable and capable of being audited, thus presenting a viable solution to the privacy issue. The system, as mentioned earlier, is a decentralized, publicly accessible database that chronologically records encrypted signatures, which are viewable by any member of the network [1,2].

7.2.1 Contact-Tracking Infrastructure Using Blockchain

Blockchain has been utilized to construct a contact-tracking infrastructure. The approach utilizes a contact tracing architecture constructed on blockchain technology to detect individuals susceptible to acquiring an infectious ailment through incidental social interactions. It is posited that initiating a novel transaction is feasible at any given time through the physical interaction of two users, whereby their respective devices detect contact via Bluetooth signals. The sole identifiers implicated in this particular scenario will be the user IDs produced by the system. Subsequently, we shall document this transaction on the local blockchain. Simultaneously, nearby medical facilities may perform diagnostic examinations on the individuals in question to detect any potential ailments. Moreover, a transaction that comprises this information is transmitted to the local blockchain. To effectively handle these transactions, it is deemed appropriate to utilize local processing methods that can provide individual prompt notifications while also transmitting the data to a master blockchain for centralized processing. The verification of transactions was conducted through a POA mechanism, which deviates from the commonly employed PoW (proof-of-work) consensus methodology. The proof-of-authority (POA) approach is considered a conventional consensus mechanism because it provides uniform incentives to all nodes to maintain the network. The employment of the POA technique mitigates the workload burden on nodes and guarantees dependable data transmission for risk management. Scholars and healthcare professionals may utilize the outcomes of statistical analysis and extensive data processing to gain insights into the dissemination of the ailment and its potential impacts, as well as to develop pre-emptive measures aimed at mitigating the transmission of the illness [1,2].

The datasets were generated using a Node.js software application named trip-simulator, which depicted the movements of multiple individuals within an urban area. Upon reception of the data, it was promptly subjected to positional alterations. The updates above furnish the user's current geographical coordinates (i.e., latitude and longitude) and the time stamp denoting the moment the update was dispatched. The converted data and subsequent position updates are processed by an algorithm that emulates the proximity detection mechanism of Bluetooth low energy (BLE). Developing an infection calculator tool is viable, considering various factors, including but not limited to the infection rate, recovery rate, and temporal aspects. The manipulation of these parameters can regulate disease transmission within a specific geographical area. The outcomes of this study have potential applications beyond the mere enumeration of individuals who have contracted the virus at a given moment. They can be employed to forecast the rate at which viral transmission will alter over time and to implement preventative measures proactively to avert an escalation of the situation. Upon undergoing encryption, hashing, and validation, the data obtained by the system is subsequently stored in the blockchain, thereby ensuring its perpetual accessibility, auditability, and immutability. The decentralized architecture of blockchain technology alleviates the workload on individual nodes, thereby augmenting the collective computational capacity of the system and significantly curtailing the processing duration [1,3].

7.2.2 Blockchain-Based Geosocial Data Sharing and Artificial Intelligence-Based Epidemic Control

Over time, many individuals have perished due to epidemics, particularly those instigated by exceedingly communicable illnesses. Consequently, there have been persistent endeavors to prevent pandemics. During an acute outbreak, strict isolation of the afflicted emerges as the most effective method of epidemic management, as demonstrated by successfully avoiding other airborne viruses, such as SARS (severe acute respiratory syndrome) and H1N1 (hemagglutinin-neuraminidase), since the entire population is at risk regardless of age. The epidemiological surveillance of verified cases remains the principal approach for identifying individuals who are unwell or may be harboring an illness. However, this approach may fail to detect infections, especially in individuals without symptoms. Preventing the spread of infectious diseases necessitates the availability of a mechanism that can promptly, efficiently, and quickly identify illnesses. Integrating social applications and artificial geospatial intelligence (GeoAI) with blockchain technology enables the prompt identification of viruses while preserving the anonymity of users. The extensive utilization of social networking applications has enabled the accumulation and retention of substantial quantities of social data, encompassing geolocation data, on blockchain technology while preserving the user's confidentiality.

In order to address these apprehensions, it is imperative to establish a secure and reliable platform for sharing information between private and public entities that safeguard users' privacy while offering valuable insights into social dynamics. The concept has put forward a new approach to managing and preventing infectious diseases that rely on social applications and GeoAI. They suggest that blockchain technology can be used to facilitate the sharing of user data. WeChat, a prominent mobile social networking application in China, is frequently cited as an exemplar. The COVID-19 pandemic has served as a starting point for integrating GeoAI methodologies with infectious disease dynamical systems, thereby facilitating the examination and control of epidemics [4].

The blockchain-based GeoAI-based epidemic control system facilitates user exchange and reception of data. The epidemic information-sharing blockchain comprises three key components: users, medical institutions, and a GeoAI analysis engine. Individuals may submit an application based on their susceptibility to infection, providing daily health metrics and progressions. Through the Internet, a medical institution can conduct diagnostic tests for infections, monitor the status of confirmed patients, securely exchange patient information, and openly disclose patient identities. The GeoAI algorithm utilizes the daily health data submitted by users. It cross-references it with the trip records of confirmed cases stored on the blockchain to identify potential cases warranting medical attention. Concurrently, the hospital's verified patient trajectory distribution is disseminated and graphically displayed on the map as a cautionary measure to other social media users. The present study employs blockchain technology to accomplish the following aims: a singular knowledge transfer, a two-tiered risk analysis, a three-tiered privacy protection, a four-tiered accountability tracing, and fifth-tiered data security and reliability [5,6].

The concept incorporates various technologies, including infectious disease dynamics modeling, social applications, GeoAI, and blockchain. The integration of GeoAI and blockchain technology enables the efficient processing and analysis of data about epidemics. Additionally, utilizing blockchain architecture ensures the preservation of privacy in data management. Concurrently, the geographical regions of confirmed patients are being delineated, and information about their symptoms is amassed. Deep learning and machine learning algorithms utilize various fundamental data types as training inputs to establish correlations between an epidemic's patient distribution, progression, and surrounding environment. The neural network model was developed using training data that underwent data pre-processing. The model's accuracy standards for practical application were achieved by regularly evaluating it through verification and testing, which incorporated the patients' distribution, trajectory, physical conditions, and the actual environment. The ultimate stage in spatial machine learning involves disseminating and implementing models. Subsequently, the model that has undergone training is utilized as a tool or service to perform the necessary computations and evaluations to ascertain the appropriate distribution of individuals affected by an epidemic [2].

7.2.3 WeChat GeoAI Blockchain-Based System

Users can submit sensitive data to the blockchain via WeChat, including medical history and travel plans. The initial task of the GeoAI susceptible-exposed-infected-recovered infectious disease dynamics model system is to measure the user's well-being. If a user believes he is a patient needing care, he can use the blockchain to request transaction confirmation. Different users will get the early warning system based on their awareness of the affected person's location, mobility, and condition. Ultimately, they use machine learning to create predictors of coronavirus infections. In addition, facilitating rapid and accurate identification of the infectious agent source may help direct the implementation of the isolation strategy. Meanwhile, blockchain technology facilitates the secure, near-instantaneous, and low-cost exchange and synchronization of patient data without compromising privacy [2].

7.3 Safety Measures Monitoring Using IoT

COVID-19 gained worldwide attention because of its fast growth and subsequent human outbreaks, but it continues to pose new challenges with each new variant that arises every few months. One of the most critical things you can do to prevent the spread of this pandemic sickness is to keep track of anybody who comes into contact with a

COVID-infected individual, including their travel history. It takes too long to collect information on others who came in touch with the afflicted person, and the current monitoring system only records travel history within the bounds of local cities. Therefore, it has to be enhanced. The IoT may be feasible for post-COVID-19 economic resuscitation using a blockchain-based secured paradigm for remote health monitoring and chain tracking. Because the IoT captures and stores sensitive information, requiring high privacy and security [16].

Traditional security and privacy solutions must often catch up when applied to intricate, public, dynamic, and decentralized topologies, exceptionally when resources are constrained. The blockchain technology used to handle its data is safe, decentralized, permanent, open, and immutable, and it has the power to solve these stated concerns. The blockchain system generates data as a series of linked blocks, each including a record of the preceding block's transactions. Numerous challenges must be handled when incorporating blockchain technology with IoT. Some examples are low scalability, large resource requirements, and traffic overhead. The research outcomes illustrate the advantages of deploying blockchain technology in a transparent environment, where all users can view and audit all transactions. Because of blockchain technology's increased efficiency and cheaper processing costs, the mechanism is more accessible to clients [16].

A blockchain-based system for controlling and tracking one's health condition, a dependable method of monitoring and tracking supervision, removes the need for intermediaries to boost employees' well-being in any place. The distributed ledger design of blockchain decreases service delivery prices for participating firms, optimizes device operations, and removes the need for many authorization levels. The concept addresses the many security and privacy concerns inherent in health monitoring and tracking technologies by lifting a blockchain load off tiny IoT-powered devices through a better network. Employers may use this method to monitor their employees' health during and after typical work hours. To facilitate economic development, this capability, which includes automatic monitoring of impacted parties' meeting records, might be made accessible via cloud computing and service providers [16].

Two distinct areas should be established on corporate property: one for workers with clean medical records and no known interactions with COVID-19 patients, and one for individuals with symptomatic records and a possibly contaminated background who have yet to be traced down. This plan is only available to employees who have previously shown symptoms in their job records. The asymptomatic COVID-19 record history will continue to be the limiting factor in the model. The approach is divided into three layers: enterprise network infrastructure, cloud computing and service provision, and superlative network [16].

7.3.1 Enterprise Network Infrastructure

The following components comprise enterprise network infrastructure.

7.3.1.1 Workers Who Use IoT-Enabled Devices

These devices, which may be worn or have rigorous carrying requirements, move from one workplace to another and remain with employees throughout the day. The devices record vital employee indicators, such as temperature, heart rate, and oxygen levels. Devices utilized in the workplace collect employees' geolocation, meeting history, and health information [16].

7.3.1.2 Buffer Zone

When someone enters the buffer zone outside the main campus, their data from the previous day's sign-out and the current day's sign-in is transferred to the local company blockchain. It is required because access to 5G networks is critical for those who utilize high speeds in the real world; when the corporate, after the global blockchain, verifies the meeting's history and the collected health data explains the symptoms, a green and orange work zone will be assigned [16].

7.3.1.3 Enterprise Blockchain

Bitcoin, which is mined, stored, and operated in secret on resource-capable computers, remains online through enterprise blockchain. Regarding corporate blockchain networks, the most often-used private blockchain is Hyperledger Caliper. All transactions involving a specific device are interlocked and linked one after the other, but control in the business BC, as in the Bitcoin BC, rests entirely with its developer [16].

7.3.1.4 Enterprise-Grade Storage

Although centralized data storage in a local repository is a costly add-on for enterprises, it enables them to operate with higher data agility and sensitivity. Consequently, there may be a more critical requirement for a nearby backup [16].

7.3.1.5 Smart Contracts

Smart contracts allow agreements to be formed on any IoT device, leading to enforcement when conditions are met. You may establish upper and lower limits for a critical situation in the workplace [16].

7.3.2 Cloud Computing and Service Provision

Rather than storing IoT healthcare facts over the blockchain, data about personnel is maintained on cloud computing servers in this situation. In other circumstances, workers may desire their company's data to be housed in the cloud, allowing an outside partner to offer easy, high-tech services. The information saved in the cloud is processed in discrete, numbered pieces. The device is identified via block numbers and a hash of the stored data. When data matches a preset block number and the hash value is detected, a customer can access the device. Information gathered from users is stored in blocks and retrieved in a FIFO (first-in, first-out) fashion using a hash key [16,17].

7.3.3 Superlative Network

Bitcoin's decentralized design is exceptionally close to that of a superlative network. A server, a mobile phone, or a tablet computer are all examples of connecting devices or nodes. According to the structure, a network comprises numerous nodes, each needing its certificate to confirm its legitimacy. A user must first upload an authentication certificate to the system to build a network profile. In this situation, the network may execute digital signatures after being granted permission by the data/transaction. To achieve the quickest possible data transmission rates and the fewest service disruptions, we divided the network into smaller "clusters," each headed by a cluster node. A node may attempt to join a different cluster if it is delayed. Although most multi-stage IoT network topologies, including the one shown earlier, are used for remote health monitoring and tracking, the concept holds in all cases. The technique might be tested for compatibility with new and existing IoT frameworks [16,18].

7.4 Disease Surveillance and Control Using AI and Blockchain

According to the latest studies on next-generation networking, users' health data and other confidential information must be handled with secure and reliable communication and networking. The adaptation of AI-enabled device allows clever and safe healthcare capable of dealing with diseases that may emerge at any moment by altering the architecture of healthcare systems. The network may allow for the safe transfer of patient information between facilities. This technique would allow for massive spying, tracking, and analysis at the periphery, thanks to the low delay and high broadband capability of 5G and beyond networks [19].

7.4.1 Data Sharing in Secure Mode Using Blockchain

Patient data will be gathered, filtered, taught, analyzed, and handled locally or via nearby nodes in a dispersed healthcare framework, necessitating a secure and private communication mechanism that is not only secure but also reliable. It will help guarantee that all deals and info are legitimate. Furthermore, local and regional healthcare groups may need constant access to patient information under a joint healthcare structure. Cooperative and dispersed systems like this one necessitate blockchain technology, in which the healthcare system comprises many entities performing various roles. It offers a safe way for the decentralized sharing and storage of private medical data. Blockchain transactions are regarded as quick and might provide a method to combine the policies of various and diverse healthcare organizations. It would allow diverse businesses to collaborate and share a particular model across various healthcare industries [19].

Because of the variety and abundance of edge and core network devices with sophisticated processing, storage, and communication capabilities, as well as the fact that decentralized and secure healthcare systems can adapt to the varying health conditions in different health districts, the adoption of a generalized AI technique that is adaptable to a wide range of devices and applications, namely, plug-and-play, is crucial. The potential for rapid advancements in AI technology and the substantial effects on the healthcare service system form the idea of a uniform and streamlined learning solution applicable to any problem or subject. Additionally, generalized AI can perform the training and fine-tuning of the model independently to offer an ideal degree of flexibility for the end products [20].

7.5 Blockchain-Based Contact Tracing

Blockchain technology has much potential for pandemic scenarios, like contact monitoring, due to its proven security and decentralization. However, the problems with current touch monitoring techniques revolve around medical privacy, data security, and transparency

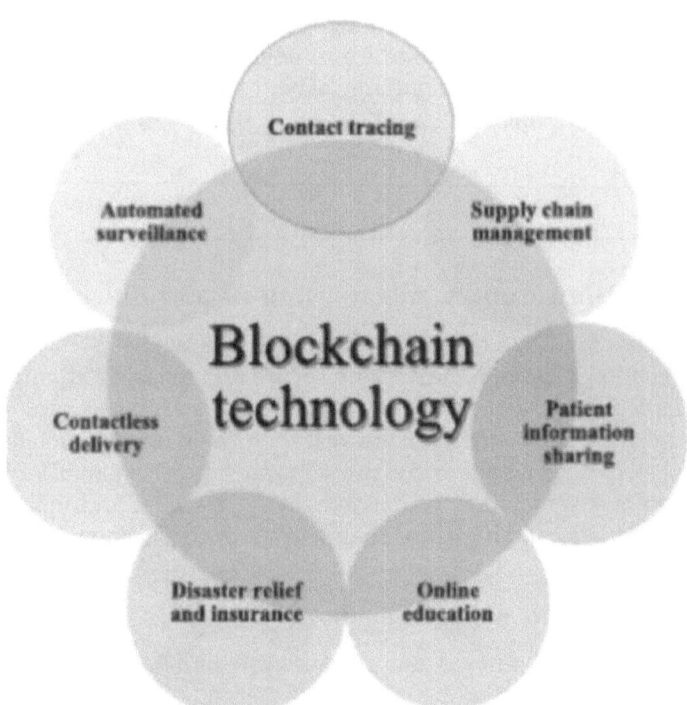

FIGURE 7.1
Applications of blockchain.

issues. The improvement in contact monitoring effectiveness, while preserving user anonymity and preventing data misuse, will be controlled using symmetric encryption in the blockchain. The approach uses IPFS, a networked file storage system, to address scalability issues. The goal is to create a contact monitoring system that is more dependable, secure, and effective and that can effectively stop the transmission of illness during an outbreak [21].

- **Contact tracing.** The process of finding, evaluating, and controlling individuals in direct contact with verified index cases is known as contact tracing. These contacts are then identified and told about their risk of receiving care and therapy in advance to stop the virus from spreading. Therefore, this technique has effectively reduced the number of cases and widespread epidemics for decades. Figure 7.1 depicts the applications of blockchain.

7.5.1 Blockchain with IoMT (Internet of Medical Things)

The information is kept in a distributed node network. The system's data is more protected because of this technological advancement. Blockchain is a distributed ledger managed, stored, and recorded by a network of individual computers known as nodes. It ensures that information may be sent between nodes in the network without interruption and stores all relevant data. A blockchain system is a distributed ledger maintained by a network of computers that allows users to conduct value transactions directly with one another without the need for a trusted third party using automated consensus. Different blockchain applications [4] include:

1. Distributed ledger technology (DLT) (which Bitcoin and other cryptocurrencies are built on) is a sort of blockchain. Get rid of centralized systems' drawbacks, such as the requirement for more security and openness. Instead of keeping the information in one central location, DLT disperses it over a network of computers.
2. A private blockchain is a blockchain implementation that can handle secure data. A network that is either private or under the jurisdiction of a single organization. Miniature compared to public blockchains. The creator of a private blockchain is aware of all the nodes from the start.
3. Hybrid blockchains combine the best features of both public and private blockchains. Businesses can now establish permissionless public and permission-based private networks to control who has access to what information on the blockchain.

When it comes to healthcare, blockchain technology is a game changer. The healthcare industry is shifting toward a patient-centered model that prioritizes service accessibility and healthcare resource availability. Thanks to blockchain technology, citizens may participate in health research initiatives, polls, and camps. Better research outcomes will result, and data sharing may benefit the general public. Protecting, sharing, and interoperating with data have been the biggest challenges in population health management. The primary purpose of blockchain technology is to improve data safety, data integrity, data sharing, and data updating in real time [4].

Blockchain ledger technology has several applications in the healthcare industry, including assisting researchers in deciphering genetic codes, ensuring the safety of patient data throughout the transfer, and organizing the distribution of medications. Blockchain is being created and applied for various excellent technical capabilities, including patient data security, electronic data management, medical records, and digitalized tracking. The whole pharmaceutical supply chain may be tracked in real time thanks to blockchain technology. With the aid of IoT and blockchain, it is possible to monitor all shipments and traffic patterns, delays, and speeds. Blockchain improves reliance and hinders dishonest bookkeeping and money transfers. You may now keep an unbreakable, decentralized, and transparent record of all patient data without the hassle of multi-factor authentication. The distributed ledger technology (blockchain) facilitates easy, around-the-clock access to data for healthcare providers, patients, and pharmacists. Companies and start-ups in the healthcare industry are working around the clock to study, experiment, discover, and develop blockchain technology. The improved data storage made possible by blockchain will one day include a patient's medical record, from diagnoses and test results to medications and sensor readings [22].

New patient data cards for physicians at different hospitals may be created using blockchain technology. Offers data transparency tools for tracking down distribution chains and stopping the proliferation of fake drugs. Researchers may keep track of information such as test outcomes, patient histories, and other factors. With the blocks accessible to professionals and patients, a medical blockchain will significantly alter the status quo of recordkeeping. Simultaneously, the patient's worries are considered while dealing with anamnesis. This blockchain's processing and approval capacity is beneficial in the healthcare sector. This innovation will improve access to individualized healthcare, expert clinical advice, and real-world scientific study. The healthcare industry may benefit from a decentralized blockchain platform in many ways, including identifying fraud, decreasing costs, generating secure employment, minimizing redundant labor, and increasing transparency. Blockchain technology can increase the trustworthiness, verifiability, and accountability of clinical trials and regulatory bodies in medical fields [23].

Blockchain is a disruptive technology that affects every market. When an agreement is reached on the status of a transaction, that information is added as a new block to the existing blockchain. A blockchain-based supply chain system guarantees medical device safety, efficiency, and on-time delivery. In order to verify therapies with the target patient and regulatory authorities, medical devices may upload patient data. It is recognized for its widespread influence in a variety of business sectors. This cutting-edge innovation streamlines the time-consuming claims procedure by doing away with unnecessary verification steps. The leakage of essential data utilized for harmful devices and other special interests is the most significant issue confronting the healthcare business. However, it can be easily solved by deploying this technology [23].

7.5.2 Blockchain in Communicable Diseases Tracking

Influenza and SARS are infectious illnesses that spread rapidly both via and outside human contact, infect large numbers of people, and take a long time to heal from. Blockchain is an innovative new technology that may be used to establish a trustworthy and decentralized ledger. Blockchain's key and time stamp mechanism ensures that records cannot be changed after entering the system. National Centers for Disease Control and Prevention (NDCP), hospitals, and other institutions may input data on infectious diseases more quickly and securely thanks to a time-stamping feature. The characteristics are highlighted in the following way [24]:

1. Transferring the central node's operations to every node to store and distribute pandemic information, like confirmed cases, suspected cases, case infection times, case infection locations, and spread directions. Get source tracing done.
2. To create a workable infectious source tracking solution, start with root source tracking and use dispersed node upkeep capabilities, hash anti-tampering capabilities, and time marking in blockchain technology.
3. Outlines how to use Python coding to create a blockchain environment for collecting, storing, querying, and tracing disease information. It also includes a simulated source-tracing scenario for testing the method.
4. Describes the information gathering, archiving, retrieval, and tracking process flow for infectious diseases.
5. Systematic information gathering on infectious diseases, confirmed and suspected cases, and the time and location of the infection in order to give infectious disease control authorities more precise data for their pandemic surveillance and response, enhancing collection [9].

Metadata tracking in the database and workflow industries was the first to use traceability technologies. Infectious illness reports data traceability was the primary research topic of this work. By continually collecting, storing, examining, and evaluating dynamic spread data and geographical distribution of infectious illnesses, epidemic information traceability allows for the timely implementation of efficient disease control measures. The scientists developed a technique to monitor the spread of highly virulent Asian avian influenza using data collected from mobile devices. Veterinarians, medical experts, and farmers from around the globe may now input data on animal health thanks to this intelligent system. Scientists monitored mosquito populations, identified their species and geographic origins, and calculated the potential spread of illness [24,25].

The goal of blockchain-based data storage during an epidemic of an irresistible disease is to make data capture and storage a reality. Data transfers are recorded on the blockchain as a hash value of a certain length, which can then be verified against a time stamp. The data may be hashed using the hash function, yielding a hash value of a predetermined length. Due to blockchain's immutable chain of records, updating data on irreversible diseases requires starting from the beginning. As soon as both parties approve the updated irresistible disease data, it will be stored on the blockchain. The renovated landmarks now have a time stamp reflecting the present. The system then sends the information to the NDCP and its administration division for final data verification and improvement. So an intelligent contract architecture was created to provide early warning of incurable diseases to detect abnormal scenarios when case numbers exceed the threshold level [24]. Every participating hub may add previously unutilized infectious disease data to the database, and the system will analyze the information to determine whether it meets the criteria for an early warning signal as specified by the blockchain smart contract. The smart contract will carry out all rulings, and the NDCP will be able to monitor and control things. Five methods for using this blockchain approach in healthcare are discussed:

1. Settings for early warning and access restrictions
2. Node-consensus data upload
3. Chain technology constructed
4. Modifying data about contagious diseases
5. Identifying the source of an outbreak by following the trail back to its beginning

The issue with the current blockchain technology is that it is still an emerging technology; hence, it still faces many challenges when applied. The disease information stored in blockchain needs to be more reliable, modifiable, and credible of data at the source. The authentication of data still needs to be implemented.

7.6 Blockchain in Patient Tracking System

On December 31, 2019, the WHO was alerted about pneumonia-like instances and patient cases rising in Wuhan, China. Blockchain is often regarded as Bitcoin's most important technical advancement since it is secure and a trustless-proof method for all network transactions. The major blockchain innovation is its use as a framework for a new system of trustless, decentralized transactions. An infected person's connections may be identified by contact tracing, which collects more information about these individuals. If the diseases are tracked at the early stages of epidemiology, tracking contacts plays an important role in finding and preventing the spread of infectious illnesses. Blockchain is essential in secure data exchange as it is a safe and efficient network. Confidential and authorized data can be exchanged securely through blockchain [26].

Two of the most often-cited difficulties are the widespread deployment of the program and the protection of sensitive patient information. Before blockchain can be widely employed in the healthcare industry to increase the efficiency of treatment and diagnostics, there are still several barriers to overcome regarding scalability and dependability. Blockchain, a distributed ledger system, might be used to record and verify healthcare business transactions. Several fields of study and development focus on improving patient care data flow, including medical records management, data gateways, blockchain, MedVault, Fatcom, BitHealth, and GemHealth. A growing number of healthcare-focused companies are conducting pilot blockchain trials. The decentralized nature of blockchain is the technology's first significant advantage. Unlike more conventional distributed database management solutions, blockchain is a decentralized system that manages data via peer-to-peer interactions. Blockchain only permits the two most basic database operations. As blockchain is a data provenance system, the only thing that can be exchanged between owners is the cryptographic protocols. Blockchain's accessibility and dependability mean the system may achieve high data redundancy with no single point of failure. The critical advantage of blockchain is the increased security and anonymity it provides via the use of cryptographic algorithms [26].

Blockchain transactions are signed using cryptography, but their details are still visible to all network users. Thus, secrecy and limited access are crucial. Request and answer form the basis of the data-sharing technique, making it such that only the recipient has access to the supplied data via the exposure of a cryptographic object. The distributed architecture, docker containers, and microservices are all built on the Ethereum platform, which enables smart contracts. The data is encrypted using a combination of two different algorithms. With blockchain, ever-evolving data can be verified instantly. Civitas and MiPasa are two of the blockchain-based options considered. With Civitas's integrated telemedicine features, physicians may monitor their patients' conditions remotely and advise on how to implement their treatment programs best. The program checks whether a person can leave the residence by comparing their government-issued ID with information stored on the blockchain. MiPasa is an IBM blockchain cloud-based data streaming platform built on Hyperledger Fabric that facilitates the exchange of trusted health and geographical information between people, government agencies, and healthcare facilities [26,27].

Intelligent testing is essential for ensuring effectiveness, and accurate records of the total number of tests conducted must be maintained. Each participant in the decentralized blockchain network has access to real-time updates to information about the number of tests conducted and the number of cases validated by laboratories at their check-in location. With blockchain technology, governments and NGOs (non-governmental organization) can monitor people's needs nationwide and coordinate lockdown procedures. The widespread use of social media facilitates the dissemination of disinformation. In order to avoid this, data may be shared over blockchain networks. A growing number of people are turning to them to combat the spread of harmful information, including rumors, conspiracy theories, false news, and offensive comments. Volunteers for COVID-19 crisis management efforts might be incentivized through a blockchain-based incentive system. The supply chain should have less disruption, and the system should keep running well. BeepTrace, a digital contact tracking tool that combines the solution with geographic information system, and Ayurveda, yoga and naturopathy, Unani, Siddha, and homeopathy are two examples of blockchain-based solutions that might be used in the aftermath of the epidemic. The current challenges in blockchain include scalability, privacy, security, and speed. The relationship between blockchain and the IoMT and their future scope and solutions will place an unremarkable position by 2040 [28].

7.6.1 Healthcare Blockchain Applications

After conducting a comprehensive literature analysis, they discovered a variety of use cases for blockchain technology, such as contact tracing, secure data sharing, and vaccination supply chain management. They also define the pros and cons of implementing blockchain technology and how further study and cooperation between stakeholders is needed to realize its potential fully. For COVID-19 and beyond, they identified and synthesized existing research on blockchain technology. They utilized predetermined inclusion and exclusion criteria to select research and then examined the selected studies qualitatively to identify important themes and conclusions. They also evaluated the included studies' overall quality using recognized quality assessment techniques. Finally, the synthesized findings provide an overview of blockchain technology's potential applications and limitations in healthcare [28,29].

7.7 Use of Blockchain and AI

Critical study criteria for measuring the vulnerability of our existing healthcare system include the sudden appearance of the novel susceptible, exposed, infected, recovered virus and its uncontrolled spread over the globe since its breakout in 2020. Integrating blockchain technology, early outbreak detection and prevention, identity protection and security, and a safe medicine supply chain are all possible at the application level. On the other hand, artificial intelligence techniques are employed to spot coronary effects before they get too serious, allowing people to avoid costly medical intervention. It covers the potential difficulties if extra manufacturing is required to establish a health monitoring system and all the conceivable new scenarios of utilizing the two technologies to combat a pandemic like COVID-19. The concept has highlighted the need for secure and efficient data sharing and management to combat the pandemic. It discusses their potential applications in healthcare and pandemic response, including tracking and monitoring the spread of the virus, developing and sharing diagnostic and treatment protocols, and facilitating the distribution and tracking of medical supplies and equipment [5].

The potential limitations and challenges of using these technologies in the pandemic response include data privacy and security concerns, interoperability issues, and the need for ethical and regulatory frameworks to govern their use. Overall, the document emphasizes the potential of blockchain and artificial intelligence technologies to overcome the coronavirus and calls for continued research and development in this area [5,23].

7.8 Blockchain in Diseases Health Surveillance

As blockchain technology enhances healthcare quality by sharing data among all parties, selecting privacy, and ensuring data security, it has great potential to alter the healthcare system in various ways radically. The benefits of blockchain over other widely used real-time and system learning methodologies are discussed, along with the basics of blockchain technology, its applications, and the quality of the user experience. Given the limitations of current real-time surveillance architectures regarding scalability, security, and interoperability, blockchain has emerged as a promising alternative. The distributed ledger technology known as blockchain has the potential to enhance global health insurance and can also guarantee the confidentiality of patient data, which may aid in healthcare research.

Recent outbreaks of re-emerging illnesses like Ebola and Zika have prompted widespread concerns about fitness protection, leading to the fortification of monitoring infrastructures. It highlights the key challenges existing disease surveillance systems face, including data fragmentation, limited interoperability, and privacy concerns. It discusses how blockchain technology can help overcome these challenges [6].

7.9 Disease Management Infrastructure Based on IoT and Blockchain

The combination of IoT and blockchain technologies addresses the challenges posed by the COVID-19 pandemic. The concept intends to make it possible to handle medical data and resources safely, openly, and effectively and improve viral monitoring and control. The concept integrates various IoT devices, such as temperature sensors, wearable devices, and health monitoring systems, which collect and transmit data to a blockchain-based platform. The concept of storing and managing the data, ensuring its integrity, privacy, and accessibility [7].

Users' vital statistics, including body temperature, heart rate, and oxygen levels, are collected via IoT sensors and recorded in an immutable ledger. The COVID-19 architecture makes use of IoT and blockchain technology. Data is analyzed to identify possible instances of COVID-19, and those who exhibit suspicious symptoms are urged to be tested [7,30].

7.10 Mobile Health Infrastructure on Blockchain (mHealth)

With an mHealth system, patients may get continuous monitoring, diagnosis, treatment, and therapy at a distance. However, there are major problems with health data privacy, security, and openness. One possibility is to implement blockchain technology. Due to their decentralized (no central authority required), immutable, traceable, and transparent nature, these technologies have found several applications in the healthcare sector; wearable sensors may communicate with a smart device that uses a peer-to-peer hypermedia protocol, the InterPlanetary File System (IPFS), for the decentralized storage of health-related data [31].

A blockchain-based framework for improving the security, privacy, and efficiency of mobile health (mHealth) systems is defined. The mHealth systems can potentially transform healthcare delivery but also present significant security and privacy challenges. The framework uses blockchain to store and manage health data, ensuring it remains secure and tamper-proof. The smart contracts are to automate some processes of managing health data, such as consent management and data sharing. The suggestion on the framework could support new applications, such as personalized medicine and population health management. The advantages of integrating blockchain technology in health systems include better data interchange and higher security and privacy. It could be used in various mHealth applications, such as telemedicine, health monitoring, and information exchange [31,32].

The medical data is saved distributively via the IPFS protocol, increasing data availability and redundancy, because blockchain activities are costly to store and process. Typically, a client–server approach would be used to construct a remote, web-based monitoring system, with the data saved in a centralized database. When a server fails or is attacked by a third party, this centralized approach is vulnerable to data loss [33].

7.11 Benefits of Blockchain

There are several advantages of using blockchain technology in healthcare, including the following:

- **Comprehensive coverage**. It offers a methodical and thorough review of the research on potential applications of blockchain technology in health maintenance.
- **High-quality analysis**. The creators used quality evaluation apparatuses to evaluate the quality of the included things, improving the discoveries' unwavering quality.
- **Practical implications**. It gives insights into the practical blockchain applications in maintaining health, which can inform the creation of real-world solutions to address difficulties connected to the COVID-19 epidemic and beyond.
- **Collaborative effort**. It was written by a team of experts from multiple institutions, enhancing the review's breadth and depth.
- **Timeliness**. Given that the COVID-19 pandemic has brought attention to the need for secure and effective healthcare data sharing and management, this article addresses a crucial and timely issue [29,34].

7.11.1 Challenges on Blockchain

The two main problems with Bitcoin are the need for interoperability and scalability. Blockchain has a limited storage capacity, so having many connection data would significantly reduce its efficiency. Off-chain holding methods would greatly reduce the burden of keeping off the blockchain. Technology can benefit some people more than others, particularly the youth. That can impact any system, but there are ways to incorporate them. Thanks to various cutting-edge technologies, they can use any system now, including movable IoT and smart technology [13,35]. Some potential limitations include the following:

- **Limited scope**. It focuses mainly on the uses of blockchain applications in healthcare during and after COVID-19 and may not cover other potential uses or applications of blockchain in healthcare.
- **Potential publication bias**. It is based on published studies, which may be subject to publication bias and may not capture unpublished studies or studies in progress.
- **Heterogeneity of studies.** The studies included in the review are heterogeneous in terms of study design, study population, and methodology, which may limit the generalizability of the findings.
- **Lack of quantitative analysis**. It is primarily qualitative and does not provide a meta-analysis or quantitative synthesis of the findings.

- **Lack of empirical evidence.** It highlights the potential uses of blockchain in healthcare, but more empirical evidence is needed to fully understand these applications' effectiveness and feasibility. Significant research and development would be needed to translate these theoretical possibilities into practical solutions. This technique consumes a lot of electricity since each transaction requires powerful hardware resources. The major problem with this technology is its inability to scale. It is because verifying that most nodes have approved the transaction takes time. Other disadvantages include blockchain's complexity and the need for an extensive user network. Another formidable obstacle is in ensuring users' privacy prior to the introduction of this technology.
- **Vulnerability analysis.** Data security is crucial for any company that values its success. The program must be safe and free of flaws that could lead to financial damage in the future. The code needs to be tested extensively to guarantee its completeness and safety. A wide variety of security study programs provides this code-testing capacity. The Oyente smart contract auto-audit tool examines smart contracts and reflects on possible defect attacks, like the well-known security attack. In January 2016, scientists from the National University of Singapore developed this. It provides studies with various features that verify the presence of security threats [5,35].

7.12 Conclusion

The studies mentioned earlier indicate that implementing blockchain technology can enhance disease surveillance systems, streamline the sharing of medical information, and furnish reliable contact tracing mechanisms. Integrating blockchain technology, artificial intelligence, and IoT can enhance the efficacy of pandemic response efforts. The utilization of IoT devices can provide instantaneous data regarding the dissemination of diseases, whereas AI has the potential to facilitate the prompt identification and forecasting of pandemics. Integrating blockchain with other emerging technologies, such as edge computing and 5G networks, may lead to additional applications in pandemic response. Issues about privacy and the necessity for regulatory frameworks to govern the utilization of blockchain technology in the healthcare sector are among the persistent obstacles. Utilizing blockchain technology in pandemic response efforts presents a promising avenue for enhancing global health outcomes, rendering it a beautiful area of research. Additional research in this domain has the potential to facilitate the development of enhanced pandemic response frameworks, thereby safeguarding individuals and societies globally.

References

1. Bleem B, Renaud J, Nguyen TTT, Bandyopadhayay S, Bandyopadhayay A, Mitra R. Anonymized blockchain-based infection tracking for disease control. In: *2021 IEEE Applied Imagery Pattern Recognition Workshop* (AIPR). 2021. pp. 1–4. https://doi.org/10.3991/ijoe.v18i06.29919.

2. Peng S, Bai L, Xiong L, Qu Q, Xie X, Wang S. GeoAI-based epidemic control with geo-social data sharing on blockchain. In: *2020 IEEE International Conference on E-health Networking, Application \& Services (HEALTHCOM)*. 2021. pp. 1–6.
3. Sharma A, Bahl S, Bagha AK, Javaid M, Shukla DK, Haleem A. Blockchain technology and its applications to combat COVID-19 pandemic. *Res Biomed Eng*. 2020;1–8.
4. Haleem A, Javaid M, Singh RP, Suman R, Rab S. Blockchain technology applications in healthcare: An overview. *Int J Intell Netw*. 2021;2:130–9.
5. Baz M, Khatri S, Baz A, Alhakami H, Agrawal A, Khan RA. Blockchain and artificial intelligence applications to defeat COVID-19 pandemic. *Comput Syst Sci Eng*. 2022;691–702.
6. Chattu VK, Nanda A, Chattu SK, Kadri SM, Knight AW. The emerging role of blockchain technology applications in routine disease surveillance systems to strengthen global health security. *Big Data Cogn Comput*. 2019;3(2):25.
7. Alam T, Benaida M. *Internet of Things and Blockchain-Based Framework for Coronavirus (COVID-19) Disease*. 2022. Available from: https://doi.org/10.3991/ijoe.v18i06.29919.
8. Capraz S, Özsoy A. A review of blockchain based solutions for fight against pandemics. In: *2021 6th International Conference on Computer Science and Engineering (UBMK)*. 2021. pp. 1–6. https://doi.org/10.1109/UBMK52708.2021.9558911.
9. Nguyen DC, Ding M, Pathirana PN, Seneviratne A. Blockchain and AI-based solutions to combat coronavirus (COVID-19)-like epidemics: A survey. *IEEE Access*. 2021;9:95730–53.
10. Chang MC, Park D. How can blockchain help people in the event of pandemics such as the COVID-19? *J Med Syst*. 2020;44:1–2.
11. Chang MC, Park D. How should rehabilitative departments of hospitals prepare for coronavirus disease 2019? *Am J Phys Med & Rehabil*. 2020;99(6):475–6.
12. Casino F, Dasaklis TK, Patsakis C. A systematic literature review of blockchain-based applications: Current status, classification and open issues. *Telemat Informatics*. 2019;36:55–81.
13. Vujičić D, Jagodic D, Ranđić S. Blockchain technology, bitcoin, and Ethereum: A brief overview. In: *2018 17th International Symposium on INFOTEH-JAHORINA, INFOTEH 2018-Proceedings*. 2018. https://doi.org/10.1109/INFOTEH.2018.8345547.
14. Bahl S, Javaid M, Bagha AK, Singh RP, Haleem A, Vaishya R, et al. Biosensors applications in fighting COVID-19 pandemic. *Apollo Med*. 2020;17(3):221.
15. Bansal A, Garg C, Padappayil RP. Optimizing the implementation of COVID-19 "immunity certificates" using blockchain. *J Med Syst*. 2020;44:1–2.
16. Gupta M, Patel RB, Jain S. Lightweight security framework for IoT enabled tracking of COVID-19 and its variants. In: *2021 2nd International Conference on Computational Methods in Science & Technology (ICCMST)*. 2021. pp. 287–92. https://doi.org/10.1109/ICCMST54943.2021.00066.
17. Zhang J, Xue N, Huang X. A secure system for pervasive social network-based healthcare. *IEEE Access*. 2016;4:9239–50.
18. Dey T, Jaiswal S, Sunderkrishnan S, Katre N. HealthSense: A medical use case of Internet of Things and blockchain. In: *2017 International conference on intelligent sustainable systems (ICISS)*. 2017. pp. 486–91.
19. Otoum S, Al Ridhawi I, Mouftah HT. Preventing and controlling epidemics through blockchain-assisted ai-enabled networks. *IEEE Netw*. 2021;35(3):34–41.
20. Torky M, Goda E, Snasel V, Hassanien AE. COVID-19 contact tracing and detection-based on blockchain technology. In: *Informatics*. 2021. p. 72. https://doi.org/10.3390/informatics8040072.
21. Bari N, Qamar U, Khalid A. Efficient contact tracing for pandemics using blockchain. *Inform Med Unlocked*. 2021;26:100742.
22. Khezr S, Moniruzzaman M, Yassine A, Benlamri R. Blockchain technology in healthcare: A comprehensive review and directions for future research. *Appl Sci*. 2019;9(9):1736.
23. Kumar T, Ramani V, Ahmad I, Braeken A, Harjula E, Ylianttila M. Blockchain utilization in healthcare: Key requirements and challenges. In: *2018 IEEE 20th International Conference on E-Health Networking, Applications and Services (Healthcom)*. 2018. pp. 1–7. https://doi.org/10.1109/HealthCom.2018.8531136.
24. Zhu P, Hu J, Zhang Y, Li X. Enhancing traceability of infectious diseases: A blockchain-based approach. *Inf Process & Manag*. 2021;58(4):102570.
25. Anderson RM, Heesterbeek H, Klinkenberg D, Hollingsworth TD. How will country-based mitigation measures influence the course of the COVID-19 epidemic? *Lancet*. 2020;395(10228):931–4.

26. Behnaminia F, Samet S. Blockchain technology applications in patient tracking systems regarding privacy-preserving concerns and COVID-19 pandemic. *Int J Inf Commun Eng.* 2023;17(2):144–56.
27. Xu H, Zhang L, Onireti O, Fang Y, Buchanan WJ, Imran MA. BeepTrace: Blockchain-enabled privacy-preserving contact tracing for COVID-19 pandemic and beyond. *IEEE Internet Things J.* 2020;8(5):3915–29.
28. Khatoon A. *Use of Blockchain Technology to Curb Novel Coronavirus Disease (COVID-19) Transmission.* Available SSRN 3584226. 2020.
29. Ng WY, Tan T-E, Movva PVH, Fang AH Sen, Yeo K-K, Ho D, et al. Blockchain applications in health care for COVID-19 and beyond: A systematic review. *Lancet Digit Heal.* 2021;3(12):e819–29.
30. Kumar A, Gupta PK, Srivastava A. A review of modern technologies for tackling COVID-19 pandemic. *Diabetes & Metab Syndr Clin Res & Rev.* 2020;14(4):569–73.
31. Taralunga DD, Florea BC. A blockchain-enabled framework for mhealth systems. *Sensors.* 2021;21(8):2828.
32. Tripathi G, Ahad MA, Paiva S. S2HS- A blockchain based approach for smart healthcare system. *Healthcare.* 2020;8(1):100391.
33. Tian S, Yang W, Le Grange JM, Wang P, Huang W, Ye Z. Smart healthcare: Making medical care more intelligent. *Glob Heal J.* 2019;3(3):62–5.
34. Gunasekeran DV, Tseng RMWW, Tham Y-C, Wong TY. Applications of digital health for public health responses to COVID-19: A systematic scoping review of artificial intelligence, telehealth and related technologies. *NPJ Digit Med.* 2021;4(1):40.
35. Syed TA, Alzahrani A, Jan S, Siddiqui MS, Nadeem A, Alghamdi T. A comparative analysis of blockchain architecture and its applications: Problems and recommendations. *IEEE Access.* 2019;7:176838–69.

8

Postmortem Concentrations: Distributed Privacy-Preserving Blockchain Authentication Framework in Cloud Forensics

Rohit Kaushik and Eva Kaushik

8.1 Introduction

Due to the blockchain's cost-effectiveness and modesty, many small businesses provide processing power and storage space to cloud storage. Each block contains the previous block's crypto-hash, time stamps, and transaction information. Blockchain is a growing collection of records connected by encryption, known as blocks. Blockchain can give immutability, ability to track, transparency, auditing ability, and accountability in addition to its security and immutable nature of the cryptographic hash linkages between blocks and instances. The gain of employing a blockchain system in digital forensics is that the administrator can supply authentication, upon which he can access digital evidence, which successfully builds verifiable evidence chains with hash functions [1]. To confirm the immutable nature, visibility, and public trust within the case examination, the blockchain uses encryption. The process of verifying that any reasonable evidence has been collected, tracked, and protected with the help of a court of law is known as the forensic report. A required stage in the forensic analysis may be the forensic report. Although it is frequently used as evidence, it must be proven that it was not tampered with during investigations for it to be accepted in a court or in legal proceedings [2][3]. Therefore, regardless of whether the evidence is used in court or not, a decent process should be followed for routine dealing and management of evidence (whether digital or not). The main branches of digital forensics are shown in Figure 8.1.

In today's situation, crime rate is high, and once it's ever-changing, the post-mortem report is quite straightforward. Cybercrime is currently emerging as one of the major crimes. The investigation will therefore go via several hierarchical levels using digital evidence. It plays a crucial function in preserving the accuracy and integrity of each document, providing transparency, and giving information clarity without tampering with the papers in the blockchain system. Their area unit has numerous strategies adopted to end life. Be it hanging, gunshot, cyanide, and forensic toxicology (poison consumption). The recreation of a crime scene after an occurrence can be challenging, because some evidence is left behind that helps investigators find the crime. For a proper analysis to be reached, it

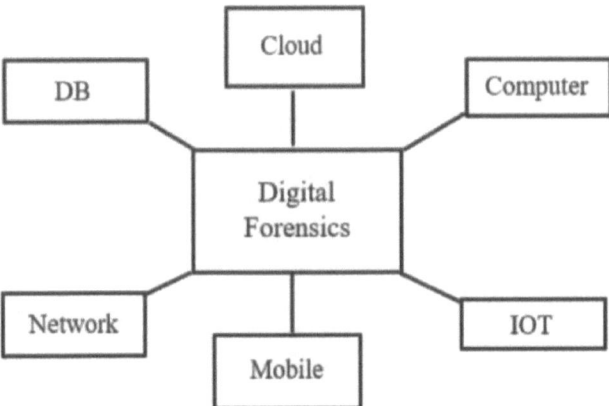

FIGURE 8.1
Main branches of digital forensics.

needs the investigation officer's skill and rhetorical understanding. To identify replicated crime scenes, meticulous analysis of the crime scene at the following points as well as an autopsy study are necessary. As numerous pieces of evidence are found at a crime scene, keep an eye out for them [4]. Drawing or image-depicting the scenario: with the suspension in place, inspection of the hanging material (noose, knot, loop, etc.); documentation of the support needed to achieve the hanging goal, ante-mortem examination of ligature material (rope) and direction of fiber on victim's body/neck; selection of swab from close to the injury (nail mark); examining the chest/throat for fingerprints and hanging-related postmortem signs; drug or alcohol use; gun fingerprints; a body shot area; and other factors evidence of dragging; suicide letter and telephone call to review decision-making history; case history, etc. When determining the cause of death, the forensic pathologist must be cautious because criminals have been known to disguise homicides as suicides in the past. The forensic pathologist's role in determining the manner of gunshot death is highlighted in the case under consideration. The downward particle distribution of the body was visible on a chest X-ray. Chest injuries caused by pellets fired from a smoothbore firearm were the cause of death. As a result of these ongoing cybercrimes that take place in the modern digital era, this proof includes a critical component of cybernetic evidence that verifies the original evidence and the evidence's relationship to the cybercrimes. It has a significant issue with Internet evidence. Managing and tracking digital evidence is done according to a custody chain approach [5]. As a result, several hierarchical layers, or top-to-bottom companies, process the forensic evidence to handle cybercrime investigations. Procedure for a cloud forensic analysis and identification: different forensic tools are shown in Table 8.1.

- The two most important procedures during the initial stage of digital forensics, case identification, are gathering data and recognizing occurrences. These two stages are essential for demonstrating the case scenario occurrence.
- The second phase is the gathering and preservation of evidence from various digital devices, such as a mobile phone, an email account, a hard drive, and other different types of digital media. The data is then secured for future processing while maintaining its integrity [6]. The security of the evidence gathered during a criminal investigation will be improved as we work to overcome

TABLE 8.1

Forensic Tools

Forensic Equipment	Information
Memory	It's been utilized to acquire the possible remains in the computer memory when no data is left on a hard drive or being erased (e.g., volatility).
Digital	It's being taken into consideration majorly to retrieve the evidence from the computer. It contains preservation, data retrieval, and identification (e.g. SANS toolkit and forensics).
Mobile devices	Evidence that is on any mobile device; nowadays, communication has made various advancements in portable devices (e.g., AXIOM and XRY, etc.).

numerous obstacles, including hacking. The evidence is kept in a safe place so that no unauthorized individuals can access it. This innovation will double the system's security.

- Examining and analyzing the devices for evidence as digital hints is part of the third stage, which is organizing the evidence. To begin, the investigator gathers the data for the case's investigation and examines the data's characteristics. In the second step, analysis, the investigator examines and connects the data to determine the truth and determine whether the evidence is conclusive.
- Presentation. The investigator then creates reports based on the investigation's findings and updates them as necessary with supporting documentation before presenting them before the court.

8.2 Problem Statement

It has been noted that forensic reports are altered frequently while an inquiry is underway. Data in forensic reports may change due to unrecognized sources. Most of the time, as a result, the needy may not receive justice, and the verdict may not be fair. Therefore, it is imperative to create a system that guarantees the security of forensics reports from the point at which they are generated to the point at which they are used in legal proceedings.

8.3 Literature Review

1. Blockchain increases trust and transparency; it has primarily been employed in the forensics of medicine. Digital evidence, which was established earlier, will play a crucial part in a blockchain-based forensic system. Numerous uses of blockchain technology are being employed to collect proof of the theory. Our database is regularly checked for alteration using a single one-way hash code and notarial service, which is regularly utilized both internally and externally. The external service, which is more trustworthy, needs to verify our network, whereas the internal service is primarily contained within the database system itself. This process

is divided into two stages: processing (during which the tuple's hash values are retrieved and notarized), as well as verification (during which all the hashes are determined repeatedly and verified with the most recent attested values) [7][8]. The presence of tampering is evident if there is any contradiction between these values. Through the blockchain system, we may discreetly monitor financial accounting systems when fraud, or the altering of accounting data, occurs. We can simply apprehend the individual who attempted to access and alter the account's data. So in this system, we can incorporate both the public and private sectors as well as the government of India institutions. The use of a blockchain system will be a protected area for owners; nevertheless, fraudulent or manipulators may use it as a means of continuing their criminal activity without being caught.

2. Investigations using digital forensics are no longer solely technical in nature. Aspects of business, systems, and law are included. The authors have developed a thorough, business- and legally oriented digital forensic framework [9]. It, as a result, developed an entirely crime-oriented architecture that will help with crime investigation.

3. Exploratory forensics on the smart contract's forensic investigation framework in this study considered a variety of tools, evidence items, data formats, and other factors. According to the study's author, hackers exploit IoT devices and other sources to steal information, and to combat this, they employ blockchain technology to create a framework for storing data and thwarting it using a variety of tactics. While we propose a framework that will aid in the prosecution of crimes like murder, they mainly focus on preventing hackers from accessing the Internet of Things.

8.4 Background of Related Work

1. **Kent, P., et al. [10].** Blockchain is a type of distributed database or ledger—one of today's top tech trends—which means the power to update a blockchain is distributed between the nodes, or participants, of a public or private computer network. Blockchain analysis is a brand-new area of study and development that only recently became popular among Bitcoin enthusiasts in 2014. This movement was primarily pushed by its decentralized and transparent nature.

2. **Akinbi, A., et al. [11].** In regard to the recognition algorithms, they first draw attention to the distinction between system characterization, which refers to the capabilities of the technology being used and the characterization of the forensic system that will give the court objective results.

3. **Bain, T., et al. [12].** Blockchains store information on monetary transactions using cryptocurrencies, but they also store other types of information, such as product tracking and other data. The review includes user access management, smart cards, mobile security, Internet/web-based security, forensics, and other existing and potential uses in an e-world. Additionally, each chapter includes an outline that explains how the book is organized.

4. **Jaquet-Chiffelle et al. [13].** Blockchain technology can store linked information in the context of a decentralized platform within a peer-to-peer (P2P) network because it is a decentralized network that depends on ledger-based transactions.

The information is kept in blocks with time stamps that are connected in an unbreakable chain, resulting in an audit system that is unchangeable, open to the public, and confirmed by a consensus-based proof-of-work.

5. **Zhihuang, W., et al. [14]**. The production and presentation of architectural evidence—relating to buildings, urban environments—within legal and political processes. The report also discusses the numerous forensics categories. The study went into the problems with forensic architecture, how to fix them, and the proper solutions They raised knowledge of cloud forensics and its issues, types of forensic techniques, and cloud architecture.
6. **Chandana, M., et al. [15]**. The authors devised the LOS algorithm to streamline the forensics procedure and proposed an upgrade composed of a number to increase the security of current digital forensics and blockchain. This algorithm enhances traceability and decreases complications.

8.5 Methodology

This suggested approach aids in reducing the amount of time needed to process an online portal. With this method, technology is used to achieve transparency, and the client can always keep track of the procedure. Hashing is used in this process to create immutability, making it impossible for anyone to alter the data stored in each node. Smart contracts are utilized to prevent delays when resolving the lawsuit. It is a safe and reliable system that aims for high quality. This work contributes to the development of a system that introduces a case study that safeguards victim reports and limits report tampering by various nodes.

It also contributes to the creation of a transparent environment for the processing of reports. Blockchain technology offers a fresh and creative perspective on how forensic applications can be used. The gathering of data, improving the data, validating the data, analyzing the data, preserving the evidence, and presenting the findings have numerous advantages for the investigative process [11]. By providing high-level consistency, openness, assurance of authenticity, and security, as well as the ability to audit digital evidence to achieve the desired purpose, blockchain digital forensic work in academic and professional fields has a significant opportunity to significantly improve forensic applications. The mechanism of forensic system with blockchain is presented in Figure 8.2.

The forensics lab will produce a victim's forensic report and transmit it to the physician or hospital. Reports are now delivered through email or copy, and the physician or any other authority can readily alter them. On the distributed and immutable blockchain network, we will post the forensic report under the proposed approach, though. The blockchain is a tremendously safe network that cannot be breached or altered. In the case that a node fails, we can also easily retrieve the data because it is stored in a dispersed manner.

The second node of the suggested system is the hospital. The diagnostics lab delivers the forensic report to the hospital. The hospital then designates a specific doctor to review the report, append his digital signature, and forward it to the law enforcement officer for extra investigation. It is hard for the doctor to modify the report since the pathology lab staff uploads it to the network using a 16-digit cryptographic hash that is static by nature [12]. The hash code changes if the report is attempted to be modified. Since the hash code should remain constant during the inquiry, we may identify the offender by determining through which node it was modified. The report is kept by the hospital in its ledger.

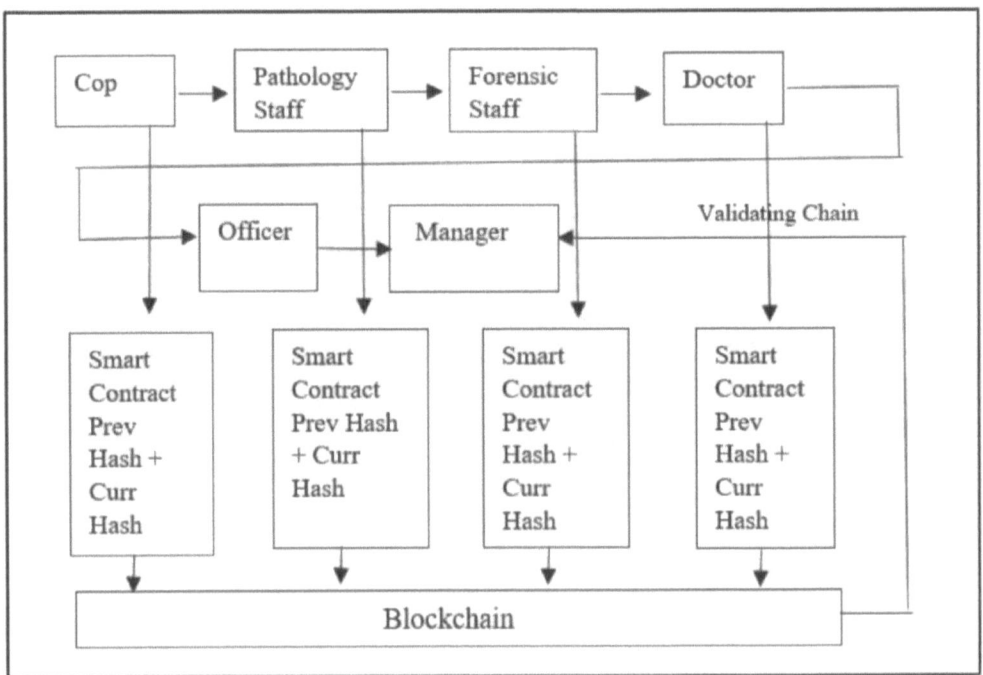

FIGURE 8.2
Mechanism of forensic system with blockchain.

The third element of the suggested system is the police department. A forensic report that has been digitally signed by the doctor will be given to the police force. The police force will then choose a policeman, whose inquiry will be based on the report. Information about the deceased who had previously been thoroughly examined and verified in the pathological lab report that has been evaluated by a doctor is provided to police detectives. As a result, the cop's job is made easier, because he only needs to focus on the investigation. If the policeman tries to edit the report, the report's hash code will be altered once more, and the policeman will be recognized because the third node is where the hash is changed.

The last node in the proposed methodology is the final report. The actual transfer record and the scope of the forensic investigation are both visible to the blockchain network administrator. The report is vandalized since it has not been attempted to be modified if the hash code obtained when the forensic lab posted the report to the Internet is static across the network. If the checksum has changed across the network, it also indicates that the report has been modified. So because the system is split up into nodes, he can easily identify the offender by following which server the digest was modified.

8.5.1 Modules

1. *Admittance management.* He or she will oversee supervising other users, including police officers, forensic experts, higher-ranking officers, and medical professionals. He or she may also name the nearest police station, the forensic team, higher officers, and physicians. He can also modify his username by typing his previous password into the interface of this module.

2. *Psychopathic officer.* The police officer receives input from all departments in this node. An officer is chosen by the department to examine a specific crime after analyzing the forensic report. The police receive all the information about the criminal or victim through the reports when the doctors successfully validate them. Therefore, the research component as well as validation and verification are trusted thanks to blockchain technology [13][14]. The hash code generated will change if somebody tries to change the data that has been collected. Chaining has allowed for its traceability. Constancy is also possible in this police department. They will have information on the crime, register it, and allow him to access forensic, pathology, and medical reports as well as add crime case logs.
3. *Crime scene staff.* They will investigate the scene of the crime, discover the samples there, and then add a description of the forensic information to produce a report.
4. *Medical staff.* Then, after carefully examining the victim's body, the examiner will write a forensic statement and transmit it to the doctor. All reports are now delivered by email or hard copy, which the physician can simply alter using a variety of techniques. As a result, once the forensic report is included, this predicted approach to the public blockchain becomes unremovable. The data can still be retrieved quickly even if one of the nodes fails, because the information is stored in a distributed fashion.
5. *Doctor.* It was created as a different kind of node in this system. The report will be examined by a specialized hospital doctor. The pathologist and forensic department's report, which was produced, is provided to the physician. Before appending their digital signature, the designated doctor confirms the data that was gathered. Therefore, he is free to read all this research and compile a summary based on their findings [15].
6. *Superior officer.* It will be straightforward for them to discover offenders who need to be brought up in front of the law for penalties, since they will check each report that is generated in their departments and can then carry out an investigation depending on those reports.

8.6 Key Terminologies

1. *Block.* Transactions are condensed into single blocks, and a fresh block of approximately 1 MB size is generated every ten minutes. In a blockchain, each block has four parts: a time stamp, a reference to the block before it, a description of the transaction it includes, and the proof-of-work [16]. Editing a block without changing the subsequent blocks is impossible, according to secure hashing. Due to two factors, no one can just join the Bitcoin network and carry out a successful transfer for millions of dollars: (1) each block requires many independent confirmations, and (2) specialized miners are needed to solve the mathematical formulas for the cryptographic challenges.
2. *Mining.* Mining is the process of validating transactions before adding their records to the blockchain ledger. It requires doing mathematical calculations on sophisticated hardware to validate transactions. Computer miners only add transactions to a secure block after first confirming their legitimacy. A blockchain is created by combining these blocks, which represent information that is in sync

across all blocks [17]. Every time a secure block is generated, a new hash is generated, and miners are paid with Bitcoins and transaction fees for each transaction they successfully confirm.

3. *Spending twice. Double spending* refers to sending a Bitcoin transaction to two separate receivers simultaneously. At all costs, you should avoid this.
4. *Proof-of-work (PoW).* Proof-of-work is a requirement that expensive computations be done to permit transactions. PoW was created to support the trustless consensus. A PoW is a block that has been hashed.
5. *Hashcash.* A PoW is an example, such as Hashcash. The PoW function of hash is used by Bitcoin. Hashcash is a PoW method that generates data that is challenging to produce computationally but simple to verify by others. For each block, miners are required to generate a hash and a "nonce number" to generate a hash with the necessary number of leading zero bits to satisfy the difficulty requirement.
6. *Nodes.* The network's nodes are dispersed computers that each hold a copy of the whole blockchain. Copies of the blockchain and access to it are disseminated as new users join the blockchain network. All the nodes in the various networks can replicate, synchronize, and share the data. There is no single node or network that has control over the data.
7. *Address.* The network's nodes are dispersed computers that each hold a copy of the whole blockchain. Copies of the blockchain and access to it are disseminated as new users join the blockchain network. All the nodes in the various networks can replicate, synchronize, and share the data. There is no single node or network that has control over the data.
8. *Smart contract.* An unchangeable, digital contract known as a *smart contract* is one that is kept on the blockchain. It specifies some logical requirements that must be met to carry out tasks, like depositing money or data [18][19]. Criteria for transferring funds to a third-party delivery team, for instance: consider a situation where a sender wants to use a third party to deliver products to a recipient, but only when the delivery is successful. Then, a smart contract might look like this: On the day when the products are loaded, the sender makes the shipment payment. Until the recipient acknowledges to the sender that the products have been received, the smart contract will withhold payment to the delivery crew.

8.7 Cloud Forensics Challenges

8.7.1 Technical

1. *Accessing logs.* The standard method of computer investigation for locating a cybercrime entails locating the log data of each action performed on the devices and then evaluating them to discover the evidence [20]. The fact that the archives reside on a distant, unidentified server makes this application of cloud computing architecture special. With cloud computing, fetching logs becomes challenging.
2. *Gathering reliable data.* The process is intended to ensure that the information contains reliable data that may be used as proof in court. As several users share the same physical location, it is very challenging to guarantee the confidentiality of data in the cloud.

3. Another significant issue with cloud forensics is the *existence of huge quantities of information* that need to be analyzed to find evidence. The traditional forensics approaches are incompatible with such enormous quantities of data. During the investigating processes, the provider of cloud services must comply.

8.7.2 Procedural

1. *Recreating the crime scene.* In some cases, the investigation process calls for re-enacting the entire criminal enterprise to find the evidence. All the actions taken at the crime scene are repeated and simulated during this process [21][22]. Cloud computing makes this more challenging because clouds are maintained as virtual machines that may be deleted after a crime to remove all traces of it and make room for recreation.
2. *Multinational laws.* The investigations are carried out in accordance with the laws of the nations where the crimes are committed. Since cloud data centers are located all over the world, many rules must be complied with when conducting investigations in the case of cloud forensics.
3. *Presentation of the evidence in court.* The case inquiry calls for the presentation of the evidence in court. It's possible that the jury members are unfamiliar with the complicated cloud computing models [23]. So presenting the evidence becomes a difficult task in cloud forensics.
4. *Crime scene reconstruction.* To investigate harmful activities, investigators often need to recreate the crime scene. Using traditional digital forensics, the investigator can quickly determine how many devices were involved in the crime or who committed it [24][25]. Reconstructing the crime scene and determining the extent of the damage is nearly impossible due to the extremely dynamic nature of the real-time, autonomous interaction in the cloud environment between multiple nodes.
5. *Evidence segregation.* In the cloud, virtualization allows for the isolation of various instances running on a single physical machine. Even though their data instances are stored on the same system, different users behave as though they are running on distinct hosts. Because of this, it is extremely challenging for CSPs and law enforcement agencies to tell them apart during investigations without endangering the anonymity of other entities who use the technology [26].
6. *Lack of user statistics anonymity.* Most cloud service providers adhere to user-friendly standards and request minimal data from clients [27]. Due to the limited information provided by the sparse user data, it is challenging for the detective to identify the guilty party.
7. *Data origin.* Unlike investigations involving traditional digital forensics, cloud-based data may originate from thousands of different user locations, making it challenging to identify who or what created and/or altered the data item there. The data's source is thus less clear.
8. *Data privacy and a lack of accountability.* In cloud services are issues that are normally handled by IaaS providers, like Cloud Servers, AWS, Microsoft Azure, iCloud, and numerous others [28]. However, a few services use common keys for disk encryption and archiving.
9. *Less control.* As opposed to digital forensics, where the investigator has more control over the access level to cloud devices, cloud forensics depends on the various service models.

8.7.3 Custody Forensic

8.7.3.1 Security, Efficiency, and Scalability Costs

The expense associated with the security management and efficacy in the chain of custody for evidence in the case is one of the main obstacles to the implementation of a blockchain network. The design enables provenance and transparency by continuously growing the distributed ledger as transactions are completed and case data from all parties are added. This enables everyone engaged, regardless of who oversaw the acts, to examine relevant case-related material at the same time [29]. Each participant's fear of sharing their operating records with the other peer group members is removed by Hyperledger.

8.7.3.2 A Lack of Uniformity

Multimedia forensics research systems employ a wide range of case investigation approaches, which add to the inconsistent chain of custody for media evidence. Digital forensics' process layer, which includes gathering evidence and preserving it, is less trustworthy. This has inescapable negative effects and offers inconsistently poor quality. Design enforces a consistent approach and raises the standard of the final product by standardizing the forensics processes. The process flow of digital forensic is shown in Figure 8.3.

8.7.3.3 Issue with Record Transparency

One of the main problems is providing data accessibility (chain of custody) in a scattered setting. We have designed Sawtooth's fully decentralized ledger verification and transaction method, as well as its consensus verification policy (PoET), to provide a solid architecture for privacy protection and security, since Sawtooth is unable to give a predetermined data transparency policy. This can also assist us in developing an architecture for forensic chain-of-custody investigations that upholds the openness and traceability of data and evidence [30][31]. We provide systems with effective document monitoring and proof administration at every layer of the smart contract by utilizing the hyper-blockchain modular platform. In comparison to the conventional technique, its comprehensive design offers superior chain security management, a better activity record case, and better outcomes.

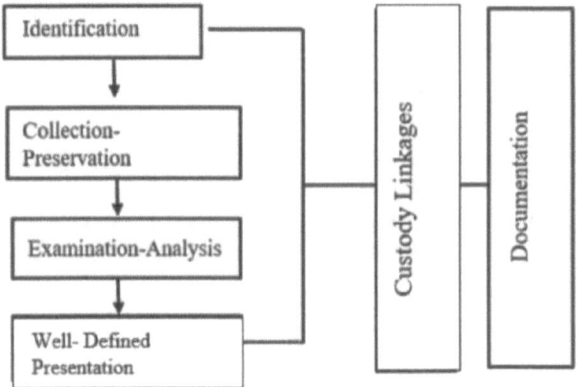

FIGURE 8.3
Digital forensic process flow.

8.7.3.4 Distributed Storage Problems and Concerns in the Chain of Custody

Because there is no viable defense against attacks using the traditional chain of custody administration, the only alternative for evidence retention is central storage, which exposes data and leaves the evidence open to modification or falsification. To overcome these constraints, we have created file coin global storage systems that interface with the suggested Sawtooth architecture and employment contracts to automatically collect, identify, inspect, analyze, report, and keep data [32]. These distributed applications use a digital contract-based method that helps the judicial process and the media forensics authority safeguard the chain of custody as well as the integrity of the evidence.

8.7.3.5 Problems with Regulatory Compliance

The normal chain of custody for collecting multimedia evidence has issues with mistakes in digital case activities, especially when records are kept on a central server and reliance is placed on external security solutions. Also, the information from portable video cameras is collected using poor and unreliable technologies before being examined and processed using various forensics techniques.

8.8 Concepts in Cloud Forensics

There are several concepts that can help identify alternative sources of evidence and significantly assist scientists working in this field, such as cloud crime types and where to conduct investigations in/on the cloud [33].

8.8.1 Kind of Crime

In that it is recognized as a crime in cloud computing, any crime committed utilizing the cloud as an object, topic, or instrument is comparable to computer crimes. Cloud computing becomes an important topic when the CSP has been the target of criminal activities, including distributed denial-of-service (DDoS) attacks, when crimes like identity theft, which happened in the Google case, are committed via the cloud environment. The cloud is finally seen as a tool when it is utilized to attack the system of another provider, such as when a dark cloud is deployed.

8.8.2 Conducting Investigations

A case supported by cloud-based evidence is known as an "in" cloud inquiry in the cloud building. Businesses must understand a CSP's incident response approach, which includes issue identification, notification, and recovery, to meet the use of contemporary digital forensics technology. Snapshots give a picture of the systems at a particular moment. It can be considered an important source of proof for services delivered by dispersed or virtual systems. Nonetheless, it is important to assess the snapshot's authenticity for forensics, given the current ways of acquiring it. As a precaution, cloud users should check whether their online reality snapshots are accessible offline and consider the frequency of these snapshots [34][35]. For instance, Elastic Compute Cloud and Amazon Elastic Block Storage (EBS) Boot Volume both offer block-level storage services (EC2). The user storage is available as snapshots via the EBS. A snapshot from a cyberattack can be later examined offline without affecting the original storage or interfering with operations. As mentioned, recording volatile data will cause modifications to the target system when examiners must access "live" systems. From our perspective, preserving an audit trail of the examiners' actions while also taking a consistent snapshot of an operational system.

8.8.3 Performing Investigation on Cloud

Recently, Dell made a forensics-as-a-service offering available. Before employing the data center's capability to image physically taken goods, Dell used the digital forensics process. A reasonable timeline of events should finally be able to be produced by the examiners. Petabytes of data cannot be photographed and analyzed, and seizing the services provider's servers will probably violate users' legitimate rights to privacy [36]. According to a speed test report from the AccessData Forensics Toolkit (FTK), it would take roughly 5.5 hours to examine a 120 GB hard drive utilizing top-of-the-line workstations. In line with that, evaluating a 2 TB hard disk would take roughly 85 hours.

8.9 Cloud Security

Before attempting to investigate the complexities of cloud forensics, it is necessary to comprehend cloud security. We go over the crucial concerns around cloud security in terms of cloud services' architecture and assaults on them.

8.9.1 Cloud Architecture

Cloud architectures are helpful for comprehending how different suggestions work together to offer a comprehensive solution [37]. Enterprises interested in cloud computing are advised to take the reference design into consideration, according to a white paper created jointly by VMware and Savvis.

The following security elements should be put in place:

1. Every level needs to have a defined security profile.
2. CSP is required to maintain the hardware and software inside a demilitarized zone (DMZ).
3. The management of operating systems and virtualization on a CSP must take place behind the DMZ.
4. The CSP is responsible for managing resource provisioning by isolating and separating VM resources.
5. Either router ACLs, a perimeter firewall, or web application security must be used to offer network security.

6. CSP must offer access routes to real-world servers that are authorized to perform the requested functionality.
7. The CSP is required to offer security authentication, authorization, and auditing (AAA).

8.9.2 Cloud Security Attacks

Some of the assaults that can occur in a cloud computing environment include the following:

1. *Wrapping attack.* When a user sends a request from his virtual machine to the browser, a SOAP (Simple Object Access Protocol) message is produced. The web server receives the request. The attackers conduct a wrapping attack by using a duplicate username and password during the login process to influence the SOAP messages sent between the web browser and server during the setup phase.
2. *Flooding attack.* The attacker creates false or harmful data, such as requests for resources or code to execute in an application. To process the virus requests, the server uses its CPU, memory, and other resources just like a genuine user would [38][39]. When the servers ultimately exhaust their capacity, they transfer the workload to another server, which causes flooding.
3. *Browser attack.* This attack compromises the signature and encryption of messages as they are transferred between the site and the web server, tricking the browser into recognizing an adversary as a legitimate user and executing all requests submitted to the web server.
4. *Malware-injection attack.* In this type of attack, the hacker creates a standard action, like deleting a user, and embeds another command, like setAdminRight, into it. Instead of following the user account deletion instructions when a user request is delivered to the server, the server divulges a user account to the attacker.
5. *Unsecured interfaces and APIs.* Businesses that provide cloud computing services make several software interfaces or APIs accessible for users to manage and interact with services that use the cloud. Reliance on a subpar set of interfaces might subject a business to certain security vulnerabilities concerning password security, availability, and secrecy [40].
6. *Rude site administrators.* The cloud services process is controlled, supervised, and maintained by site administrators. By default, they have access to all the data, papers, and restricted corporate assets. In revenge or for other reasons, administrators may wind up leaking or allowing the leak of critical information.
7. *Data theft.* One of the most serious unrecognized security flaws with virtualized data is that system administrators can take any amount of data without leaving a trail of proof. A virtual machine can be replicated with just three easy steps: logging in as the superintendent's administrator, mounting the disk image, and unmounting the original copy.
8. *Breach of data.* The term "data leakage" refers to the transfer of data from one client to another. When a customer deletes their disk and a new client starts a new drive, data leakage is a concern [41][42]. The physical disks again for old and new drives can have some overlapped portions. Hence, the new customer might attempt to image from written tons of data.

8.10 The Necessity of Digital Forensics

A digital forensic examination is a planned, methodical process used to identify, collect, examine, and present digital information for use as testimony in court. Maintaining a chain of custody throughout the electronic inquiry process is crucial for achieving that. For the digital evidence used in the inquiry to be admitted as evidence in a court of law, the chain of custody (CoC) protocol must be documented, recorded, and archived. Obviously, we need to stop CoC from being altered or destroyed. The end goal is to demonstrate that the information gathered is reliable, accurate, and pertinent to the conduct under investigation.

Because it can provide immutable blockchain technology for maintaining data blocks in a chain structure, blockchain has been widely embraced and employed in a range of security applications. This enables the storing of hashed encrypted data with electronic signatures on the permissionless public blockchain to prevent unwanted alterations [43]. Throughout the forensic investigation, the immutable ledger technology suggested in the blockchain architecture helps with the proper controls to manage and maintain digital information in a secure and accessible manner. The three key aspects of blockchain are as follows:

1. Anybody who joins the public blockchain and participates in accessing the events on the ledger has access to this technology. With an open application interface, consumers may utilize the public blockchain.

2. By relying on a global and decentralized P2P packet forwarding paradigm, where all parties involved have equal utilization of the system and participation rights, blockchain eliminates the requirement for a third platform and solution providers.

3. To create an immutable ledger for preserving the private information (evidence) crucial to the case being investigated, each block in a secured chain of blocks has an encrypted hash code that is derived from the hash of a transaction that was previously saved. We employ agreements, where all the fundamental functionality is defined and put into practice, to do this. The blocks are later stored in the ledger chain after being verified and approved.

A (suspected) security event must typically be investigated further, which may necessitate the gathering, evaluating, and interpreting of evidence. These findings may finally be provided in the form of expert reports, court proceedings, and testimony in any legal or civil procedures. This analysis may then help shape the interpretation and attribution. The procedures (including the instruments and methods used in the acquiring as well as analysis of evidence) and results of a digital forensic inquiry must be accurately documented in the investigative report for it to be admitted into evidence in a court of law, unlike most cyber safety incident investigations [44][45]. Yet the absence of defined procedures makes it challenging for forensic investigators, particularly those employed by local law enforcement organizations, to generate high-quality forensics reports that may be utilized as evidence in court cases. As a result, there are variations in the methods used to develop and convey forensic results to different stakeholders after an investigation is complete. While developing and putting into practice standardized methods and specifications for producing forensic reports, it is necessary to consider the vast range of procedures indicated in current investigation models and standards, such as the ISO/ISEC 27043:2015 international standard.

It is crucial to ensure a sound and accurate forensic document every step of the digital forensic analysis process in a forensic report to reduce the likelihood that evidence won't be accepted into evidence in a court of law. Conventional procedures in digital forensic inquiry are thus required to address the issues and discrepancies related to the creation and use of forensic findings in any court or legal proceedings. The fundamental objective of the ISO/IEC 27043 standard was to define and put into practice some standardized inquiry concepts and processes that would produce consistent outcomes for different investigators working in related situations. These guidelines must be followed by any forensic investigation procedure to be reproducible and repeatable. The ISO/IEC 27043 guideline also seeks to provide openness and simplicity in each procedure's results for each distinct procedure throughout the investigation process. It is vital to keep in mind that when writing a forensic report, it should accurately represent the scope of the digital evidence inquiry process [46]. The relevance of the digital forensic investigation must be expressly underlined at this point, because the information contained in the inquiry cannot be recovered without adhering to the established procedures. This makes it possible to inform pertinent parties about the inquiry in a transparent manner. The use of blockchain to guarantee the reliability of the data used in the report could also be investigated.

8.11 Case Studies

Detection of IOT intrusions

To identify potential threats in a network, intrusion detection systems frequently use anomaly-based techniques, the latter of which depends on monitoring the behavior of network devices. Detecting corrupted IoT devices is designed to help automatically detect anomalies in an IoT ecosystem by using an identity framework to categorize devices based on their categories and produce normal profiles that are then used to detect deviations. A privacy-preserving framework known as Siotome was designed to defend smart home environments from highly decentralized attacks by rogue IoT devices. By applying machine learning approaches to determine the ideal operational configurations, the scheme can monitor, detect, and evaluate IoT-based risks as well as provide a suitable security basis. Because of their frequent use for private and sensitive functions, which makes them particularly valuable and attractive targets for attackers, phones are a special kind of device in a smart home environment [47]. The investigation processes are done using part of this in the event of any crime scene, including the utilization of Internet of Things (IoT) devices to provide a suitable way for recognizing the evidence that can be submitted in court proceedings. Every forensic method used in the IoT setting usually follows a few standard investigative methods. The problem scenario must be established, information must be gathered, crime scenes must be investigated, and the evidence must be assessed. Among the approaches available for digital forensics inquiry is the extended model of cybercrime investigation (EMCI), abstract digital forensic model (ADFM), and computer forensics research workshop (CFRW). The confluence of these qualities emphasizes the necessity of an organized DF approach to occurrences. Direct access to items of forensic interest (OOFI) in the IoT domain (or appropriate, such as pacifiers) would not always be possible. This is the rationale behind the next best thing triage (NBT) strategy of approaching the Internet of Things investigations. Yet in these instances, it is necessary to identify and consider the next greatest source of pertinent evidence. It might be possible to develop a process for selecting what the next best thing is with the help of further research.

Public Transaction Ledger Solutions

Blockchain technology can be used in new platforms to support today's electronic forensic and incident response (DFIR). For instance, incident responders should be aware of the advantages these new "digital witnesses" (DW) can bring to aid in their inquiry. It is generally known that the Internet of Things (IoT) has increased intricacy in cyberspace. IoT device logs can help with event reconstruction, but their integrity and admissibility can only be achieved if a chain of custody (CoC) is maintained within the wider context of a current digital investigation. Stakeholder communication is enhanced in a similar way to how transitioning to electronic documentation improves data accessibility, readability, and note-taking capabilities. These data, however, could be fabricated in the absence of validating evidence. For instance, it is necessary to uphold many current (and new) laws and norms pertaining to authoring, auditing, and the security of patient history in an application field like eHealth. The absence of data control can result in system abuse, fraud, and serious service quality compromises. An online CoC can be implemented to allay these worries [48][49]. In this study, we explore the benefits and practical applications of integrating blockchain technology into contemporary DFIR systems. We show how blockchain technology benefits the use of digital evidence models and go through why police forces and event responders need to be familiar with it. Additionally, chronological recording is necessary for digital forensics to be admissible in a court of law. Hence, we talk about how a distributed ledger can support the CoC. To show the value of this strategy for introducing forensic preparedness to computer networks and enabling improved police interventions, we give a real-world example involving eHealth. In various applications, including eHealth industries and voting, blockchain has lately emerged as a groundbreaking technology to ensure increased security and privacy. A peer-to-peer network replicates a decentralized, shared, and tamper-proof record known as a blockchain. Bitcoin Blockchain was initially successfully employed in the virtual currency system Bitcoin. The fundamental data unit of the blockchain is a transaction. A certain number of transactions make up a block. Blockchain nodes broadcast the block to create the block's final hash code. Proof-of-work is the name given to this method.

Embezzlement Forensic Model

The environment of financial crime is changing as financial services become more digital. Laws and forensic procedures are unable to keep up with the rapid development of new technology, which results in the late adoption of legislation and legal gaps, creating favorable conditions for bad actors. In this sense, the immutability, verification, and authentication properties provided by blockchain technology increase the robustness of fiscal forensics. This study presents the comprehensive state-of-the-art of Bitcoin digital forensic approaches as well as a taxonomy of the common financial investigative techniques. Additionally, we develop and put into practice a framework for forensic investigations based on standardized practices and record the appropriate approach for investigations into embezzlement schemes. Our strategy is feasible and flexible enough to be applied to various forms of fraud investigations as well as routine internal audits. In addition to integrating standardized forensic flows and custody chain preservation techniques, we offer a working Ethereum-based implementation [50]. In addition to the management implications and potential future study areas, we also examine the difficulties of the symbiotic relationship between blockchain and financial investigations.

Cloud of Things

There are several industries that use digital forensics. Investigators may stumble across a variety of devices, including various electrical equipment, like computers, washers, and mobile phones, while searching an Internet of Things (IoT) enabled crime scene. It is essential to include all digital technologies in the forensics for the cloud platform. There are several difficulties in the investigative process due to the many types of devices in an IoT criminal investigative scenario. Like how neurons in our brain connect to one another, different sorts of technologies can be seen interacting with one another in our environment. A standard digital forensics investigation often involves significantly fewer devices than an IoT digital forensics study.

As more gadgets, including those used in people's daily lives, are connected to the Internet because of the introduction of IoT into society, the volume of data will grow exponentially. When expected, the volume of data will increase by nearly 40,000 trillion gigabytes. The distinction between local area networks (LANs) and wide area networks (WANs) will become less clear as there are more devices on the network.

Data Exchange

Over the past ten years, cybercrime has grown to be a serious menace. Despite the various efforts made by national and supranational agencies, the complexity of the fight against cybercriminals for judicial forces and all parties involved in the investigation process has increased due to differences in rules and the decentralization of information networks. In this article, we analyze how blockchain technology can assist to secure the custody chain throughout the flow of forensic analyses, with the purpose of increasing the security level of the players involved in court procedures and ensuring the appropriate gathering and integrity of digital evidence [51][52]. Similarly, we identify further initiatives to increase the exchange of digital evidence between all entities participating in the inquiry, in addition to the effective mechanisms pushed by the EU targeted at enabling cross-border data interchange. In this context, we draw attention to the strategy put forth by the EU project LOCARD, which offers a distributed platform for collaboration and automation of the management of digital evidence using blockchain technology, thus ensuring the transparency and integrity of the passing chain of custody.

Problems with Regulatory Compliance

Two problems with the conventional multimedia evidence collection chain of custody include flaws in the digital case process, particularly with documents in the central server and relying on outside security solutions. Also, the information from portable multimedia devices is gathered utilizing subpar and unreliable tools before being looked at and processed using different forensics procedures.

8.11.1 Traditional Forensics vs. Cloud Forensics

The evidence is handled by the investigator in a traditional investigation; in a global investigation, it is handled by several cloud service providers. To support or assist in the recreation of allegedly criminal events or to foresee illegal activities that have been shown to be challenging to plan tasks, *digital forensics* is defined as the application of experimentally determined, proven techniques to identify, validate, interpret, try to gather, preserve, present, and document evidence of the data gathered from electronic devices obtained from high-tech hotspots. The term "cloud computing" refers to an access model that permits global, on-demand system access to a collection of shared reconfigurable computational power, including systems, servers, storing, apps, and presidencies, that can be rapidly procured and discharged with organizational effort or skilled organizational collaboration [53]. Therefore, cloud crime scene investigation can be defined as the use of tried-and-true methods for the preservation, collection, approval, differentiating proof, inquiry, transcription, documentary evidence, and introduction of sophisticated proof from dispersed, having to register frameworks so that it is sufficient for admittance in court in a formal courtroom. A foundation for carrying out efficient criminological investigations has been supplied by a computerized informed model. Even though there isn't a single advanced quantitative technique model that can be applied to all computer criminological examinations, a traditional procedure design can be applied to a wide range of rigorous science examinations without considering the technologies being used.

8.12 Way Forward/Solutions

8.12.1 Traditional

As was already stated, log administration is an essential problem in cloud computing. A variety of models can be applied to cloud computing monitoring. One recommendation is to save logs of any operations that alter an instance's status using special transport layer protocols before delivering the information to a central cloud log storage site.

Retrieval of cloud data on a specific plane. The difficulty of data collecting in the forensic investigation can be lessened by granting the investigators access to a distinct plane for controlling the data retrievals they require. This level of cloud infrastructure requires trustworthy parties to keep it up-to-date.

The issue of the absence of a legislative framework for cloud forensics can be solved by creating a special service-level agreement (SLA) between customers and cloud service providers (CSPs) that stipulates the laws to be followed in the case of felony investigative activities. Table 8.2 shows the difference in traditional and cloud forensic tools.

TABLE 8.2

Traditional vs. Cloud Forensic Tools

Traditional	Cloud
SANS SIFT	Offline windows analysis and data extraction
FTK Imager	eDiscovery using access data
Prodiscover	eDiscovery using EnCase

8.12.2 Blockchain-Based

In several applications, including eHealth, industries, and voting, blockchain has lately made strides in terms of technology. Blockchain describes a peer-to-peer network that replicates a decentralized, shared, and tamper-proof ledger. A virtual monetary system called Bitcoin was the first to successfully utilize blockchain. Transactions are the fundamental unit of data in blockchain. A block is made up of a specified number of transactions. To create the target hash code for the block, the blockchain nodes broadcast the block. If it is implemented into the present forensics system, blockchain technology can advance the current digital forensics and incident response (DFIR). Storage of evidence and the reliability of evidence are the two main issues considered in cloud forensics [54][55]. To address these issues, the authors propose a blockchain-based data storage and integrity management architecture for cloud forensics. As a result, it contrasts the proposed network's effectiveness with that of other cryptocurrencies based on blockchain. More transactions could be handled by the proposed architecture than current permissionless-based blockchains while still maintaining data integrity.

The existing system's output evaluation does, however, have the limitation that it cannot do the actual review by comparing the observed concluding values to the expected data size. To reconstruct the network and determine how long it will take to solve using Hyperledger, Sniff is used to collect network data. The blockchain infrastructure as a service (IaaS) cloud solution addresses the problem of centralized evidence gathering and storage. The evidence is acquired, stored in the chain, and distributed across numerous peers in the proposed forensic architecture. To protect the device from unauthorized users, a system known as Secure Ring Verification-Based Authentication (SRVA) has been developed. The secret keys are generated using the Cuckoo Search Optimization (HSO) method in a way that benefits the cloud environment. Depending on the level of sensitivity, all information is protected using the Sensitivity Sensitive Deep Elliptic Curve Cryptography (SA-DECC) technique and stored on a cloud server. Each piece of cloud data is given its own block by the SDN controller, and the history of personal information is stored as metadata. Each block of the Safe Hashing Algorithm-3 (SHA-3) method has a Merkle hash tree. Users can maintain track of their data thanks to the incorporation of fuzzy-based smart contracts (FCS) in the framework. Researchers were finally able to study the proof thanks to the establishment of the logical evidence graph (LGoE) on the blockchain. Following a thorough analysis, it can be concluded that the suggested forensic design needs to perform admirably regarding response time, evidence implant placement time, proof having checked time, overhead interplay, hash data processing time, key rate of reproduction, cryptographic time, decryption, and as a whole change rate [56]. If blockchain is incorporated into the existing forensics system, it can support the digital forensic and event response system in use today (DFIR). Even though logs from IoT devices and cloud services might help reconstruct events, only a chain of custody can guarantee their validity and, consequently, their admission. On the Bitcoin computer forensics system, CoC is preserved. Researchers have developed a framework for a forensic investigation that makes use of the distributed, tamper-proof structure of the blockchain. To address the challenges of cloud forensics, we addressed a few current works on cryptography.

The extent of the proof and data storage are the two main factors in cloud forensics. To solve these issues, the authors propose a Bitcoin data store and asset integrity solution for cloud forensics. As a result, it contrasts the suggested network's effectiveness with that of other currencies. The proposed system would ensure data integrity while managing more operations than the existing permissionless blockchains. However, the current system's output evaluation is limited in that it cannot be done by just comparing the measured result values to the expected data size. To do a simulation and compute tps using the blockchain network for this study's future iterations, network data is obtained using Snort. A cryptographic-based identification privacy solution is introduced, along with comprehensive information on the method and an explanation of the device's architecture. Smart contracts are used for a wide variety of transactions that are suitable for these forensic inspection applications. The issue of identifying privacy is improved by using a modified symmetric key mechanism to hide the proof's submitter from the public. The controllers create a block each time a piece of data is saved to the cloud, and the past of the data is recorded as metadata. The protection of logs generated during cloud data activities is given careful consideration. Even though different security concerns (such as flawed operations, cyberattacks, etc.) can damage and abuse cloud data, log analysis remains one of the most popular techniques for tracking incidents. Log file privacy must be upheld to complete the incident's monitoring. The public model presented in this study relies on a third auditor to confirm the veracity of cloud logs. The log block tags gathered using the standard Merkle hash tree structure is used to form the root of the trees that will be kept inside the blockchain, guarding against tampering with log data. The open audit of the planned scheme, however, has discovered no leaks of any kind [57][58]. The framework can effectively raise the security evaluation of cloud logs in respect of overhead computing complexity, which is higher than the prior, based on the theoretical analysis and empirical analysis. The main purpose of the elliptic curve hashing algorithm is to create log block tags.

8.13 Future Scope

The study's discussions mostly center on the security difficulties and problems that arise when cloud computing and digital forensics are combined. These security difficulties and problems can be addressed in a future project as a means of creating a safe network. By moving cloud services, additional security measures can be put in place. A comprehensive and realistic scenario can be created to encompass all the many parts of the cloud forensic difficulties to better understand and address them [59][60]. A framework that has additional capabilities can also be developed to facilitate the production of reliable forensic evidence. The current digital forensics models are not suitable for cloud systems since they do not meet the necessary standards. The multiple attackers make ongoing attempts to use the network's weaknesses to their advantage and seize control.

8.14 Conclusion

Blockchain is the ideal option for the administration and traceability of the forensic custody chain since it is designed to ensure legitimacy, accountability, protection, authenticity, and audibility. With such assurance, blockchain contributes to the reduction of friction and so offers the forensic culture its true potential. The goal of this project is to create a comprehensive Java-based smart digital forensic chain, by creating a group of restricted end users who oversee the forensics investigation, and by constructing a forensics evidence system and obtaining optimization. Ethereum is used to construct blockchain technology.

Additionally, this method prevents single-point failures. When a complaint is filed, a new block will be appended to that block in the chain. If someone modifies the block after it is created, we may determine it using a specific block. They will be labeled as "nullified blocks." As a result, immutability is less likely. Additionally, victims can track the complaint's progress, which promotes transparency. Therefore, all criminal situations may be simply prevented by utilizing blockchain technology, which achieves safety, coherence, and transparency.

8.15 Discussion

To protect submitted forensics report submissions, it employs a blockchain-based technique. The software, analytical staff, pathology staff, cops, doctors, and higher officers are just a few of the numerous nodes in this system. To accomplish transparency and immutability, they are individually given the go-ahead. So that individuals with their confidential credentials can see all the records that they submit and start to observe in line with the given work, forensic and pathology staff members create new reports [61]. The application component node at a node can add any detail. Senior police can therefore view a graph of the number of crimes reported at their specific locations.

References

[1] 3205–2023 – IEEE standard for blockchain interoperability data authentication and communication protocol. (2023). IEEE.https://standards.ieee.org/ieee/3205/10237/ (accessed on May 2023).

[2] Chapple, M., & Seidl, D. (2023). *(ISC)2 CCSP Certified Cloud Security Professional Official Study Guide*. John Wiley and Sons.

[3] Prieto, J., Luis, B. M. F., Ferretti, S., Guarde, D. A., & Nevado-Batalla, P. T. (2023). *Blockchain and Applications 4th International Congress*. Springer International Publishing.

[4] Mukhopadhyay, D. (2023). *Blockchain for IOT*. Chapman & Hall/CRC Press.

[5] Garg, R. (2023). *Blockchain for Real World Applications*. John Wiley & Sons, Incorporated.

[6] Wang, J. (2022). *Encyclopedia of Data Science and Machine Learning*. IGI Global.

[7] Albano, C. (2022). *Out of Breath: Vulnerability of Air in Contemporary Art*. University of Minnesota Press.

[8] Cao, B. (2022). *Wireless Blockchain: Principles, Technologies and Applications*. John Wiley & Sons, Inc.

[9] P3205/d5.0, Aug 2022 – IEEE draft standard for blockchain interoperability – Data authentication and communication protocol. (n.d.). IEEE. https://blockchain.ieee.org/standards (accessed on April 2023).

[10] García-Corral, F. J., Cordero-García, J. A., de Pablo-Valenciano, J., et al. (2022). A bibliometric review of cryptocurrencies: How have they grown? *Financial Innovation*, 8(2), 1–31. https://doi.org/10.1186/s40854-021-00306-5

[11] Akinbi, A., MacDermott, Á., & Ismael, A. M. (2022). A systematic literature review of blockchain-based internet of things (IOT) forensic investigation process models. *Forensic Science International: Digital Investigation*, 42–43, 301470. https://doi.org/10.1016/j.fsidi.2022.301470

[12] Kent, P., & Bain, T. (2022). *Bitcoin. For Dummies®*, Wiley.

[13] Jaquet-Chiffelle, D.-O., Casey, E., & Bourquenoud, J. (2022). Corrigendum to "Tamperproof timestamped provenance Ledger using blockchain technology*" [Forens. Sci. Int.: Digit. Invest. 33 (2020) 300977]. *Forensic Science International: Digital Investigation*, 40, 301332. https://doi.org/10.1016/j.fsidi.2022.301332

[14] Zhihuang, W., Qing, Z., Changjie, G., & Kaimin, Y. (2022). Building a blueprint for forensic supervision with blockchain innovation. *Criminal Justice Science & Governance*, 3(1), 84–88. https://doi.org/10.35534/cjsg.0301012

[15] Chandana, M., & Vidya Raj, C. (2022). Reliability reinforcement of forensic affirmation using blockchain. *International Journal of Scientific Research in Computer Science, Engineering and Information Technology*, 8(6), 357–362. https://doi.org/10.32628/cseit228644

[16] Agbedanu, P., & Jurcut, A. D. (2022). Bloff. In *Research Anthology on Convergence of Blockchain, Internet of Things, and Security*, IGI Global; 738–749. https://doi.org/10.4018/978-1-6684-7132-6.ch040

[17] Goyal, R. (2021). Blockchain technology in forensic science. A bibliometric review. *2021 3rd International Conference on Advances in Computing, Communication Control and Networking (ICAC3N)*, Greater Noida, India, 2021, pp. 1570–1573. https://doi.org/10.1109/icac3n53548.2021.9725660

[18] Singh, S. K., Roy, P., Raman, B., & Nagabhushan, P. (2021). *Computer Vision and Image Processing 5th International Conference, CVIP 2020*. Springer.

[19] Tanwar, R., Choudhury, T., Zamani, M., & Gupta, S. (2021). *Information Security and Optimization*. C&H\CRC Press.

[20] 2020 7th IEEE international conference on cyber security and cloud computing (cscloud)/2020 6th IEEE international conference on edge computing and scalable cloud (EdgeCom): Cscloud-edgecom 2020: New York, (2020). IEEE. https://www.proceedings.com/55552.html

[21] Billard, D. (2020). Tainted digital evidence and privacy protection in blockchain-based systems. *Forensic Science International: Digital Investigation*, 32, 300911. https://doi.org/10.1016/j.fsidi.2020.300911

[22] Shi, N. (2020). *Architectures and Frameworks for Developing and Applying Blockchain Technology*. Engineering Science Reference.

[23] Liyanage, M., Braeken, A., Kumar, P., & Ylianttila, M. (2020). *IOT Security: Advances in Authentication*. John Wiley & Sons, Inc.

[24] Lusetti, M., Salsi, L., & Dallatana, A. (2020). A blockchain based solution for the custody of digital files in Forensic Medicine. *Forensic Science International: Digital Investigation*, 35, 301017. https://doi.org/10.1016/j.fsidi.2020.301017

[25] Jaquet-Chiffelle, D.-O., Casey, E., & Bourquenoud, J. (2020). Tamperproof timestamped provenance ledger using blockchain technology. *Forensic Science International: Digital Investigation*, 33, 300977. https://doi.org/10.1016/j.fsidi.2020.300977

[26] Shang, H., & Qiang, H. (2020). Electronic data preservation and storage of evidence by blockchain. *Journal of Forensic Science and Medicine*, 6(1), 27. https://doi.org/10.4103/jfsm.jfsm_21_19

[27] Burri, X., Casey, E., Bollé, T., & Jaquet-Chiffelle, D.-O. (2020). Chronological independently verifiable electronic chain of custody ledger using blockchain technology. *Forensic Science International: Digital Investigation*, 33, 300976. https://doi.org/10.1016/j.fsidi.2020.300976

[28] Chen, S., Zhao, C., Huang, L., Yuan, J., & Liu, M. (2020). Study and implementation on the application of blockchain in electronic evidence generation. *Forensic Science International: Digital Investigation*, 35, 301001. https://doi.org/10.1016/j.fsidi.2020.301001

[29] Nuzzolese, E. (2020). Electronic health record and blockchain architecture: Forensic chain hypothesis for human identification. *Egyptian Journal of Forensic Sciences*, 10(1), 1–5. https://doi.org/10.1186/s41935-020-00209-z

[30] Aparecido Petroni, B. C., Gonçalves, R. F., Sérgio de Arruda Ignácio, P., Reis, J. Z., & Dolce Uzum Martins, G. J. (2020). Smart contracts applied to a functional architecture for storage and maintenance of digital chain of custody using blockchain. *Forensic Science International: Digital Investigation*, 34, 300985. https://doi.org/10.1016/j.fsidi.2020.300985

[31] Quan, Y., Li, C.-T., Zhou, Y., & Li, L. (2020). Warwick image forensics dataset for device fingerprinting in multimedia forensics. *2020 IEEE International Conference on Multimedia and Expo (ICME)*. Publisher: IEEE. https://doi.org/10.1109/icme46284.2020.9102783

[32] Nyaletey, E., Parizi, R. M., Zhang, Q., & Choo, K.-K. R. (2019). BlockIPFS – blockchain-enabled interplanetary file system for forensic and trusted data traceability. *2019 IEEE International Conference on Blockchain (Blockchain)*. Publisher: IEEE. https://doi.org/10.1109/blockchain.2019.00012

[33] Senkyire, I. B., & Kester, Q.-A. (2019). Validation of forensic crime scene images using watermarking and cryptographic blockchain. *2019 International Conference on Computer, Data Science and Applications (ICDSA)*. Publisher: IEEE. https://doi.org/10.1109/icdsa46371.2019.9404235

[34] Fabian, M. L. (2016). Analyzing the bitcoin network: The first four years. *Future Internet*, 8(1), 1–40. https://doi.org/10.3390/fi8010007

[35] Nelson, B., Phillips, A., & Steuart, C. (2019). *Guide to Computer Forensics and Investigations*. Cengage.
[36] Pérez-Solà, C., Navarro-Arribas, G., Biryukov, A., & Garcia-Alfaro, J. (2019). *Data Privacy Management, Cryptocurrencies and Blockchain Technology ESORICS 2019 International Workshops, DPM 2019 and CBT 2019*. Springer International Publishing.
[37] Joshi, J., Nepal, S., Zhang, Q., & Zhang, L.-J. (2019). *Blockchain – ICBC 2019: Second International Conference, Held as Part of the Services Conference Federation, SCF 2019*. Springer International Publishing.
[38] Meng, W., & Furnell, S. (2019). *Security and Privacy in Social Networks and Big Data: 5th International Symposium, SOCIALSEC 2019*. Springer Singapore.
[39] Ras, D. J. (2019). *Digital Forensic Readiness Architecture for Cloud Computing Systems*. https://repository.up.ac.za/handle/2263/70644
[40] Verdoliva, L., & Bestagini, P. (2019). Multimedia forensics. *Proceedings of the 27th ACM International Conference on Multimedia (MM '19)*. Association for Computing Machinery, New York, NY, USA, 2701–2702. https://doi.org/10.1145/3343031.3350542
[41] Qiu, M. (2018). *Smart Blockchain: First International Conference, SmartBlock 2018*. Springer International Publishing.
[42] Urquhart, A. (2016). The inefficiency of bitcoin. *Economics Letters*, 148, 80–82. https://doi.org/10.1016/j.econlet.2016.09.019
[43] Urquhart, A. (2018). What causes the attention of bitcoin? *Economics Letters*, 166, 40–44. https://doi.org/10.1016/j.econlet.2018.02
[44] Bashir, I. (2017). *Mastering Blockchain: Deeper Insights into Decentralization, Cryptography, Bitcoin, and Popular Blockchain Frameworks*. Packt Publishing Ltd.
[45] Barni, M., & Tondi, B. (2017). Threat models and games for adversarial multimedia forensics. *Proceedings of the 2nd International Workshop on Multimedia Forensics and Security* (MFSec '17). Association for Computing Machinery, New York, NY, USA, 11–15. https://doi.org/10.1145/3078897.3080533
[46] Sebastian, L. (2017). *Bitcoin: The Bitcoin Basics*. Createspace Independent Press.
[47] Atiquzzaman, M., Choo, K.-K. R., Wang, G., & Yan, Z. (2017). *Security, Privacy, and Anonymity in Computation, Communication, and Storage Spaccs 2017 International Workshops*. Springer International Publishing.
[48] Van Alstyne, M. (2014). Why bitcoin has value. *Communications of the ACM*, 57(5), 30–32. https://doi.org/10.1145/2594288
[49] Vrochidis, S. (2017). Session details: Multimedia forensics and verification. *Proceedings of the 2nd International Workshop on Multimedia Forensics and Security* (MFSec '17). Association for Computing Machinery, New York, NY, USA.. https://doi.org/10.1145/3248728
[50] De, D. (2016). *Mobile Cloud Computing: Architectures, Algorithms and Applications*. Taylor & Francis.
[51] Ravindran, U., Rai, B. K., & Sharma, S. (2018). A review paper on regulating bitcoin currencies. *International Journal for Research in Applied Science and Engineering Technology*, 6, 4136–4140. https://doi.org/10.22214/ijraset.2018.4682
[52] Satapathy, S. C., Mandal, J. K., Udgata, S. K., & Bhateja, V. (2016). *Information Systems Design and Intelligent Applications: Proceedings of Third International Conference*. Springer India.
[53] de Vries, A. (2018). Bitcoin's growing energy problem. *Joule*, 2(5), 801–805. https://doi.org/10.1016/j.joule.2018.04.016
[54] Miller, M. (2015). *The Ultimate Guide to Bitcoin*. Que.
[55] Worring, M. (2015). Multimedia analytics for image collection forensics. In *Handbook of Digital Forensics of Multimedia Data and Devices*. Wiley; 305–327. https://doi.org/10.1002/9781118705773.ch8
[56] Wang, J., & Kissel, Z. A. (2015). *Introduction to Network Security: Theory and Practice*. Wiley.
[57] Wright, P. M. (2014). *Protecting Oracle Database 12C*. Apress.
[58] Simou, S., Kalloniatis, C., Kavakli, E., Gritzalis, S. (2014). Cloud Forensics: Identifying the Major Issues and Challenges. In: Jarke, M., et al. *Advanced Information Systems Engineering*. CAiSE 2014. Lecture Notes in Computer Science, vol 8484. Springer, Cham. https://doi.org/10.1007/978-3-319-07881-6_19
[59] Ruan, K. (2013). *Cybercrime and Cloud Forensics: Applications for Investigation Processes*. Information Science Reference.
[60] Pearson, S., & Yee, G. (2013). *Privacy and Security for Cloud Computing*. Springer.
[61] Rogers, M. K., & Seigfried-Spellar, K. C. (2013). *Digital Forensics and Cyber Crime: 4th International Conference, ICDF2C 2012*. Springer.

Authors' Biography

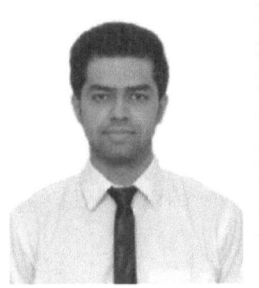

Rohit Kaushik Rohit is a graduate student at the University of Illinois, majoring in data analytics. His research interests lie in the fields of machine learning, mathematical computation, statistical analysis, artificial intelligence, and data mining. His previous research has focused on the integration of technology to diminish societal issues, leading to betterment. Rohit has enormous potential and a burning desire to accomplish his pursuits, along with a creative mind filled with new ideas.

Adding new heights to his research, he has been selected by the Illinois Department of Public Health (IDPH) to research the motor vehicle data linkage project in collaboration with the Illinois Department of Transportation (IDOT). He has been awarded the title of director of technology at "DREAMtorous," a business networking conclave and brand of Global Conflux of Stalwarts (GCS). His dynamic personality leads him to new opportunities, like getting invited as a guest speaker at the IEEE Student Branch (2021) to deliver a session on data science, machine learning, and deep learning. He has amazing analytical and management skills, which directed him to serve as a community manager at a non-profit community to support and enhance their development using precise statistical data insights.

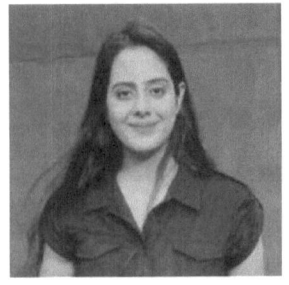

Eva Kaushik* Eva Kaushik is an IT professional with extensive experience in research. As a researcher, she is well-versed in varied domains, including fintech, haptics, astrophysics, financial economics, bioinformatics, and genomics. She has published research manuscripts, book chapters, and articles in renowned journals supporting her interest. She has been a founding pioneer at Dexigner, a co-founder at FiCord community, and even augmented the fintech niche via various initiatives.

Her belief in hard work and perfection has led her to prominent positions. She has served as the chairperson of IEEE ADGITM, an educational activist in IEEE USA, a core committee member of the IEEE QT3 Series, an editorial coordinator at IEEE WIE DS, and a public speaker at YPLO. She was chosen by Microsoft for the start-up program "Binance Build for Bharat" and received the IEEE WIE Affinity Group Award. She is serving as an advisor at FrontForumFocus (a non-profit organization). She has volunteered with MHRD, WWF, IEEE MOVE India, and the World Youth Alliance. Along with this, she is at spreading cognition about technology at different platforms for the advancement of society.

Precisely, being a woman of serious potential, she believes in achieving accuracy and perfection.

9
Blockchain in Tracing and Securing Medical Supplies

Tamanna Rai, Rishabha Malviya, Niranjan Kaushik, and Pramod Kumar Sharma

9.1 Introduction

The blockchain technology and its fundamental characteristics of decentralization, transparency, and anonymity came into being simultaneously with the launch of the Bitcoin cryptocurrency in 2008 [1]. Bitcoin, which has had close to 400 million transactions successfully completed as of March 19, 2019 [2], provides a compelling example of how blockchain technology might be put to use. The potential utility of blockchain technology in other data-driven industries, such as healthcare, has been the subject of much discussion and suggestion as a result [3]. IBM found that 70% of healthcare leaders believe that blockchain's biggest impact in the health domain will be in enhancing regulatory compliance, clinical trial management, and creating a decentralized platform for sharing electronic health records (EHR) [4]. In addition, it is anticipated that by the year 2022, the market for blockchain applications in healthcare will have exceeded $500 million [5]. Despite widespread optimism about blockchain's potential to enhance healthcare IT [3], the existing body of research offers just a limited overview of the applications that have been created, evaluated, or implemented, and the recent excitement surrounding this technology has been accompanied by the promotion of ideas and strategies that are unrealistically idealistic. When considering blockchain technology's potential uses in healthcare, biomedicine, and health education (together called "the healthcare domain"), it's important to determine if present research meets expectations. However, it has also found applications in a variety of other industries, including finance, logistics, energy, commodity trading, healthcare, and many others. Utilizing blockchain technology can provide a secure and unalterable system of drug provenance and traceability, which would be beneficial in the fight against the proliferation of counterfeit pharmaceuticals. Distributed shared data platforms, built on blockchain technology, can be used by several parties in the supply chain to securely store and trade transaction records. This is made possible by the use of cryptographic methods, which ensure that only authorized parties have access to the ledger and keep unauthorized parties from accessing it. It provides a means for preventing the distribution of counterfeit medications across the pharmaceutical supply chain. This method monitors and controls the dissemination of counterfeit medications. This chapter examines the use of blockchain technology for tracking drugs, explores its benefits and potential drawbacks, and investigates the many alternatives available for safeguarding the pharmaceutical supply chain [6].

9.2 Background

Blockchain can be thought of as a decentralized, immutable ledger that records transactions. It eliminates the need for a trusted third party to mediate communications between parties. The blockchain stores a growing list of records, or "blocks," which are added to sequentially. After these blocks are added to the blockchain, cryptographic procedures are used to link them to the blocks that came before and those that will come after [7]. When implemented as intended, blockchain makes it possible for anybody to read, write, and verify the integrity of a block of data. This paves the way, for instance, for distributed ledgers and databases. Because of these features, blockchain is being considered for a wide range of uses. Blockchain technology also makes smart contracts, which do not require third-party supervision, possible [8].

9.2.1 Blockchain Technology in Brief

9.2.1.1 A Concise Introduction to Blockchain as It Applies to Medical Care

This section introduces the topic by discussing the reasons behind adopting blockchain technology in healthcare. We also introduce and analyze the core ideas behind blockchain.

9.2.1.1.1 The Important Role That Technology Plays in the Field of Healthcare

The healthcare industry is becoming more dependent on help from other sectors, including computer science, which can make important contributions in this field [9]. This encompasses a wide range of fields, from genomics and gene prediction to electronic health records and illness diagnostic tool development [10–12]. The systems employed by public health organizations (and commercial ones) hold large volumes of patient data daily, which begs the question of what to do with it all. In recent years, a trending concept known as "big data analysis" has been put to use in order to circumvent this impediment. "Big data analysis" is a term that refers to a group of unique techniques that are applied to extraordinarily huge and difficult datasets, for which the conventional methods of data analysis are insufficient [13]. Improvements in healthcare diagnostic prediction, MRI analysis, and other areas could result from the use of big data in medicine [14]. Since computer science is interdisciplinary, it may be used in many other areas of study to improve and streamline the relevant processes. The application of computers and the technologies connected with them can be utilized in the field of medicine to assist with a broad variety of problems. Healthcare systems may benefit from increased quality, efficiency, and reduced costs as a result [15].

9.3 The Blockchain Technology

Bitcoin and other cryptocurrencies introduced a novel technology called blockchain circa 2008–2009 [16,17]. Currently, it provides a range of activities in the domains of banking, healthcare, transportation, and government, among others. With the help of this modern innovation, we can keep track of our possessions in a more organized and safe fashion than ever before [18]. It operates on decentralized P2P networks with a duplicated and distributed ledger [19,20]. This article describes the ideas behind how blockchain might be used to track and secure medical supplies.

9.4 Blockchain's Benefits: Blockchain Technology's Advantages Make It Suited for Medical Record Management [21]

- **Accessibility**. Users of apps that are enabled with blockchain technology have the ability to access their medical records in a way that is safe, convenient, and effective.
- **Interoperability**. Conventional methods make use of centralized data storage, which contributes to the friction that exists in the interoperability of patients' records. These issues can be circumvented thanks to the fact that blockchain technology does not necessitate the existence of a centralized database; as an alternative, all nodes are able to communicate with one another.
- **Authentication**. Use of a unique private key in conjunction with a publicly available key is how blockchain's block-based data authentication system works.
- **Decentralized storage**. Blockchain's decentralized nature makes it ideal for archiving large amounts of data in multiple locations. Better data quality, quicker access to medical data, and higher levels of security are all made possible by decentralized storage.

9.5 Blockchain Networks

Blockchain can be broken down into several categories which have their own characteristics and whose actions mirror those of the network as a whole. We can classify these blockchains based on the features mentioned by Zheng et al. [22] and Alhadhrami et al. [23].

9.5.1 Public Blockchain

There are no issues preventing any node from having access to the transaction data. After a transaction has been recorded in a blockchain, any node in the network can use the consensus processes to validate it. This node is not limited in any manner, and it is not familiar with the network in advance. Because of this configuration, the nodes in the network are able to collaborate on their efforts and offer one another assistance. A network like this is the foundation upon which cryptocurrencies like Bitcoin and Ether are formed [22].

9.5.2 Permissioned Blockchain

The nodes that are permitted into the structure as well as the transactions that take place within it are under the authority of an organization [22]. Because the design of this network requires user verification before allowing access to the content, it's more private and discreet than conventional approaches. The name MultiChain describes one such platform [24].

9.5.3 Consortium Blockchain

Given that it is typically managed by a group and participation in the network necessitates authentication, it has several features in common with permissioned blockchains. In this network configuration, only a subset of nodes is equipped with the necessary capabilities to validate a transaction in advance. Select nodes in this network must agree, generate a new block, and complete the transaction validation procedure [25].

9.6 Blockchain's Verification Procedure

By the standards of certain algorithms, such as proof-of-work, the blockchain validation procedure is also known as mining. A consensus method is used to execute this function, and it also determines the rules that the nodes must follow in order to validate the blocks. By adhering to the proper sequence of transactions, the consensus protocol guarantees that all validating nodes will receive a good result. It's up to them to determine whether or not to add the block to the chain [26]. Consensus methods are developed specifically for the purpose of validating blocks on a blockchain, making the network more secure. Here is a summary of the most important blockchain-related healthcare protocols that have been published so far.

9.6.1 Practical Byzantine Fault Tolerance (PBFT)

The network's nodes can be broken down into two groups: clients and servers. The client node initiates communication with the server node by submitting a request, the server node distributes the transaction to the other server nodes, and the accepted server node notifies the other server nodes that it is ready to process the transaction. The PBFT uses this method to verify the transactions. In order for a transaction to be considered validated, (1) it must be confirmed by a majority of nodes (also referred to as a "confirmation alert"), (2) each validated node must broadcast a message to the network attesting its action, and (3) the sender node must receive the answer [27,28].

9.6.2 Proof-of-Stake (PoS)

Each validation is selected from the pool of network users. Therefore, the greater the node's coin supply, the more probable it is that it will be used to verify blocks and thus serve as the final arbiter of block legitimacy [29].

9.6.3 Proof-of-Work (PoW)

The validating nodes (also known as "miners") engage in a race to the bottom to decipher a cryptographic challenge. When a transaction needs to be implemented in a new block, the right to do so goes to the node that finds the solution first. It's also important to remember that the winner of the PoW algorithm in some implementations (like Bitcoin) receives a prize [17].

9.7 Insights into Blockchain-Based Tracking Methods

The problem of phony or counterfeit pharmaceuticals is growing rapidly within the healthcare business. A patient's health could be jeopardized if they took those counterfeit medications. The company producing the pills and any other parties involved will suffer as a result of the spread of these counterfeit medications [30–32]. Therefore, a secure system for medicine tracing needs to be designed to address the problem of drug counterfeiting. Governments around the world are making significant efforts to improve drug tracking systems. By using a protected drug traceability system, patients and other stakeholders may easily track where a drug is in the drug supply chain and check that it is genuine [33–36]. There are crucial elements missing from the current drug tracking systems that are necessary for the pharmaceutical supply chain. It is possible that the lack of openness that exists in the current healthcare system contributes to the problems of drug shortages, opioid misuse, and counterfeit pharmaceuticals. Because the drug supply chain is not transparent, it is difficult for patients and other stakeholders to track where their drugs are at any given time. This is a problem because patients' lives may depend on the medications.

9.7.1 The Aims of Drug Traceability

- Using the tools provided in this treaty and protocol, we can protect public health, stop the spread of fake pills, and win the fight against them on a national and local scale.
- In order to devise a standard and coordinated strategy for getting rid of the fake tablets, and to create standardization in terms of definitions, information resources, and tools.
- So as to put an end to the production of fake pharmaceuticals.
- In order to raise awareness of the problem of counterfeit drugs, which necessitates a higher level of protection against the theft of legitimate pharmaceutical products [37].

9.8 The Need for Blockchain in Medication Traceability Is Described by the Issues That Follow Conventional Techniques of Tracking Drugs [21]

9.8.1 Consenting to Regulations

It is necessary to import a sizable quantity of pharmaceutical ingredients from other countries in order to produce a significant quantity of pharmaceuticals. Drug supply chain laws apply to the entire process, beginning with manufacturing and ending with distribution.

9.8.2 Cold Chain Shipping

Numerous medications are extremely delicate and must be kept in a temperature-controlled space. However, in the present applications, such cold-chain shipment details are stored in centralized databases, making them extremely susceptible to hacking and manipulation.

9.9 Using Blockchain Technology to Track Pharmaceuticals

We'll examine two blockchain-based technologies and discuss how each could help the pharmaceutical sector meet pressing medication supply chain management needs. Hyperledger Fabric and Hyperledger Besu are employed because they provide superior trust, security, data integrity, decentralization, transparency, privacy, adoption, modularity, and scalability than blockchain frameworks. These frameworks allow a single expert or a consortium of experts and stakeholders to register, control, and regulate pharmaceutical stakeholders and end users.

9.9.1 Hyperledger Besu Architecture

Businesses interested in blockchain solutions that are compatible with Ethereum will find all they need in the forthcoming Hyperledger Besu drug traceability architecture. Hyperledger Besu is gaining traction in the business world because of its promise to aid in the construction of networks that can handle private transactions and connect with public blockchains (Ethereum) without sacrificing architectural flexibility or transaction throughput. The proposed Hyperledger Besu architecture for the pharmaceutical supply chain connects private and public blockchains to develop high-performance, scalable applications on private peer-to-peer networks while ensuring data privacy and complex permissioning management [38].

Hyperledger Besu makes use of the private transaction manager (PTM) Orion to ensure the confidentiality of all transactions conducted by its users. The state and transactions of a smart contract can be encrypted using PTMs that adhere to the Enterprise Ethereum Alliance (EEA) Client Specification, restricting access to the contract's shared business logic to the intended parties. PTMs include the Hyperledger Besu fork known as Orion. Launching an Orion node for each Hyperledger Besu node is necessary for a safe transaction network configuration. Hyperledger Besu is an open-source Ethereum client. JSON-RPC APIs handle Hyperledger Besu nodes and transactions. The Hyperledger Besu architecture can store private and public drug transaction data for pharmaceutical supply chain drug traceability [39].

9.9.2 Hyperledger Fabric Architecture

Hyperledger Fabric is a distributed ledger framework with a modular architecture that offers high levels of privacy, security, reliability, adaptability, and scalability. Built on blockchain technology, it is an enterprise-grade distributed ledger that uses smart contracts to maintain mutual trust among its numerous users. While keeping important aspects of blockchain-based cryptocurrencies such as Bitcoin and Ethereum, Hyperledger Fabric eliminates the need for miners. Among these features are immutable blocks, a predictable sequence of events, and the elimination of double spending. It has been demonstrated that Hyperledger Fabric can handle tens of thousands of transactions per second [38]. Channels distinguish Hyperledger Fabric. Protecting sensitive data and proprietary business processes may be difficult when multiple users access the same database. Hyperledger Fabric's built-in, crash-fault-tolerant transaction sequencing allows deterministic event recording, secure communication, and trustworthy medication-related transactions across untrusted stakeholders. This helps create a dependable PSC drug track-and-trace system to combat fakes. The suggested blockchain design uses a new modular mechanism for adaptability, resilience, scalability, and confidentiality.

In conclusion, the Hyperledger Fabric design relies on peer nodes and the ordering service (OS). Peers operate smart contracts, authenticate transactions, and commit them. The client apps accept the endorsed transactions, organize them into blocks, and cryptographically sign them. The committed peers in the blockchain network validate the endorsement policies [40].

9.10 Steps Involved during the Transaction in Drug Safety

- Each party to a transaction will need to have a public key and digital signature, as well as the public key of the recipient and the data being delivered.
- The information about each participant will be put into a QR code that can only be read with the public key of the person who is supposed to get it.
- All links in the medical supply chain will verify the sender's public key.
- When a transaction is finalized, all involved parties receive a copy.

9.11 Proposed Method for Blockchain in Personal Health Records

Emergency personnel may not have access to a patient's PHR. PHR historical record management is important due to sensitive patient data. Blockchain-based healthcare management systems with security policies enable tamper-resistant software. These standards specify scalable auditing, tamper-resistant protections, and emergency access restrictions. It supports Hyperledger Fabric and Composer. Blockchain-based smart contracts were built by a collaboration to give patients security controls over healthcare stakeholders' access laws. The technology provides historical records for critical care patient audits. If they are recovered (by doctors), they will follow the recordings of other participants. We tested our framework on Hyperledger Composer. Our research shows that immutability, auditing, and emergency access control safeguard PHR data exchange [41]. Figure 9.1 defines the brief overview of the access control for personal health records (PHR) in an emergency.

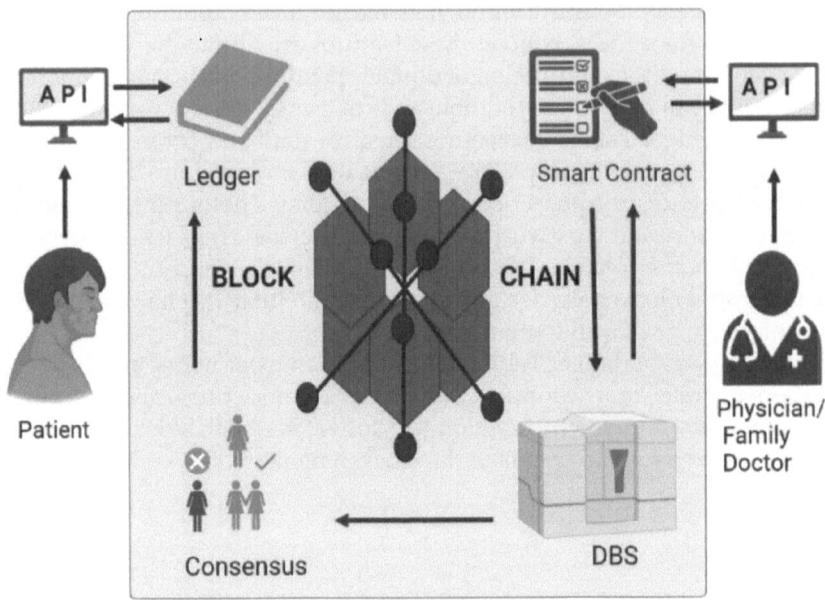

FIGURE 9.1
Proposed framework for personal health record (PHR) access control in an emergency.

9.12 Applying Blockchain to Healthcare Supply Chains

All businesses that provide goods, services, and products must practice effective supply chain management since, when poorly managed, supply networks may quickly fail and create production delays [42]. The term "supply chain" (SC) refers to the network of businesses, facilities, and workers involved in producing a good or service for consumers. Stakeholder coalitions are one way in which stakeholders add value to the market [43]. In this way, a supply chain can be thought of as the coordination of material and content that circulates among producers, distributors, and end users [44]. Supply-and-demand regulation is the SC's main focus. SCs ensure patients get access to the correct instruments and treatments for their recovery. Manufacturers, distributors, hospitals, pharmacies, and insurance companies comprise the SCHM supply chain [45]. Delays in therapy, lower levels of patient satisfaction, and higher overall expenditures can all result from SCs that are less than optimal. The success of an SCHM hinges on the cooperation and coordination of all involved participants to make sure that the appropriate products are shipped to the right locations at the right times. Logistics software and inventory management systems can be used to monitor and control the flow of items inside the SC [46]. To reduce healthcare spending, we must increase the effectiveness of SC and boost outcomes. This idea has gained traction in recent years. In order to better understand and address the requirements of patients and clinicians, there are ongoing attempts to streamline operations, enhance inventory management, and utilize data analytics. Healthcare organizations can boost patient care and provider satisfaction by learning more about and effectively managing their SC. The goals of an SCHM are to reduce healthcare expenses without compromising the quality of care provided to patients or the safety of healthcare providers [47,48]. Providers incur greater expenses and are more reliant on third parties while managing an SCHM than in other sectors [49]. Furthermore, an SCHM has its own set of difficulties because it is typically decentralized, lacks established procedures between physicians, hospitals, and patients, and is subject to regulatory constraints. The primary stakeholders in SCHMs are often policymakers, medication manufacturers, the pharmaceutical sector, and other organizations and structures like hospitals, clinics, and pharmacies. An SC is responsible for the distribution of both industry- and patient-derived products, such as pharmaceuticals and medical equipment [50]. Figure 9.2 suggest the steps in the healthcare supply chain for DMDs and BOTs, which include the general flow of a pharmaceutical SC, as follows: raw material, manufacture, distribution to pharmacies and hospitals, and patient; and it also consists of the BOT flow, as follows: donor, storage, transit, quality inspection, and patient usage.

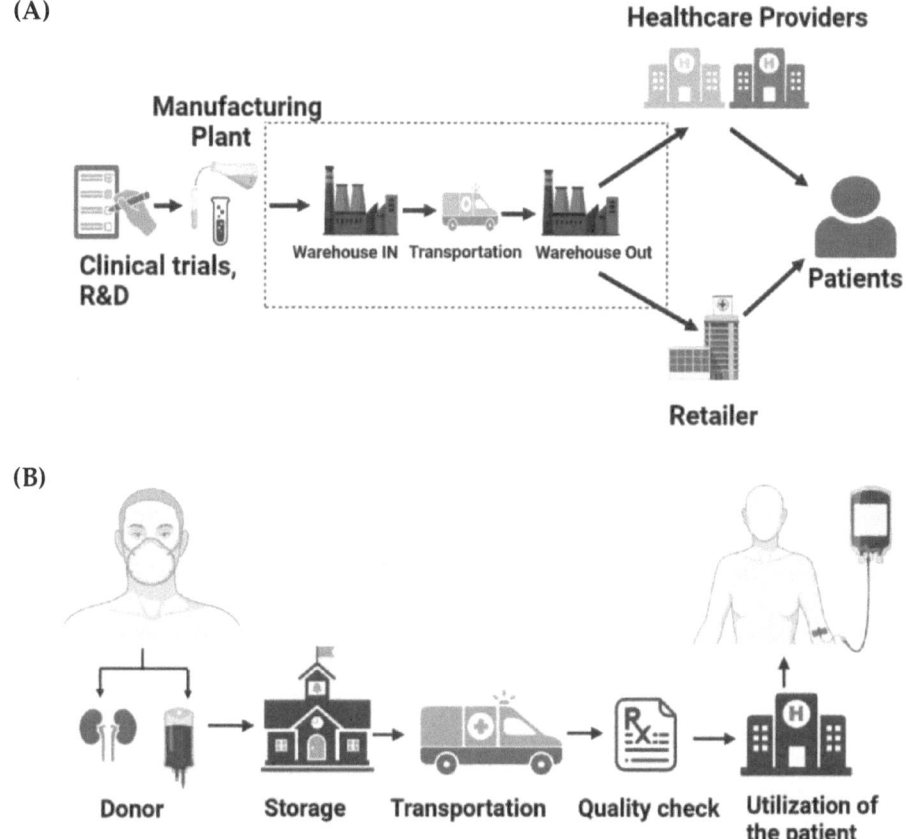

FIGURE 9.2
Steps of the supply chain in healthcare, specifically for DMDs (A) and BOTs (B). (A) A pharmaceutical SC's general flow: from the raw material to the manufacturers, to the distribution to pharmacies and hospitals, and to the patient; (B) general flow of BOT: from the donor to storage transportation, quality check, and utilization for the patient.

Blockchain technology has the potential to radically alter the healthcare industry because of its ability to increase data security and interoperability and to track and trace data and information. A great issue in the healthcare sector is the lack of acceptable data storage and retrieval systems that are trustworthy, safe, and secure. The blockchain technology provides a workaround for this problem by allowing users to record transactions in an immutable distributed ledger that is immune to tampering. Additionally, the use of blockchain technology may enhance interoperability across several existing healthcare systems and institutions, leading to more streamlined communication and the exchange of data. Since many healthcare systems are becoming more siloed and employing technologies that are incompatible with one another, it becomes difficult for various providers to access and exchange data. Better care coordination and outcomes are feasible when healthcare professionals can quickly access and exchange pertinent information stored in a shared, decentralized database. One possible use of blockchain technology in the medical profession is verifying the legitimacy of medical supplies and equipment, such as medications and surgical tools. By keeping tabs on patients' SCs with blockchain technology, patients will have a better idea of whether or not the medications they are receiving are safe, effective, and of high quality. As a result, blockchain technology is finding increasing use in the medical field [51], and furthermore, it may aid in resolving SC issues [52]. One major benefit of distributed systems is that they make it easier to share information and hold entities accountable even when their interests are at odds. As a result, blockchain technology has the potential to increase the SCs' reliability, authenticity, safety, and scalability. Blockchain technology's traceability characteristics can be used by businesses all along the supply chain to maintain track of critical data in a decentralized ledger that validates it without the need for third-party involvement. This, along with governmental and private sector alerts, creates a checking mechanism capable of identifying and reporting unauthorized or artificial drugs [53].

9.13 Blockchain and IoT for Supply Chain

Transmission of actual data and checking in on possessions along the supply chain are only two examples of the many uses for IoT technology [54]. Integrating blockchain with IoT may improve asset security. Modum, whose main focus is this area, is used to demonstrate how merging varied technology can increase performance. Sensors that may be integrated into compact devices to monitor patient health and create reports for analysis are attracting attention in the healthcare business. Hospitals that use the Internet of Things to streamline administrative tasks for medical staff are intriguing [55]. For example, Kshetri cites the Modum Corporation as an example of how blockchain and IoT may be used together, which originated from a cooperative effort between the university and local community in Zurich. The companies' ultimate goal is to develop a blockchain-based system for the distribution of pharmaceuticals. The company's goal is to use Internet of Things (IoT) principles to track how the medications are holding up over time, according to Kshetri [56] and Campbell. The system checks if specific shipping conditions are met to guarantee the items arrive undamaged. The Modum platform, built on Ethereum and operated by a smart contract, routinely checks that the drug's quality is up to code. If there's a problem with the transaction, the medication won't be given, and an alert will be issued to the control panel [57]. Modum must keep an eye on things like temperature because it deals with the transport of pharmaceuticals. This means the consumer can track the shipment of their medication from the time it leaves the manufacturer all the way to the time it arrives at its final destination, thanks to the distributed ledger technology known as blockchain. Here are the nuts and bolts of how the Modum platform is put together, so you know exactly what you're getting: (1) an Ethereum-based blockchain network; (2) Bluetooth sensors for Internet of Things devices; (3) a PostgreSQL database to keep track of asset information; (4) a REST API platform to service JSON; (5) an intelligent contract to define transactional milestones; and (6) a mobile app to scan drug barcodes and perform quality assurance checks [58].

9.14 Conclusion

This systematic literature study on blockchain technology to support SCs in healthcare found researchers worldwide using this new technology for industry-derived items, like pharmaceuticals and medical devices, and patient-derived products. Blockchain-based traceability technology may make supply chains more transparent and trackable. Blockchain-based traceability solutions are growing in popularity across all supply chains, according to a survey of published articles. The food and pharmaceutical sectors employ them most, according to the literature. Smart contracts and IoT integration are greatly expanding blockchain's uses. Surprisingly, blockchain will not replace current methods. Blockchain-based supply chain transparency needs to be proven.

References

1. Nakamoto S. Bitcoin: A peer-to-peer electronic cash system. *Decentralized Business Review*. 2008 Oct 31:21260.
2. Hasselgren A, Kralevska K, Gligoroski D, Pedersen SA, Faxvaag A. Blockchain in healthcare and health sciences—A scoping review. *International Journal of Medical Informatics*. 2020 Feb 1;134:104040.
3. Mettler M. Blockchain technology in healthcare: The revolution starts here. In *2016 IEEE 18th International Conference on E-Health Networking, Applications and Services (Healthcom)*, 2016 Sep 14 (pp. 1–3). IEEE.
4. Yun D, Chen W, Wu X, Ting DS, Lin H. Blockchain: Chaining digital health to a new era. *Annals of Translational Medicine*. 2020 Jun;8(11).
5. Rupa C, MidhunChakkarvarthy D, Patan R, Prakash AB, Pradeep GG. Knowledge engineering—based DApp using blockchain technology for protract medical certificates privacy. *IET Communications*. 2022 Sep;16(15):1853–64.
6. Bocek T, Rodrigues BB, Strasser T, Stiller B. Blockchains everywhere-a use-case of blockchains in the pharma supply-chain. In *2017 IFIP/IEEE Symposium on Integrated Network and Service Management (IM)*, 2017 May 8 (pp. 772–7). IEEE.
7. Raikwar M, Gligoroski D, Kralevska K. SoK of used cryptography in blockchain. *IEEE Access*. 2019 Oct 11;7:148550–75.
8. Buterin V. A next-generation smart contract and decentralized application platform. *White Paper*. 2014 Jan 14;3(37):2–1.
9. Wechsler R, Anção MS, Campos CJ, Sigulem D. A informática no consultório médico. *Jornal de Pediatria*. 2003;79:S3–12.

10. Azaria A, Ekblaw A, Vieira T, Lippman A. Medrec: Using blockchain for medical data access and permission management. In *2016 2nd International Conference on Open and Big Data (OBD)*, 2016 Aug 22 (pp. 25–30). IEEE.
11. De Aguiar EJ, Faiçal BS, Krishnamachari B, Ueyama J. A survey of blockchain-based strategies for healthcare. *ACM Computing Surveys*. 2020;53(2):1–27; Article 27 (March 2021).
12. Kalil D, Spak T, Godoi W, Santos R, Faria A, Siqueira P, Rosendo M, Gruber Y. *Artificial neural networks as a technique for risk assessment of training critical activities by means of a virtual environment*. 2018. Available from: https://www.sbgames.org/sbgames2018/files/papers/ComputacaoShort/188251.pdf
13. Lee CH, Yoon HJ. Medical big data: Promise and challenges. *Kidney Research and Clinical Practice*. 2017 Mar;36(1):3.
14. Otero P, Hersh W, Ganesh AJ. Big data: Are biomedical and health informatics training programs ready? *Yearbook of Medical Informatics*. 2014;23(1):177–81.
15. Chaudhry B, Wang J, Wu S, Maglione M, Mojica W, Roth E, Morton SC, Shekelle PG. Systematic review: Impact of health information technology on quality, efficiency, and costs of medical care. *Annals of Internal Medicine*. 2006 May 16;144(10):742–52.
16. Mukhopadhyay U, Skjellum A, Hambolu O, Oakley J, Yu L, Brooks R. A brief survey of cryptocurrency systems. In *2016 14th Annual Conference on Privacy, Security and Trust (PST)*, 2016 Dec 12 (pp. 745–52). IEEE.
17. Hughes A, Park A, Kietzmann J, Archer-Brown C. Beyond bitcoin: What blockchain and distributed ledger technologies mean for firms. *Business Horizons*. 2019;62(3):273–81.
18. Swan M. *Blockchain: Blueprint for a New Economy*, 2015 Jan 24 (pp. 1–152). O'Reilly Media, Inc.
19. Rifi N, Rachkidi E, Agoulmine N, Taher NC. Towards using blockchain technology for eHealth data access management. In *2017 fourth international conference on advances in biomedical engineering (ICABME)*, 2017 Oct 19 (pp. 1–4). IEEE.
20. Dinh TT, Liu R, Zhang M, Chen G, Ooi BC, Wang J. Untangling blockchain: A data processing view of blockchain systems. *IEEE Transactions on Knowledge and Data Engineering*. 2018 Jan 4;30(7):1366–85.
21. Kumari K, Saini K. Data handling & drug traceability: Blockchain meets healthcare to combat counterfeit drugs. *International Journal of Scientific & Technology Research*. 2020 Mar;9(3):728–31.
22. Zheng Z, Xie S, Dai HN, Chen X, Wang H. Blockchain challenges and opportunities: A survey. *International Journal of Web and Grid Services*. 2018;14(4):352–75.
23. Alhadhrami Z, Alghfeli S, Alghfeli M, Abedlla JA, Shuaib K. Introducing blockchains for healthcare. In *2017 International Conference on Electrical and Computing Technologies and Applications (ICECTA)*, 2017 Nov 21 (pp. 1–4). IEEE.
24. Greenspan G. *Multichain Private Blockchain-White Paper*. 2015 Jul;85. www.multichain.com/download/MultiChain-White-Paper.pdf.
25. Zhang Q, Cherkasova L, Smirni E. A regression-based analytic model for dynamic resource provisioning of multi-tier applications. In *Fourth International Conference on Autonomic Computing (ICAC'07)*, 2007 Jun 11 (p. 27). IEEE.
26. Pîrlea G, Sergey I. Mechanising blockchain consensus. In *Proceedings of the 7th ACM SIGPLAN International Conference on Certified Programs and Proofs*, 2018 Jan 8 (pp. 78–90). https://doi.org/10.1145/3167086
27. Castro M, Liskov B. Practical byzantine fault tolerance. In *OsDI*, 1999 Feb 22 (pp. 173–86). https://pmg.csail.mit.edu/papers/osdi99.pdf
28. Mingxiao D, Xiaofeng M, Zhe Z, Xiangwei W, Qijun C. A review on consensus algorithm of blockchain. In *2017 IEEE International Conference on Systems, Man, and Cybernetics (SMC)*, 2017 Oct 5 (pp. 2567–72). IEEE.
29. King S, Nadal S. Ppcoin: Peer-to-peer crypto-currency with proof-of-stake. *Self-Published Paper*. 2012 Aug 19;19(1).
30. Clauson KA, Breeden EA, Davidson C, Mackey TK. Leveraging blockchain technology to enhance supply chain management in healthcare: An exploration of challenges and opportunities in the health supply chain. *Blockchain in Healthcare Today*. 2018;1:1–12. https://doi.org/10.30953/bhty.v1.20.
31. Naen MF, Adnan MH, Yazi NA, Nee CK. Development of attendance monitoring system with artificial intelligence optimization in cloud. *International Journal of Artificial Intelligence*. 2021 Dec 23;8(2):88–98.

32. Sylim P, Liu F, Marcelo A, Fontelo P. Blockchain technology for detecting falsified and substandard drugs in distribution: Pharmaceutical supply chain intervention. *JMIR Research Protocols*. 2018 Sep 13;7(9):10163.
33. Dimitrov DV. Blockchain applications for healthcare data management. *Healthcare Informatics Research*. 2019 Jan 31;25(1):51–6.
34. Arpitha MJ, Binduja B, Jahnavi G, Mohanchandra K. Brain computer interface for emergency virtual voice. *International Journal of Artificial Intelligence*. 2021 Jun 22;8(1):40–7.
35. Chamarajan G, Charishma Y. Alzheimer's disease: A survey. *International Journal of Artificial Intelligence*. 2021 Jun 22;8(1):33–9.
36. Desai V, Singh M, Mohanchandra K. Survey on early detection of Alzheimer's disease using capsule neural network. *International Journal of Artificial Intelligence*. 2020 Apr 23;7(1):7–12.
37. Kamath V, Lahari Y, Mohanchandra K. Blockchain based framework for secure data sharing of medicine supply chain in health care system. *International Journal of Artificial Intelligence*. 2022 Jun 9;9(1):32–8.
38. Uddin M, Salah K, Jayaraman R, Pesic S, Ellahham S. Blockchain for drug traceability: Architectures and open challenges. *Health Informatics Journal*. 2021 Apr;27(2):14604582211011228.
39. Nevile C, Polzer G, Coote R, Noble G, Burnett D, Hyland-Wood D. Enterprise ethereum alliance client specification v6. *Enterprise Ethereum Alliance*. 2020. Available from: https://entethalliance.org/wp-content/uploads/2020/11/EEA_Enterprise_Ethereum_Client_Specification_v6.pdf
40. Sousa J, Bessani A, Vukolic M. A Byzantine Fault-Tolerant Ordering Service for the Hyperledger Fabric Blockchain Platform. In *2018 48th Annual IEEE/IFIP International Conference on Dependable Systems and Networks (DSN)*, 2018 (pp. 51–58). https://doi.org/10.1109/DSN.2018.00018
41. Rajput AR, Li Q, Ahvanooey MT. A blockchain-based secret-data sharing framework for personal health records in emergency condition. In *Healthcare*, 2021 Feb 14 (vol. 9, no 2, p. 206). MDPI.
42. Ellram LM, Tate WL, Billington C. Understanding and managing the services supply chain. *Journal of Supply Chain Management*. 2004 Sep;40(3):17–32.
43. Lin FR, Shaw MJ. Reengineering the order fulfillment process in supply chain networks. *International Journal of Flexible Manufacturing Systems*. 1998 Jul;10(3):197–229.
44. Samaranayake P, Toncich D. Integration of production planning, project management and logistics systems for supply chain management. *International Journal of Production Research*. 2007 Nov 15;45(22):5417–47.
45. Schneller ES, Smeltzer LR. Strategic management of the health care supply chain. *Jossey-Bass*. 2006 Feb 17. Available from: https://www.wiley.com/en-us/Strategic+Management+of+the+Health+Care+Supply+Chain-p-9781118193426
46. Choi TY, Li JJ, Rogers DS, Schoenherr T, Wagner SM. *The Oxford Handbook of Supply Chain Management*, 2021. Oxford University Press.
47. Turhan SN, Vayvay Ö. A non traditional vendor managed inventory: A service oriented based supply chain modeling in health services. In *International Conference on Industrial Engineering and Operations Management Istanbul, Turkey*, 2012 (pp. 1526–35). https://ieomsociety.org/ieom2012/pdfs/366.pdf
48. Dobrzykowski D. Understanding the downstream healthcare supply chain: Unpacking regulatory and industry characteristics. *Journal of Supply Chain Management*. 2019 Apr;55(2):26–46.
49. Saeed H, Malik H, Bashir U, Ahmad A, Riaz S, Ilyas M, Bukhari WA, Khan MI. Blockchain technology in healthcare: A systematic review. *PLoS ONE*. 2022 Apr 11;17(4):0266462.
50. Elangovan D, Long CS, Bakrin FS, Tan CS, Goh KW, Yeoh SF, Loy MJ, Hussain Z, Lee KS, Idris AC, Ming LC. The use of blockchain technology in the health care sector: Systematic review. *JMIR Medical Informatics*. 2022 Jan 20;10(1):17278.
51. Sanmarchi F, Toscano F, Fattorini M, Bucci A, Golinelli D. Distributed solutions for a reliable data-driven transformation of healthcare management and research. *Frontiers in Public Health*. 2021;9:944.
52. Maher A.N. Agi, Ashish Kumar Jha, Blockchain technology in the supply chain: An integrated theoretical perspective of organizational adoption, *International Journal of Production Economics*, Volume 247, 2022,108458:1–15. https://doi.org/10.1016/j.ijpe.2022.108458.
53. Longo F, Nicoletti L, Padovano A, d'Atri G, Forte M. Blockchain-enabled supply chain: An experimental study. *Computers & Industrial Engineering*. 2019 Oct 1;136:57–69.

54. Yan B, Huang G. Supply chain information transmission based on RFID and internet of things. In *2009 ISECS International Colloquium on Computing, Communication, Control, and Management*, 2009 Aug 8 (vol. 4, pp. 166–9). IEEE.
55. Rahmani AM, Gia TN, Negash B, Anzanpour A, Azimi I, Jiang M, Liljeberg P. Exploiting smart e-Health gateways at the edge of healthcare Internet-of-Things: A fog computing approach. *Future Generation Computer Systems*. 2018 Jan 1;78:641–58.
56. Kshetri N. 1 Blockchain's roles in meeting key supply chain management objectives. *International Journal of Information Management*. 2018 Apr 1;39:80–9.
57. Öz S, Gören HE. Application of blockchain technology in the supply chain management process: Case studies. *Journal of International Trade, Logistics and Law*. 2019 Jun 12;5(1):21–7.
58. Bocek T, Rodrigues BB, Strasser T, Stiller B. Blockchains everywhere-a use-case of blockchains in the pharma supply-chain. In *2017 IFIP/IEEE Symposium on Integrated Network and Service Management (IM)*, 2017 May 8 (pp. 772–7). IEEE.

10

Leveraging Blockchain in Sharing and Managing Health Record Credential

Atul B. Kathole, Sonali D. Patil, Vinod V. Kimbahune, and Avinash P. Jadhav

10.1 Introduction

The informatization of more and more healthcare facilities is leading to an increase in the amount of medical data that is being collected [1]. It is absolutely necessary to encourage the sharing of electronic medical data if one wishes to achieve improved resource integration as well as higher diagnostic and treatment efficacy. The patient's medical records, on the other hand, include a plethora of personally identifiable information that must be safeguarded. Issues about data privacy leaks and misuse in the interchange of medical data pose a significant risk to the lives and possessions of patients. In the context of data sharing, concerns regarding data security and privacy are, as a result, of utmost significance. In addition, there are information islands as a result of the dispersion of medical records among numerous medical facilities as well as the utilization of a variety of data storage formats. A medical health record (MHR) is an electronic version of a patient's medical history that is stored on a computer (MHR). Electronic health records are playing an increasingly important part in the healthcare profession in this day and age of information. Despite this, there are concerns over the security and confidentiality of the medical records of patients [1], [2]. The transition to cloud-based systems and Ethereum blockchains, which enable global connections to be made between patients and clinicians, is being pursued by a number of organizations in an effort to overcome these issues [3]. The patient has full control over their own data and can provide access to parties whom they have determined to be reliable [4]. In this day and age, we are able to share virtually anything with a mobile device, including images, movies, texts, and even access to our investment accounts; but medical records continue to be inaccessible. This is as a result of the fact that the environment surrounding healthcare is becoming more complicated as an increasing number of parties become involved in the process of generating intricate and essential data connections. Because of this, there is the potential for privacy breaches, security breaches, and a decrease in operational efficiency. Hence, there has been no progress made in solving the problem of incompatible health data [5]. In 2008, Nakamoto wrote a paper describing Bitcoin and is credited with having invented the blockchain system. It's a network that allows different computers to communicate and share information with one another [6]. A blockchain is a complex data system that stores ever-expanding archives in individual blocks [7]. As a consequence of this, each newly contributed block of information in the blockchain is connected to the block that came before it. The use of a hash price renders it unchallengeable; all recorded processes are time-stamped, giving it a unique identity, and the models are disseminated to each node in the participating system, guaranteeing that the information's veracity is preserved even after terminations occur without any outside interference [8]. The InterPlanetary File System (IPFS) is a distributed data storage system that operates in a manner that is analogous to that of the peer-to-peer (P2P) bit torrent protocol. Its purpose is to build a network in which all digital devices have access to the same data file structure, which in this instance would be helpful for storing vast quantities of medical data [9]. The Internet of Things (IoT) is ubiquitous in the modern world; however, it has had a particularly rapid growth in the field of medicine since [10]. Because the Internet of Things (IoT) and wearable devices are gaining popularity in the medical industry, the quality of therapy that is offered has improved as a result. Wearable technology has the capability of collecting a person's health data and transmitting it to medical facilities or physicians [11]. The information that is gathered by wearable Internet of Things devices in the realm of medicine is both essential and confidential. Because of the potential influence that this information can have on a person's life, it is of utmost significance that it be protected [12]. Blockchain technology allows for the secure storage of sensitive patient information that has been collected by a wide variety of Internet of Things devices.

The following is a list of important takeaways from this article:

> (1) To explain the concept behind blockchain technology, how the distributed ledger technology (blockchain) impacts (2) the confidentiality of patient records. (3) Information about each requester is stored in the form of a collection of attributes within a smart contract. Hence, smart contracts can automatically implement access control if the appropriate data is provided [13].

10.2 Literature Review

A basic organization is responsible for managing, leading, and guiding the system in a centralized design, such as those that support old-style EHR systems. This organization is also responsible for ensuring that the system is functioning properly. With a distributed architecture, each lump is managed separately from any dominant specialized one that may be present. Following that, we will offer a concise summary of the EHR framework as well as our blockchain expertise [14].

10.2.1 EHR Structures

A lot of people consider the electronic health record, sometimes known as an EHR, to be a database that stores patients' medical histories (such as electronic medicinal records—EMRs). Electronic health records (EHR) can benefit from the information contained in electronic medical records (EMRs), which are kept primarily by medical professionals, such as physicians and nurses. The patient's private health record (PHR) now contains the health information that was acquired by the patient's own wearable devices. The patient is now able to provide their PHR to the healthcare professionals who are treating them (patients). Information can be continuously transmitted among authorized users (for example, medical doctors who are granted permission to view a specific patient's information in order to assist in research), and the EHR structure should guarantee the confidentiality of the data entered as well as its accessibility and integrity. In addition to this, if done correctly, the development of such a framework has the ability to eliminate the possibility of redundant data as well as the danger of files becoming lost [15]. Yet the growing interconnectedness of these networks makes the problem of protecting information while it is in transit or while it is stored within these kinds of systems even more difficult (e.g., more probable outbreak vectors).

10.2.2 Blockchain

Blockchain technology, which sprang to prominence as a result of Bitcoin's success, enables users to carry out reliable and secure communications across an untrusted system without relying on a centralized third party. In this part of the guide, we'll discuss the fundamental components of blockchain that put it all together. Blockchain technology is the best option for creating comprehensive and effective contract records [16].

The following information is contained within the block header:

- Prior block hash: the value of the hash function computed on the previous block.
- Time stamp: the point in time at which the current block was generated.

Before calculating the hash value, miners will alter an arbitrary four-byte field that is known as a "nonce." This is done so that they can solve mining problems that need proof-of-work. The value of the Merkle tree root hash that was formed by the transactions in the main body of the blockchain; For a new effective block, the target hash is the value cutoff. The target hash will decide the level of difficulty of the proof-of-work problem. The transactions that took place inside a specified window of time and have had their validity verified are what constitute the block body. The hash value of the related divisions can be used to validate the validity of any contract in such a tree assembly, giving it a reliable mechanism for demonstrating the integrity and continuing existence of a transaction. This is in contrast to the entire Merkle tree, which cannot be used for this purpose. In the meantime, every time there is a change to the agreement, a new hash value will be generated in the leading deposit, which will result in the root hash being compromised. In addition, the maximum number of contracts that a block is able to carry is determined not only by the parameters of each individual contract but also by the parameters of the block as a whole [17]. For the purpose of linking and composing these blocks, a cryptographic hash function and an append-only assembly are utilized. Because it is not possible to alter or remove information that has previously been confirmed, any new information that is contributed must be done so in the form of supplemental blocks that are linked to earlier blocks. Each time a block was modified, a new hash value and link connection would be generated. This was something that had been stated previously. Because of this, we have achieved both immutability and safety.

10.2.2.1 Smart Agreement

Smart contracts are protocols that are built on blockchain technology and have the ability to execute themselves. These contracts have found applications in a broad variety of fields, including government, healthcare, and the financial sector. A system like this one is able to carry out complicated programming tasks, provided that it receives the contract invocation signal in the appropriate agreement discourse [18]. The smart agreement will automatically put the predetermined terms into effect inside a safe container. Ethereum is the first blockchain platform that is publicly available, and it features the world's first library of revolutionary agreement dialects. These dialects are Turing complete, and they can be used to install any kind of distributed request system (DApps).

10.2.2.2 Nomenclature of Blockchain Structures

There are essentially three different kinds of blockchain systems, which can be separated from one another based on the accuracy of the data that is authenticated by the nodes that make up the network: a public ledger that is shared. To participate in the community blockchain as a miner or a significant node at any moment, anyone who meets the requirements can do so in exchange for tokens [19]. Bitcoin and Ethereum are two of the most well-known public blockchain systems; however, there are numerous other public blockchain systems as well.

10.2.2.3 Private Blockchain

Participants need to submit an application for participation in the decentralized blockchain network and then be granted permission to do so before they may join. Isolated blockchain topologies are some instances, and GemOS and MultiChain are two that come to mind. Ledger that is distributed contextually. The association blockchain is considered to be a "semi-private" blockchain, which allows it to bridge the gap between local and decentralized networks. It is presented to recognized institutions who have demonstrated a dedication to fostering an innovative culture for the betterment of their workforce. A business consortium conceived up and created the blockchain infrastructure known as Hyperledger Fabric MultiChain [20]. Moreover, consortium blockchains can be created more easily with Ethereum's help.

10.3 Blockchain-Based EHR Systems

There will be a purpose for private data, and only users who have been given permission will be able to access the data that has been requested. Privacy, veracity, and access are all assured, which contribute to the system's overall level of safety. The information is encrypted, and only people who have been authorized to see it can view it.

- *Accuracy*. In order to guarantee that the information is accurate, it must be transferred without being altered by any third parties.
- *Accessibility* ensures that data and property are not unlawfully withheld from legitimate users of the system.
- *Auditability*, a crucial component of information security. Review logs, for instance, are primarily made up of information on who accessed which electronic health record (or individual personal health record) and for what cause, in addition to the time-stamping of all activities carried out over the entirety of the life cycle.

In the case that improper behavior was observed, the individuals involved will be held accountable through the use of auditing methods. Because of concerns about privacy, there are no external signals that can be used to determine who or what an entity is. Being fully invisible to others is not an easy task. Research on healthcare applications of blockchain technology is now concentrating its efforts in the following areas, with the end goal of achieving the goals outlined earlier: preserving the confidentiality and safety of the records [21]. The blockchain is a reliable and validated database that may be used for keeping track of a wide variety of confidential medical records. In addition to the construction of secure storage, the privacy of the data must also be guaranteed. In contrast, healthcare datasets are usually extremely vast and intricate in practice. Having said that, another problem that needs to be solved is how to store vast volumes of data without causing a blockchain network to become sluggish.

A fair and balanced presentation of the data. The responsibility of data stewardship is placed on service providers in the majority of contemporary forms of healthcare delivery. The idea of self-sovereignty is the driving force behind a movement that is moving toward returning control of one's medical records to the individual, who should be free to disclose or withhold that data as he sees fit [22]. This change is expected to take place in the next several years. It is essential for ensuring honest communication between companies and industries, as well as between industries and sectors.

Auditing of data. By checking audit logs, requestors can be held responsible for their usage of electronic health records (EHRs) when disagreements emerge (EHRs). Several systems rely on blockchain technology and smart contracts to maintain activity logs, which enables auditing of those systems. Any transaction or request will be able to undergo instant verification thanks to the distributed ledger.

Leadership that is both dynamic and original. Verifying the identities of all the system's operators is essential to ensuring that everything runs well. Only authorized operators are allowed to make the necessary wishes in order to maintain the integrity of the structure, as well as to avoid any kind of malicious activity. Following this, we will examine the current procedures for data archiving, data sharing, data auditing, and identity management to gain a better understanding of these topics.

10.3.1 Information Storage

10.3.1.1 How to Accomplish Safe Information Storage

Using blockchain technology is one of the many potential approaches that may be taken in order to improve the EHR system's already-impressive level of security. Nonetheless, in the absence of encryption or authentication, sensitive data that is kept in a blockchain database may be open to statistical attacks. Encoding, anonymization, and contact switch instruments are a few examples of ways for maintaining secrecy that are both cryptographic and non-cryptographic in nature. According to the recommendations made by Zheng et al., data should be encoded by employing the symmetrical essential approach as well as a threshold encoding strategy before being saved in the cloud (2018). Using Shamir's top-secret distribution method, the symmetrical key will be cut up into a large number of pieces, each of which will be given to a separate key holder [23]. Deciphering the ciphertext is only possible if the requester has access to a sufficient number of key stocks. A breach that affects less than the predetermined minimum number of essential keepers would not result in the loss of data. Yue et al. came up with the idea for the Healthcare Data Gateway in 2016, which is a mobile application that makes use of blockchain technology as well as MPC (HDG). Guo et al. also proposed an attribute-based healthcare blockchain autograph technique that would include many organizations (2018) (MA-ABS). The signature used in this system does not serve to attest to the one-of-a-kind nature of the individual who gives final approval to a message; rather, it serves to indicate a right (such as an access strategy) to the characteristics that he possesses as determined by some higher authority. In other words, the signature does not serve to authenticate the uniqueness of the individual. The network is made more resistant to collisions when the secret seeds for the pseudorandom function (PRF) are dispersed throughout a number of different companies [24]. In order for healthcare infrastructures to be able to withstand violent assaults, their encoding keys for typical operations need to be continuously updated (such an arithmetical attack). In order to understand specific old content, many historical keys will need to be put in a secure location; as a result, the expense of keeping and administering these historical keys will increase. This will be especially true for applications that only have a limited amount of processing resources and/or pricey storage devices.

10.3.1.2 How to Store Extensive Healthcare Information

The blockchain may one day be utilized by electronic health record (EHR) systems to facilitate the archiving of medical records and other types of data. If this information were to be directly stored in the blockchain network, it would result in an increase in both the computational cost and the storage load. This is because the blockchain has a secure and restricted block extent. Yet there is a risk that one's privacy could be compromised [25] by such information. Zheng et al. (2018) came up with the idea of cloud packing in order to demonstrate how machine learning could benefit from health records that have been stored on the blockchain [26]. Data that is kept in the cloud can be decrypted, but only if the buyer meets certain requirements and has sufficient replacement components. Using a distributed storage architecture, Juneja and Marefat (2018) have developed a solution to the problem of the packing constraint imposed by blockchain as well as the inability to carry out correct rollbacks when the number of false alarms increases. This approach can now be implemented. In addition, Azaria et al. (2016) utilized offline data stores in order to save data associated with medicine in a cache that was located behind firewalls. If Gatekeeper is given permission to do so, it is possible for it to provide the result of a query [18]. Liu et al. have devised a method for the safe storage of medical records in the cloud that is based on CP-ABE for hospital admission control (2018) (CCAC). By integrating cloud-based data with corresponding extraction signatures, data requesters are able to validate the reliability and authenticity of the data being requested. According to the idea put forth by Sun et al., the newly developed SignedEHR is legally bound by the attribute-based signatures of healthcare donors and is kept in a reliable third-party database to preserve the privacy of patients (2018). Before the document can be uploaded to the blockchain system, the doctors need to verify its authenticity by using a decentralized attribute-based sign (DABS) [19]. This is necessary for the blockchain system to be able to approve the application for the proposal record. The address of the applicable SignedEHR is the most important component of the request that must be provided. Verifying the user's signature is required in order to determine whether or not the person requesting access to the data is who they claim to be. Data pertaining to medical care can be documented using a variety of mediums, such as text, photographs, and electronic medical records. Because of its small block size, blockchain is not ideal for high-capacity data storage; as a consequence, healthcare systems will need to study alternative methods of storing huge amounts of data [20]. Blockchain's limited block size renders it unsuitable for high-capacity data storage. Nguyen et al. (2019) developed a system that integrates smart agreements with IPFS to enable decentralized cloud packing and regulated information delivery. This was done with the intention of enhancing operator and contact monitoring.

10.3.2 Information Sharing

There is essential data that is used to assist the healthcare industry located in a variety of locations, including hospitals, clinics, and laboratories, among other locations. The storing, retrieval, and updating of healthcare data is essential to the provision of medical treatment. Because different businesses employ a variety of data formats, there are complications that arise when attempting to communicate medical data in this manner [21]. We will begin by talking about interoperability, which is a requirement for data interchange and requires a thorough investigation of the data collected by each organization before it can be used by other businesses.

10.3.2.1 Contact Control Instrument with an Intelligent Agreement for Information Distribution

Patients should not have to go through the inconvenience and inefficiencies of transporting their hefty paper medical records from one healthcare facility to another. By improving the way in which information is shared, both the quality of healthcare services and the cost of treatment can see significant improvements. Current EHR systems certainly give a great deal of convenience; yet, there are still a great many barriers in the healthcare data formats that are used, which limit the safe and ascendable exchange of information across a variety of settings. As was indicated previously, one of the hazards associated with a centralized system is the potential for data loss as well as attacks directed at a single location. When patients share their information with a trusted third party, they have little choice but to give up control of their personal information. This might leave the door open for businesses to abuse the confidence they have earned in the community [22]. Not only that, but the difficulty of organizations that compete with one another to create trustworthy links with one another and share information is a barrier to the expansion of information sharing. Because of this, it is essential to reinstate consumer control over their data and increase privacy laws in order to make communication more accessible. It will be more challenging to safely share health information across several domains, but it will be much simpler to manage issues of safety and confidentiality when the information is contained within a single institution. In the meanwhile, it is necessary to investigate different strategies to improve collaboration within the healthcare industry. A secure access control system, which demands that only approved firms transmit information, is a standard solution that is commonly used. An ACL is a list of requestors who may need admission information and the associated consents (read, inscribe, apprise) to detailed information. The admission policy in this method typically includes an ACL related to the information owner. An ACL is a list of requestors who may need admission information and the associated consents (read, inscribe, apprise). The process by which legally operating enterprises are given permission to enter restricted regions in a manner that is in conformity with the standards that have been set forth for admittance is referred to as an "endorsement" [23]. The step that requires authentication happens first, always before the one that requires authorization. The access rules that govern this mechanism place a primary emphasis on determining who makes what changes to what data item and why they make those changes. A third party is responsible for the implementation, administration, and operation of the traditional methods of regulating access to the exchange of electronic health records. Users typically rely on third parties (such as cloud servers) to reliably check and accept their information use preferences. This is because third parties have more access to the user's information. In point of fact, however, the server is sociable and inquisitive. When blockchain technology is combined with an admission control apparatus, it may be possible to generate a reliable framework within which companies may handle their data in a manner that is both confidential and secure between themselves [24]. The fact that individuals are able to maintain control over their data even as they use smart contracts on the blockchain to establish access permissions (grant, deny, revoke), actions (read, inscribe, apprise, delete), and durations (read, inscribe, apprise, delete) is one of the most important aspects of this new paradigm (read, inscribe, apprise, remove). A smart agreement can be implemented on the blockchain if the conditions are met, and it can also be used as a tool for auditing any demand that has been recorded there. If the prerequisites are not met, the smart agreement cannot be completed. There is an increasing amount of research on the use of smart contracts to ease safe exchange of healthcare information, and there is also a growing demand for this.

10.3.2.2 Cryptography Knowledge for Information Sharing

When it comes to electronic health record (EHR) systems, the use of encryption can further improve the level of safety offered to the transmission of data as well as the admittance of patients. This is because encryption can prevent unauthorized parties from reading the data. In the research paper that Dubovitskaya and her colleagues published in 2017, they advocated that the management and dissemination of electronic medical records (EMRs) for cancer patients should make use of an architecture that was based on symmetrical encryption. Patients have the ability to generate symmetrical encoding keys, which can then be used in secure communication with their respective healthcare practitioners. These keys can be utilized for the purpose of transmitting sensitive information. In accordance with the access regulations that were established [25], the medical professionals will each receive a new key after the procedure, for re-encrypting the proxy has been finished and is considered complete. This whole thing hinges on whether or not the symmetric key is willing to cooperate.

The information that is stored on the reliable cloud service. Patients have the ability to utilize smart contracts to safely set access restrictions and exchange symmetric keys in order to protect the confidentiality of their data and prevent unauthorized access. This can be accomplished by preventing unauthorized access. A method for validating operator identities and distributing keys to unlock limited content from a shared database of sophisticated data was developed by Xia et al. (2017). This method was published in 2017. Creating a method to check operator identities and distribute keys was necessary in order to achieve this goal. Only authorized operators will be able to make information requests to the system as a result of the combination of the user–issuer protocol, which is used to create the association confirmation and contract keys, and the user–verifier process, which is used to verify the authenticity of the association. Both of these protocols are used to ensure that the association is genuine. The combination of these two techniques makes this accomplishment feasible. Ramani et al. (2018) created a large number of lightweight cryptographic methods that were requested by the community as part of an attempt to boost the level of security provided by authorization checks (affix, retrieve). When patient information is maintained on a private blockchain, only the patient themselves can make changes to that information, and they will be notified before the alteration is made public.

10.3.3 Information Audit

In the event that there is a disagreement regarding the users' contacts with the patient history, audit logs can be used as proof in order for users to continue to bear responsibility for those interactions. The immutable community ledger and smart contracts offered by blockchain technology have the potential to produce immutable records for all admissions requirements, thereby creating both responsibility and traceability in the process. The information that is documented in the audit log must be both vital and easily comprehended in order to be valid. The user ID for a recorded event's request for data owner ID is obtained as part of an accomplishment type, indicating the impact of authentication requirements [26].

10.3.4 Identity Manager

Before allowing access to any resources, the first step in verifying the safety of any structure is to establish the structure's associations. The access control system that was just described always performs identity verification prior to releasing any sensitive data. This is done with the intention of ensuring that only genuine data requestors are provided access to sensitive information. Examples of typical types of operator verification include pass-through verification, biometric verification, and individuality confirmation through the use of community basic cryptography. The master patient index (MPI) is the central component that acts as the backbone for managing discrete information in traditional electronic health record (EHR) systems. It ensures the authenticity and one-of-a-kindness of each record while also facilitating the appropriate connections between files. Users that wish to join the blockchain network are required to offer an explanation, which must include a community key and a remote key. The remote key is used for marking transactions, while the community key is used for operator documentation. The shared-world component of this asymmetric key pair then describes the characteristics of each distinct entity. When it comes to identifying information, the blockchain relies on an address rather than a person's actual name [27]. Identity management, issuance of registration, and contract documents for contributing nodes were all taken care of by the Hyperledger Fabric Association Facility Benefactor (MSP). Al Omar and his colleagues were the ones who came up with the idea of uniqueness oversight registration (2017). When a celebration makes its first attempt to enter the building, it is required to register once, and it must keep its ID and PWD in order to log in and have access to secure channels on subsequent occasions.

10.4 Future Movements

10.4.1 Big Information

The immutability, security, and traceability of the technology known as blockchain may provide the solution to the problem of how to handle the security flaws in the big data approach. According to Otero et al. (2014), comprehensive data may be able to maximize the exploitation of all healthcare information assets to support essential changes. These changes include predicting in the healthcare diagnostics field, assessing magnetic resonance imaging, and other claims. In most cases, *information management* and *data investigation* are the appropriate umbrella terms to use when discussing extensive data analysis. There is potential for blockchain technology to be used in the administration of patient data in the healthcare industry. This would protect the privacy of patients' personal information. In terms of data analysis, it is feasible to filter through records and conversations that are based on blockchain technology in order to find indications of prospective commercial activity.

10.4.2 Machine Learning

Methods of machine learning have the potential to be helpful in both the optimization of healthcare systems and the delivery of intelligent services. Figuring out how to collect, transmit, and train sensitive information in a secure manner is one of the most significant challenges that real-world machine learning systems face. Using machine learning with blockchain is becoming increasingly popular as a strategy to enhance the datasets' level of privacy and data security. Sharing data across several computer nodes can be an effective way to machine learning that is referred to as linked learning, provided that appropriate precautions are in place. By sharing their encrypted datasets, many hospitals and other healthcare organizations can collaborate to develop prediction algorithms that are extraordinarily precise. It is possible that blockchain technology might be utilized as a controller to record training-related communications that cannot be disputed and are completely transparent, so ensuring accountability and trustworthy collaboration. This will make it easier for medical administrations and researchers to communicate encoded datasets, which will ultimately lead to improvements in both medical care and public health. Because blockchain has the capacity to maintain users' confidentiality, the data that is fed into machine learning algorithms may be relied upon. The purpose of Yaji et al.'s work is to make it easier for academics to share massive datasets with one another who are working in a variety of subjects (2018). Gentry claims that there is current research being done toward homomorphic encryption in order to perform machine learning on encrypted data (2009). Nonetheless, homomorphic encryption does in fact result in a significant loss of processing capacity. In the not-too-distant future, it may be able to protect critical data in smart buildings without obstructing the process of machine learning. In the event that inaccurate predictions are made with a high rate, rollback models could be saved in the blockchain. The references that retrained models use to access their necessary data are saved in an immutable and secure format in blockchain [22]. Moreover, AI might be used to automate the development of intelligent interactions, which would both increase the safety of operations and their degree of adaptability.

10.4.3 Internet of Things (IoT)

There is a rising need to enhance protections for the privacy of sensitive data acquired by sensors as their use becomes more widespread in a diverse array of applications. These sensors capture a lot of personal information. The majority of data in the Internet of Things is exchanged between low-powered devices using unsecured wireless networks, making it susceptible to being intercepted and changed by hostile actors. As we have seen, the blockchain-based technologies that we have been discussing up to this point provide a secure information access control framework and distributed critical supervision that can be used to build a secure IoT device message. This can be accomplished by distributing critical supervision across multiple nodes. 5G would be the next generation of message networks, and it would be characterized by a high throughput, an enormous storage capacity, and the ability to scale. The field of next-generation intelligent healthcare will benefit from 5G IoT in a variety of ways, including improved reliability, decreased latency, and increased throughput, to name just a few. A 5G wireless smartphone system was proposed to be used in the future for the long-term care of people who suffer from chronic illnesses. Patients suffering from diabetes were evaluated and monitored in the same manner as before by Min et al. (2018). Both the system slice agent and the 5G system supervision layer may stand to gain from the application of blockchain technology within the framework of this design.

10.5 Conclusion

This study demonstrates that the blockchain technology holds significant promise for bringing about significant change within the conventional healthcare system. There are, however, a few scientific and practical obstacles that need to be cleared away before existing EHR institutions would be able to participate fully in blockchain-based knowledge sharing. It is necessary for a patient to go through a lengthy and involved procedure in order to have access to his or her medical records. Electronic health records, also known as EHRs, might very well provide the foundation for an increase in the monitoring of digital health records in the near future. Information security techniques and approaches may be utilized in order to provide digital care in a variety of areas, including banking, economics, supply chain supervision, public media, and the Internet of Things. During the course of our investigation, we focused more closely on a few of these difficulties and talked at length about them. After that, we identified a number of intriguing research gaps in a variety of fields, one of which was the Internet of Things (IoT). We have high hopes that our analysis will lead to a greater knowledge of how to develop and execute EHR structures for the benefit of our (ageing) species in the generations to come, and we expect that this will come about as a direct result of our efforts.

References

[1] Ahram T., Sargolzaei A., Sargolzaei S., Daniels J., Amaba B. *2017 IEEE Technology & Engineering Management Conference (TEMSCON)*. IEEE; 2017. Blockchain technology innovations; pp. 137–41.

[2] Ahsan M.A.M., Wahab A.W.B.A., Idris M.Y.I.B., Khan S., Bachura E., Choo K.-K.R. CLASS: Cloud log assuring soundness and secrecy scheme for cloud forensics. *IEEE Trans. Sust. Comput.* 2021;6(2):184–96. https://doi.org/10.1109/TSUSC.2018.2833502.

[3] Al Omar A., Rahman M.S., Basu A., Kiyomoto S. *International Conference on Security, Privacy and Anonymity in Computation, Communication and Storage*. Springer; 2017. Medibchain: A blockchain based privacy preserving platform for healthcare data; pp. 534–43.

[4] Dai W., Dai C., Choo K.R., Cui C., Zou D., Jin H. SDTE: A secure blockchain-based data trading ecosystem. *IEEE Trans. Inf. Forens. Secur.* 2020;15:725–37.

[5] Feng Q., He D., Liu Z., Wang D., Choo K.-K.R. Multi-party signing protocol for the identity-based signature scheme in IEEE p1363 standard. *IET Inf. Secur.* 2020;1(99):1–10.

[6] Feng Q., He D., Zeadally S., Khan M.K., Kumar N. A survey on privacy protection in blockchain system. *J. Netw. Comput. Appl.* 2019;126:45–58. [Google Scholar]

[7] GemOS: The blockchain operating system; 2020 [online]. Available: https://enterprise.gem.co/.

[8] He D., Zhang Y., Wang D., Choo K.-K.R. Secure and efficient two-party signing protocol for the identity-based signature scheme in the IEEE P1363 standard for public key cryptography. *IEEE Trans. Dependable Secure Comput.* 2018;1(99):1–10.

[9] Ho S.Y., Guo X., Vogel D. Opportunities and challenges in healthcare information systems research: Caring for patients with chronic conditions. *Commun. Assoc. Inf. Syst.* 2019;44(1):39.

[10] Hardjono T., Pentland A. Verifiable anonymous identities and access control in permissioned blockchains. *arXiv preprint arXiv:1903.04584.* 2019.

[11] Huang H., Chen X., Wang J. Blockchain-based multiple groups data sharing with anonymity and traceability. *Sci. China Inf. Sci.* 2020;63:130101. https://doi.org/10.1007/s11432-018-9781-0.

[12] Hyperledger Fabric; 2020 [online]. Available: www.hyperledger.org/.

[13] Jiang S., Cao J., Wu H., Yang Y., Ma M., He J. *2018 IEEE International Conference on Smart Computing (SMARTCOMP).* IEEE; 2018. Blochie: A blockchain-based platform for healthcare information exchange; pp. 49–56.

[14] Lin C., He D., Huang X., Khan M.K., Choo K.-K.R. Dcap: A secure and efficient decentralized conditional anonymous payment system based on blockchain. *IEEE Trans. Inf. Forensics Secur.* 2020;15:2440–52.

[15] Liu J., Li X., Ye L., Zhang H., Du X., Guizani M. *2018 IEEE Global Communications Conference (GLOBECOM).* IEEE; 2018. BPDS: A blockchain based privacy-preserving data sharing for electronic medical records; pp. 1–6.

[16] Lloret J., Parra L., Taha M., Toms J. An architecture and protocol for smart continuous ehealth monitoring using 5g. *Comp. Netw.* 2017:S1389128617302189.

[17] Miah S.J., Gammack J., Hasan N. Methodologies for designing healthcare analytics solutions: A literature analysis. *Health Inform. J.* 2019:1460458219895386.

[18] Min C., Yang J., Zhou J., Hao Y., Youn C.H. 5g-smart diabetes: Toward personalized diabetes diagnosis with healthcare big data clouds. *IEEE Commun. Mag.* 2018;56(4):16–23.

[19] Morelli U., Ranise S., Sartori D., Sciarretta G., Tomasi A. *International Workshop on Security and Trust Management.* Springer; 2019. Audit-based access control with a distributed ledger: Applications to healthcare organizations; pp. 19–35.

[20] MultiChain: Open platform for building blockchains; 2020 [online]. Available: www.multichain.com/.

[21] Pussewalage H.S.G., Oleshchuk V.A. *2018 IEEE International Conference on Internet of Things (iThings) and IEEE Green Computing and Communications (GreenCom) and IEEE Cyber, Physical and Social Computing (CPSCom) and IEEE Smart Data (SmartData).* IEEE; 2018. Blockchain based delegatable access control scheme for a collaborative e-health environment; pp. 1204–11.

[22] Qi X., Sifah E.B., Asamoah K.O., Gao J., Du X., Guizani M. Medshare: Trust-less medical data sharing among cloud service providers via blockchain. *IEEE Access.* 2017;5(99):14757–67.

[23] Sun Y., Zhang R., Wang X., Gao K., Liu L. *2018 27th International Conference on Computer Communication and Networks (ICCCN).* IEEE; 2018. A decentralizing attribute-based signature for healthcare blockchain; pp. 1–9.

[24] Tovanich N., Heulot N., Fekete J.-D. Isenberg P. Visualization of blockchain data: A systematic review. *IEEE Trans. Vis. Comput. Graph.* 2021;27(7):3135–52. https://doi.org/10.1109/TVCG.2019.2963018.

[25] Yaji S., Bangera K., Neelima B. *2018 IEEE 25th International Conference on High Performance Computing Workshops (HiPCW).* IEEE; 2018. Privacy preserving in blockchain based on partial homomorphic encryption system for ai applications; pp. 81–5.

[26] Yang G., Li C. *2018 IEEE International Conference on Cloud Computing Technology and Science (CloudCom).* IEEE; 2018. A design of blockchain-based architecture for the security of electronic health record (ehr) systems; pp. 261–5.

[27] Yang R., Yu F.R., Si P., Yang Z., Zhang Y. Integrated blockchain and edge computing systems: A survey, some research issues and challenges. *IEEE Commun. Surv. Tutor.* 2019;21(2):1508–32.

11

Healthcare Record Management for Healthcare 4.0 via Blockchain: A Review of Current Applications, Opportunities, Challenges, and Future Potential

Shalom Akhai

11.1 Introduction to Healthcare 4.0: Embracing Digital Transformation in Healthcare

The healthcare sector has undergone considerable transformations from the initial days of industry 1.0 to the current HC 4.0 era [1]. The integration of novel technologies and digitalization has led to more streamlined, productive, and patient-oriented healthcare delivery [2]. This chapter discusses the development of healthcare delivery, the features and definition of HC 4.0, and the major factors that enable this change, along with the hinderances which need to be addresses for more effective implication.

11.1.1 The Progression of Healthcare Delivery: From Industry 1.0 to Healthcare 4.0

The healthcare sector has experienced several phases of growth throughout its history, beginning with industry 1.0, which introduced steam power and mechanization. Industry 2.0 brought mass production and assembly-line techniques, while industry 3.0 saw the rise of automation and computerization. Currently, we have entered the age of HC 4.0, which integrates state-of-the-art technologies, such as the Internet of Things (IoT), into healthcare delivery, with the goal of creating a better capable, useful, and patient-focused medical assistance structure [3–5]. From manual to digital, from reactive to proactive, from isolated to interconnected—the progression of healthcare delivery is transforming lives in the era of healthcare 4.0. **Figure 11.1** illustrates the essential technologies driving the industry 4.0 revolution in the manufacturing sector. The figure includes icons that represent computer-aided manufacturing, factories, technology, and related concepts, all of which play a crucial function in the transformation of healthcare delivery in the era of HC 4.0.

Figure 11.2, on the other hand, illustrates the intersection of emerging technologies and patient-centered care in the healthcare industry. This figure depicts various technologies that are transforming the delivery of healthcare, such as blockchain, telemedicine, and artificial intelligence, among others. The figure emphasizes the importance

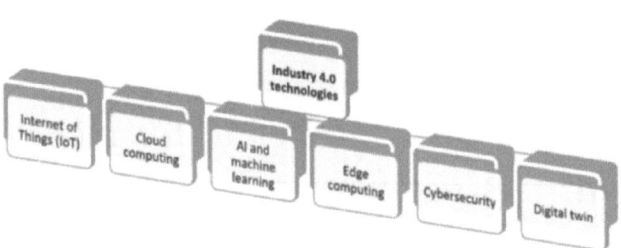

FIGURE 11.1
Industry 4.0 technologies.

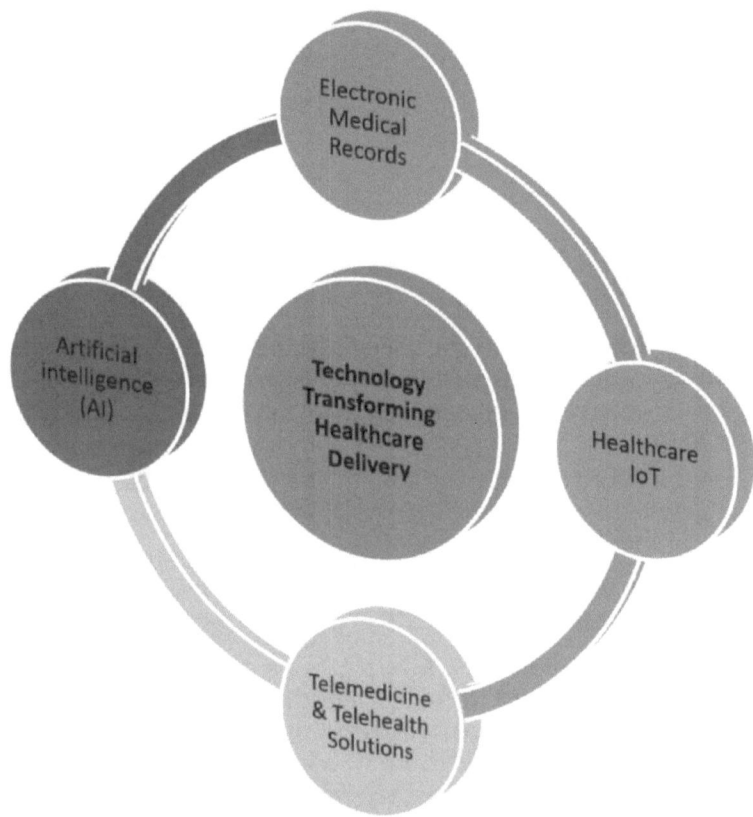

FIGURE 11.2
The intersection of emerging technologies and patient-centered care.

of patient-centricity in healthcare, where patients are at the center of care delivery and emerging technologies are used to enhance their experiences and outcomes.

11.1.2 Healthcare 4.0: Definition, Characteristics, and Goals

HC 4.0 represents a new era of healthcare delivery, marking the fourth industrial revolution. This phase is distinguished by the incorporation of digital technologies, including

IoT, artificial intelligence (AI), big data analytics, and blockchain, into the healthcare system [6–8]. The primary objective of HC 4.0 is to enhance healthcare delivery by improving efficiency, effectiveness, and patient-centered care.

- One of the essential elements of HC 4.0 is the emphasis on personalized medicine. With the help of digital technologies, healthcare providers can collect and analyze patient data to tailor treatments to individual patients. This personalized approach to healthcare delivery can lead to better patient outcomes and improved overall healthcare system efficiency [9].
- Another important characteristic of HC 4.0 is the use of digital tools to enhance communication and collaboration between healthcare providers, patients, and other stakeholders. Digital technologies, such as telemedicine and remote patient monitoring, can facilitate real-time communication and information sharing between patients and providers, regardless of their physical location [10].

Goals. Healthcare 4.0 has several objectives, including providing individualized care to patients by utilizing data analytics, machine learning, and AI to recognize trends, anticipate outcomes, and personalize treatments. In addition, it aims to connect patients, providers, and payers through digital technologies, like telemedicine, mobile health, and wearable devices, which can enhance access to care, lower expenses, and improve patient results. Healthcare 4.0 also aims to improve population health by leveraging data and analytics to detect health trends, develop targeted interventions, and assess the efficacy of these interventions. Moreover, it seeks to shift toward a value-based care model where compensation is linked to outcomes rather than the number of services provided. This can encourage providers to concentrate on quality and efficiency, resulting in reduced expenses and improved patient outcomes. Finally, healthcare 4.0 aims to encourage innovation in healthcare by fostering the development and acceptance of new technologies and care models. This can lead to better patient outcomes, reduced costs, and improved access to care.

11.1.3 Key Drivers of Healthcare 4.0

There are several key drivers of HC 4.0 [11–13], which are discussed here.

- One of the most important is the increasing demand for better healthcare services and outcomes. With an aging population and rising healthcare costs, there is a need to find more efficient and effective ways to deliver healthcare services.
- The accessibility and affordability of digital technologies, such as IoT, AI, etc., have become a crucial driver of HC 4.0. These technologies are now more widely available, making it easier for healthcare providers to adopt them into their systems.
- HC 4.0 is also being propelled by regulatory changes that are encouraging the use of digital technologies in healthcare delivery. Governments worldwide are introducing the latest guidelines and laws to support the endorsement of such technologies. One such example is the General Data Protection Regulation of the European Union, which mandates stringent needs for data privacy and protection, prompting the adoption of the BcT in healthcare [14].

Now that our population is increasing on a daily basis and our resources are limited, there is a strict competition in quality improvement along with no compromise in the cost for the expense of that quality. This is because, in order to provide better facilities in terms of medical amenities for our growing population, we need to provide better facilities. This transformation for the betterment of healthcare is ongoing, and in healthcare 4.0, this is accomplished by integrating technology and advancements for serving the patients as well as hospitals, by bridging them through a connection of Internet of Things and advanced digital technology. This transformation for the betterment of healthcare is never-ending. Digital connections are made between workers, patients, and their healthcare data, and this data is then analyzed so that healthcare solutions may be provided in a way that is both simpler and better and more accurate. Digital technologies such as IoT and AI have become more accessible and affordable, making it easier for healthcare providers to adopt them into their systems. Thus, HC 4.0 is driven by the need to provide better healthcare services and outcomes, at optimum healthcare costs.

11.2 Blockchain Technology and Its Application in Health Record Management

BcT is a decentralized, distributed digital ledger system that is recognized for its immutability, transparency, and security. Its potential to revolutionize various industries, including healthcare, is enormous. Among the most advantageous implementations of blockchain in healthcare is health record management. Health records contain patients' confidential and sensitive personal health information (PHI) and are presently stored in centralized databases that are vulnerable to cyberattacks, data breaches, and unauthorized access. With its decentralized and secure platform, BcT can address these challenges and provide a secure and immutable platform for health record management [15–18].

Here are some ways BcT can be applied in health record management.

11.2.1 Decentralized Storage

By using BcT, patients can store their health records in a decentralized network of computers, which withdraws the requirement for a central control to manage health records. This can greatly improve data privacy, security, and accessibility as patients will have full control over who can explore their health records and how they are shared. Additionally, BcT provides a tamper-proof record of all transactions, ensuring that the data is trustworthy and cannot be altered or deleted without proper authorization.

11.2.2 Improved Data Security

By utilizing BcT, healthcare providers can benefit from a highly secure and tamper-resistant system for managing health records. The use of cryptography guarantees that only authorized parties have access to the data, and any changes made to it are recorded and cannot be altered without leaving a trace. Additionally, BcT can be implemented as a decentralized ledger, which can provide a means for verifying the authenticity of transactions.

11.2.3 Interoperability

BcT can allow different healthcare providers to share health records in a secure and standardized manner. This can improve patient care coordination and reduce the duplication of medical tests and procedures.

11.2.4 Patient Control

BcT can give patients more control over their health records. Patients can choose who has access to their health records and can revoke access at any time.

11.2.5 Research and Analytics

BcT can enable researchers to access health records in a secure and privacy-preserving manner, allowing for more accurate and comprehensive analysis of health data.

11.3 BcT Advantages and Challenges in Healthcare Delivery

BcT is poised to revolutionize healthcare delivery, bringing about better patient outcomes, lower costs, and enhanced data privacy and security. However, integrating this technology in the healthcare sector comes with various challenges. In the following paragraphs, we will examine the benefits and drawbacks outlined in the literature [19–26] of employing BcT in healthcare delivery.

11.3.1 Benefits

11.3.1.1 Enhanced Data Security and Privacy

Blockchain, as a distributed ledger technology, provides a secure and tamper-resistant platform for storing and exchanging data, which can contribute to safeguarding sensitive patient information. By doing so, it can help prevent data breaches and ensure patients' privacy is protected.

11.3.1.2 Improved Data Management and Interoperability

BcT can allow healthcare providers to securely share patient data across different platforms and systems. This can improve data management and interoperability, leading to better patient outcomes.

11.3.1.3 Faster and More Accurate Diagnoses

BcT can help improve the accuracy and speed of diagnoses by providing doctors with access to more comprehensive and up-to-date patient data.

11.3.1.4 Streamlined Clinical Trials and Research

BcT can enable researchers to access and analyze large volumes of patient data in a secure and privacy-preserving manner. This can streamline clinical trials and lead to more accurate research findings.

11.3.1.5 Cost Savings

By improving data management and interoperability, BcT can help reduce healthcare costs by eliminating duplicative tests and procedures and improving efficiency.

11.3.2 Challenges

11.3.2.1 Complexity of Implementation and Maintenance

The technical complexity of BcT can pose a challenge as its implementation and maintenance require specialized knowledge and expertise.

11.3.2.2 Legal and Regulatory Frameworks

The absence of comprehensive legal and regulatory frameworks governing the implementation of BcT in healthcare can lead to hesitancy and discourage adoption.

11.3.2.3 Interoperability and Data Standardization

While BcT can enhance data interoperability, there is a requirement for a consistent standardization of data formats and protocols to ensure seamless data sharing across various systems.

11.3.2.4 Patient Privacy Concerns

While BcT can enhance data security and privacy, there are concerns about how patient data will be used and who will have access to it.

11.3.2.5 Scalability

BcT can be resource-intensive and may not be scalable enough to support large volumes of data and transactions.

11.4 Healthcare Use Cases for Blockchain Technology

Following are some healthcare use cases that have been discussed in the literature [27–36] for the implementation of BcT.

11.4.1 Patient-Centered Health Data Management

A patient-centric health data management system can be created using BcT, giving patients control over their medical records. The data can be stored in a decentralized network, allowing patients to share their medical records with healthcare providers and researchers when necessary. Patients can also manage their own data, deciding who has access to it. This can enhance data privacy, security, and accessibility while also allowing for more accurate and comprehensive analysis of health data.

11.4.2 Clinical Trials and Research

BcT can streamline clinical trials and research by providing a secure and privacy-preserving platform for storing and sharing patient data. Researchers can access data from multiple sources in a standardized manner, allowing them to conduct more precise and comprehensive analysis of health data. This can help speed up drug discovery and enhance patient outcomes.

11.4.3 Supply Chain Management

BcT can monitor the movement of medical devices, drugs, and supplies, ensuring they are authentic, safe, and free from tampering. This can reduce the risk of counterfeit drugs and medical devices entering the market, ensuring that patients receive high-quality products.

11.4.4 Claims and Payment Processing

BcT can improve the claims and payment processing system in healthcare by using smart contracts and blockchain-based systems, automating the claims processing and payment settlement process. This reduces the administrative burden on healthcare providers and enhances the accuracy and efficiency of the process.

11.4.5 Telemedicine

BcT can enhance telemedicine by providing a secure and privacy-preserving platform for storing and sharing patient data. Patients can utilize telemedicine services to remotely consult with healthcare providers, and the data collected during these consultations can be stored safely in a blockchain-based system, enabling more accurate and comprehensive analysis of health data.

11.5 Legislative and Ethical Concerns Surrounding Blockchain in Healthcare

As BcT continues to be integrated into healthcare, there are ethical and legislative concerns that must be addressed. Here are some of the primary concerns [37–42].

11.5.1 Data Protection and Privacy

The decentralized nature of blockchain systems makes it challenging to control access to personal health information. It is crucial to ensure that patient data is safeguarded and that the technology is compliant with regulations such as HIPAA and GDPR.

11.5.2 Security and Ownership

While blockchain provides a tamper-proof record of transactions, there are concerns about the ownership and control of the data stored on a blockchain-based system. It is important to establish clear ownership rights to ensure that patients retain control over their personal health information.

11.5.3 Interoperability and Standardization

The lack of interoperability and standardization of data formats and protocols can impede the adoption of BcT in healthcare. Collaboration between stakeholders is necessary to develop standardized protocols that enable data exchange and interoperability between different blockchain-based systems.

11.5.4 Regulatory Compliance

Blockchain in healthcare raises legal and regulatory compliance concerns. It is essential to ensure that the technology adheres to regulations such as HIPAA and GDPR, and that it does not breach ethical or legal principles.

11.5.5 Informed Consent

Patients must be informed about BcT in healthcare, and they must give their consent for their data to be used in this manner. It is crucial to ensure that patients are fully conscious of the risks and benefits of using BcT in healthcare and that they have the right to opt out of having their data stored on a blockchain-based system.

11.6 Obstacles and Future Directions for Blockchain in Healthcare

The COVID-19 pandemic has accelerated the necessity for healthcare to swiftly adapt and evolve to meet the ever-changing needs of the world [43–45]. HC 4.0, incorporating the integration of BcT, holds the potential to revolutionize health record management and enable more streamlined and secure data sharing across providers. Nonetheless, concerns like the correlation between myocardial injury after non-cardiac surgery and mortality still need to be addressed [46]. In navigating the complexities of the pandemic, it is crucial to prioritize patient safety and harness the capabilities of innovative technologies to enhance healthcare outcomes. While embracing HC 4.0 and blockchain offers an opportunity to build a more resilient healthcare system that can better cope with future challenges, it also faces a multitude of obstacles and challenges. Here are some of the significant barriers and future directions for blockchain in healthcare [47–53].

11.6.1 Interoperability and Standardization

Blockchain in healthcare is the lack of interoperability and standardization of data formats and protocols. This makes it difficult for different blockchain-based systems to communicate with each other and limits the potential benefits of the technology. Future directions for blockchain in healthcare should focus on developing standardized protocols that enable data exchange and interoperability between different blockchain-based systems.

11.6.2 Adoption and Implementation

The adoption and implementation of BcT in healthcare are still in the initial level. There is a need for further education and awareness about the potential benefits of the technology and for stakeholders to collaborate to develop and implement blockchain-based solutions that address specific healthcare challenges.

11.6.3 Cost and Complexity

The cost and complexity of implementing BcT in healthcare can be a barrier to adoption. The development and implementation of blockchain-based systems require significant investment in technology infrastructure, talent, and resources. Future directions for blockchain in healthcare should center on reducing the cost and complexity of implementing blockchain-based systems to increase their adoption.

11.6.4 Regulatory Compliance

This technology in the medical sector raises legal and regulatory compliance issues. There is a necessity for precise policies and regulations for the use of blockchain in healthcare to ensure that it is compliant with regulations such as HIPAA and GDPR. Future directions for blockchain in healthcare should focus on developing clear regulatory frameworks that govern the use of BcT in healthcare.

11.6.5 Trust and Security

The decentralized nature of BcT makes it difficult to control access to personal health information and raises concerns about data protection, privacy, and security. Future directions for blockchain in healthcare should focus on developing secure and trustworthy blockchain-based systems that protect patient data privacy and security.

11.7 Conclusions

From the preceding discussion, it can be concluded that BcT has the potential to transform healthcare delivery through innovative solutions for health record management, in the context of the emerging concept of HC 4.0.

- HC 4.0 is transforming healthcare delivery by leveraging digital technologies to improve efficiency, effectiveness, and patient-centered care. With the integration of technologies such as IoT, artificial intelligence, big data analytics, and BcT, healthcare providers can offer personalized medicine and real-time communication between patients and providers. The key drivers of HC 4.0 include the demand for better healthcare outcomes, the availability of new technologies, and regulatory

changes. As we move forward, HC 4.0 is poised to revolutionize healthcare delivery and improve patient outcomes.
- BcT has the potential to revolutionize health record management by providing a secure, decentralized, and interoperable platform for storing and sharing health records. It can improve patient privacy, security, and control, while also enabling more accurate research and analytics. However, it is important to consider the legal, ethical, and technical challenges associated with implementing BcT in healthcare.
- BcT can transform healthcare delivery by improving patient outcomes, reducing costs, and enhancing data security and privacy. However, there are also several challenges that need to be addressed, including technical complexity, legal and regulatory frameworks, interoperability and data standardization, patient privacy concerns, and scalability.
- BcT has several use cases in healthcare, including patient-centered health data management, clinical trials and research, supply chain management, claims and payment processing, and telemedicine. By leveraging the benefits of BcT, it is possible to improve patient outcomes, reduce costs, and enhance data security and privacy in healthcare.
- There are several legislative and ethical concerns surrounding the use of BcT in healthcare, including data privacy and security, regulatory compliance, interoperability and data standardization, informed consent, and bias and discrimination. These concerns need to be addressed through collaboration between stakeholders to ensure that the use of BcT in healthcare is ethical, legal, and beneficial for all.
- The adoption and implementation of BcT in healthcare face several obstacles and challenges, including interoperability and standardization, adoption and implementation, cost and complexity, regulatory compliance, and trust and security.

Future directions for BcT in healthcare should focus on addressing these challenges to realize the potential benefits of the technology for healthcare delivery and patient outcomes.

11.8 Research Directions for Blockchain in Healthcare

The HC 4.0 technology revolution has the potential to enhance both the quality of care provided to patients as well as the effectiveness of that treatment. Since it provides a safe as well as a decentralized method for managing medical records, BcT is a key player in this change because it offers a secure and decentralized way to manage medical records.

The future scope of this chapter includes exploring how BcT can be used to make healthcare data more interoperable, which will enable healthcare providers and the patients to access and exchange essential medical data securely, leading to more accurate diagnoses and personalized treatments by data monitoring and interpolation.

- Another potential topic of investigation is the use of BcT to increase the transparency and accountability of healthcare supply chains. BcT can provide a trustworthy and open ledger that monitors the flow of medicinal supplies from the producer to the patient, leading to a decrease in the number of fake pharmaceuticals and medical equipment and improving patient safety.

- BcT can also be used to improve the delivery of patient-centered healthcare by allowing patients to securely store and manage their own healthcare data, giving them more control over their healthcare journey.
- Lastly, ethical and legal considerations should also be explored when adopting BcT in healthcare to ensure that patients' privacy and safety concerns are addressed. Research in the future could focus on developing ethical and legal frameworks that ensure the benefits of BcT are realized while minimizing any negative impact on patients.

In conclusion, this chapter's future scope is extensive, offering several possibilities for research and innovation in healthcare record administration using BcT. It lays a solid foundation for future research and identifies potential areas for investigation that contribute to the growth of this rapidly developing field. This will result in an improvement not only to the quality of life but also to the efficiency and effectiveness of the hospital's and the patient's interactions with one another. Thus, by unlocking the power of blockchain for healthcare record management, we can revolutionize the way we store, share, and secure health data in the era of healthcare 4.0.

References

[1] Tanwar, S., Parekh, K., & Evans, R. (2020). Blockchain-based electronic healthcare record system for HC 4.0 applications. *Journal of Information Security and Applications, 50*, 102407.
[2] Warraich, H. J., Califf, R. M., & Krumholz, H. M. (2018). The digital transformation of medicine can revitalize the patient-clinician relationship. *NPJ Digital Medicine, 1*(1), 49.
[3] Chanchaichujit, J., Tan, A., Meng, F., Eaimkhong, S., Chanchaichujit, J., Tan, A., ... & Eaimkhong, S. (2019). An introduction to HC 4.0. *Healthcare 4.0: Next Generation Processes with the Latest Technologies*, 1–15.
[4] Li, J., & Carayon, P. (2021). Health Care 4.0: A vision for smart and connected health care. *IISE Transactions on Healthcare Systems Engineering, 11*(3), 171–80.
[5] Chanchaichujit, J., Tan, A., Meng, F., & Eaimkhong, S. (2019). *Healthcare 4.0*. Springer.
[6] Shrivastava, A., Krishna, K. M., Rinawa, M. L., Soni, M., Ramkumar, G., & Jaiswal, S. (2021). Inclusion of IoT, ML, and blockchain technologies in next generation industry 4.0 environment. *Materials Today: Proceedings, 80*(3), 3471–75. https://doi.org/10.1016/j.matpr.2021.07.273
[7] Chanchaichujit, J., Tan, A., Meng, F., & Eaimkhong, S. (2019). An Introduction to healthcare 4.0. In *Healthcare 4.0*. Palgrave Pivot. https://doi.org/10.1007/978-981-13-8114-0_1
[8] Paul, S., Riffat, M., Yasir, A., Mahim, M. N., Sharnali, B. Y., Naheen, I. T., ... & Kulkarni, A. (2021). Industry 4.0 applications for medical/healthcare services. *Journal of Sensor and Actuator Networks, 10*(3), 43.
[9] Roy, S., Meena, T., & Lim, S. J. (2022). Demystifying supervised learning in healthcare 4.0: A new reality of transforming diagnostic medicine. *Diagnostics, 12*(10), 2549.
[10] Dal Mas, F., Massaro, M., Rippa, P., & Secundo, G. (2023). The challenges of digital transformation in healthcare: An interdisciplinary literature review, framework, and future research agenda. *Technovation, 123*, 102716.
[11] Al-Jaroodi, J., Mohamed, N., & Abukhousa, E. (2020). Health 4.0: On the way to realizing the healthcare of the future. *IEEE Access, 8*, 211189–210.
[12] Aceto, G., Persico, V., & Pescapé, A. (2020). Industry 4.0 and health: Internet of things, big data, and cloud computing for healthcare 4.0. *Journal of Industrial Information Integration, 18*, 100129.

[13] Kishor, A., & Chakraborty, C. (2022). Artificial intelligence and internet of things based healthcare 4.0 monitoring system. *Wireless Personal Communications, 127*(2), 1615–31.

[14] Larrucea, X., Moffie, M., Asaf, S., & Santamaria, I. (2020). Towards a GDPR compliant way to secure European cross border healthcare industry 4.0. *Computer Standards & Interfaces, 69*, 103408.

[15] Kumar, A., Krishnamurthi, R., Nayyar, A., Sharma, K., Grover, V., & Hossain, E. (2020). A novel smart healthcare design, simulation, and implementation using healthcare 4.0 processes. *IEEE Access, 8*, 118433–71.

[16] Tanwar, S., Parekh, K., & Evans, R. (2020). Blockchain-based electronic healthcare record system for healthcare 4.0 applications. *Journal of Information Security and Applications, 50*, 102407.

[17] Ahmad, R. W., Salah, K., Jayaraman, R., Yaqoob, I., Ellahham, S., & Omar, M. (2021). The role of blockchain technology in telehealth and telemedicine. *International Journal of Medical Informatics, 148*, 104399.

[18] Bodkhe, U., Tanwar, S., Bhattacharya, P., & Verma, A. (2021). Blockchain adoption for trusted medical records in healthcare 4.0 applications: A survey. In *Proceedings of Second International Conference on Computing, Communications, and Cyber-Security: IC4S 2020* (pp. 759–74). Springer.

[19] Attaran, M. (2022). Blockchain technology in healthcare: Challenges and opportunities. *International Journal of Healthcare Management, 15*(1), 70–83.

[20] Sharma, A., Kaur, S., & Singh, M. (2021). A comprehensive review on blockchain and Internet of things in healthcare. *Transactions on Emerging Telecommunications Technologies, 32*(10), e4333.

[21] Tandon, A., Dhir, A., Islam, A. N., & Mäntymäki, M. (2020). Blockchain in healthcare: A systematic literature review, synthesizing framework and future research agenda. *Computers in Industry, 122*, 103290.

[22] Siyal, A. A., Junejo, A. Z., Zawish, M., Ahmed, K., Khalil, A., & Soursou, G. (2019). Applications of blockchain technology in medicine and healthcare: Challenges and future perspectives. *Cryptography, 3*(1), 3.

[23] Hussien, H. M., Yasin, S. M., Udzir, S. N. I., Zaidan, A. A., & Zaidan, B. B. (2019). A systematic review for enabling of develop a blockchain technology in healthcare application: Taxonomy, substantially analysis, motivations, challenges, recommendations and future direction. *Journal of Medical Systems, 43*, 1–35.

[24] Zheng, Z., Xie, S., Dai, H. N., Chen, X., & Wang, H. (2018). Blockchain challenges and opportunities: A survey. *International Journal of Web and Grid Services, 14*(4), 352–75.

[25] Garcia-Teruel, R. M. (2020). Legal challenges and opportunities of blockchain technology in the real estate sector. *Journal of Property, Planning and Environmental Law, 12*(2), 129–45.

[26] Mackey, T. K., Kuo, T. T., Gummadi, B., Clauson, K. A., Church, G., Grishin, D., . . . & Palombini, M. (2019). 'Fit-for-purpose?'—Challenges and opportunities for applications of blockchain technology in the future of healthcare. *BMC Medicine, 17*(1), 1–17.

[27] Ahmad, R. W., Salah, K., Jayaraman, R., Yaqoob, I., Ellahham, S., & Omar, M. (2021). The role of blockchain technology in telehealth and telemedicine. *International Journal of Medical Informatics, 148*, 104399.

[28] Colón, K. A. (2018). Creating a patient-centered, global, decentralized health system: Combining new payment and care delivery models with telemedicine, AI, and blockchain technology. *Blockchain in Healthcare Today, 1*. https://doi.org/10.30953/bhty.v1.30.

[29] Hylock, R. H., & Zeng, X. (2019). A blockchain framework for patient-centered health records and exchange (HealthChain): Evaluation and proof-of-concept study. *Journal of Medical Internet Research, 21*(8), e13592.

[30] Jabarulla, M. Y., & Lee, H. N. (2021, August). A blockchain and artificial intelligence-based, patient-centric healthcare system for combating the COVID-19 pandemic: Opportunities and applications. In *Healthcare* (Vol. 9, No. 8, p. 1019). MDPI.

[31] Reda, M., Kanga, D. B., Fatima, T., & Azouazi, M. (2020). Blockchain in health supply chain management: State of art challenges and opportunities. *Procedia Computer Science, 175*, 706–9.

[32] Haleem, A., Javaid, M., Singh, R. P., Suman, R., & Rab, S. (2021). Blockchain technology applications in healthcare: An overview. *International Journal of Intelligent Networks, 2*, 130–9.

[33] Yaqoob, I., Salah, K., Jayaraman, R., & Al-Hammadi, Y. (2021). Blockchain for healthcare data management: Opportunities, challenges, and future recommendations. *Neural Computing and Applications*, 1–16.

[34] Bazel, M. A., Mohammed, F., & Ahmed, M. (2021, August). Blockchain technology in healthcare big data management: benefits, applications and challenges. In *2021 1st International Conference on Emerging Smart Technologies and Applications (eSmarTA)* (pp. 1–8). IEEE.

[35] Ali, O., Jaradat, A., Ally, M., & Rotabi, S. (2022). Blockchain technology enables healthcare data management and accessibility. *Blockchain Technologies for Sustainability*, 91–118.

[36] Katuwal, G. J., Pandey, S., Hennessey, M., & Lamichhane, B. (2018). Applications of blockchain in healthcare: Current landscape & challenges. *arXiv preprint arXiv:1812.02776*.

[37] Kumar, R. L., Wang, Y., Poongodi, T., & Imoize, A. L. (Eds.). (2021). *Internet of things, artificial intelligence and blockchain technology*. Springer.

[38] Liu, W., Zhu, S. S., Mundie, T., & Krieger, U. (2017, October). Advanced block-chain architecture for e-health systems. In *2017 IEEE 19th International Conference on e-Health Networking, Applications and Services (Healthcom)* (pp. 1–6). IEEE.

[39] Odeh, A., Keshta, I., & Al-Haija, Q. A. (2022). Analysis of blockchain in the healthcare sector: Application and issues. *Symmetry*, 14(9), 1760.

[40] Srivastava, V., Mahara, T., & Yadav, P. (2021). An analysis of the ethical challenges of blockchain-enabled E-healthcare applications in 6G networks. *International Journal of Cognitive Computing in Engineering*, 2, 171–9.

[41] Nehme, E., Salloum, H., Bou Abdo, J., & Taylor, R. (2021). AI, IoT, and blockchain: Business models, ethical issues, and legal perspectives. In *Internet of things, artificial intelligence and blockchain technology* (pp. 67–88). Springer International Publishing.

[42] Galetsi, P., Katsaliaki, K., & Kumar, S. (2022). Exploring benefits and ethical challenges in the rise of mHealth (mobile healthcare) technology for the common good: An analysis of mobile applications for health specialists. *Technovation*, 102598.

[43] Akhai, S., Mala, S., & Jerin, A. A. (2021). Understanding whether air filtration from air conditioners reduces the probability of virus transmission in the environment. *Journal of Advanced Research in Medical Science & Technology (ISSN: 2394–6539)*, 8(1), 36–41.

[44] Akhai, S., Mala, S., & Jerin, A. A. (2020). Apprehending air conditioning systems in context to COVID-19 and human health: A brief communication. *International Journal of Healthcare Education & Medical Informatics (ISSN: 2455–9199)*, 7(1&2), 28–30.

[45] Ng, W. Y., Tan, T. E., Movva, P. V., Fang, A. H. S., Yeo, K. K., Ho, D., . . . & Ting, D. S. W. (2021). Blockchain applications in health care for COVID-19 and beyond: A systematic review. *The Lancet Digital Health*, 3(12), e819–e829.

[46] Mala, S. (2021). Myocardial injury after non-cardiac surgery and its correlation with mortality: A brief review on its scenario till 2020. *International Journal of Preventive Cardiology*, 1(1), 29–31.

[47] Durneva, P., Cousins, K., & Chen, M. (2020). The current state of research, challenges, and future research directions of blockchain technology in patient care: Systematic review. *Journal of Medical Internet Research*, 22(7), e18619.

[48] Atlam, H. F., Alenezi, A., Alassafi, M. O., & Wills, G. (2018). Blockchain with internet of things: Benefits, challenges, and future directions. *International Journal of Intelligent Systems and Applications*, 10(6), 40–8.

[49] Deepa, N., Quoc-Viet Pham, Dinh C. Nguyen, Sweta Bhattacharya, Prabadevi, B., Thippa Reddy Gadekallu, Praveen Kumar Reddy Maddikunta, Fang Fang, & Pubudu N. Pathirana. (2022). A survey on blockchain for big data: Approaches, opportunities, and future directions. *Future Generation Computer Systems*, 131, 209–26. https://doi.org/10.1016/j.future.2022.01.017

[50] Jan, M. A., Cai, J., Gao, X. C., Khan, F., Mastorakis, S., Usman, M., . . . & Watters, P. (2021). Security and blockchain convergence with internet of multimedia things: Current trends, research challenges and future directions. *Journal of Network and Computer Applications*, 175, 102918.

[51] Abdelmaboud, A., Ahmed, A. I. A., Abaker, M., Eisa, T. A. E., Albasheer, H., Ghorashi, S. A., & Karim, F. K. (2022). Blockchain for IoT applications: Taxonomy, platforms, recent advances, challenges and future research directions. *Electronics*, 11(4), 630.

[52] Akhai, S. (2023). *From black boxes to transparent machines: The quest for explainable AI*. Available at SSRN 4390887.

[53] Krishnamoorthy, S., Dua, A., & Gupta, S. (2023). Role of emerging technologies in future IoT-driven healthcare 4.0 technologies: A survey, current challenges and future directions. *Journal of Ambient Intelligence and Humanized Computing*, 14(1), 361–407.

12
Benefits and Roles of Blockchain in Genomics

Dablu Kumar

12.1 Introduction

Researchers are using genomic databases to extract details on the molecular causes of human diseases and to find genetic changes that cause particular diseases. The human genome is made up of approximately 3 billion base pairs of nucleotides. The prospects of genomics have great potential to improve healthcare. Using high-throughput sequencing (HTS) and genomic data can give unique information about health that can't be gotten from other technologies, non-invasive and critical to the advancement of precision medicine [1].

The unwillingness of people to directly share the necessary data is a barrier to genomics. For instance, by looking at a person's entire genome, it is possible to identify the person or perhaps learn more about his ancestry. Transactions are saved using their hash values in blockchain systems rather than their original data. Furthermore, people simply exchange metadata, which comprises broad data information. Editing personal access permissions is possible with blockchain [2]. Data management, which addresses the four severe issues listed in what follow, presents another difficulty in this area. A collection, a store, a share, and an ownership. Blockchain can reduce analytics costs for genomics and healthcare applications. Contrary to current methods, allowing data owners to speak with their clients directly without middlemen lowers the cost of analysis and increases data owner earnings [3]. Both academic and industrial communities have become interested in blockchain in genomics, each with a different agenda for applying this technology. Commercial genomic customers have become more numerous in recent years as direct-to-consumer (DTC) businesses have begun to commercialize DNA sequencing. This is because technological developments have made genome sequencing considerably more accessible and quicker. The chosen studies on blockchain's non-commercial uses mostly concentrate on sharing genomic data to promote science. Data sharing, analysis, storage, and their access control are some of the use cases that this research fits into [4,5]. Platforms that are built on blockchain technology are addressing important issues, such as the governance of sharing genetic data, among other issues. The end objective is to make sure that organizations and people may exchange data while maintaining their privacy using algorithms that make it easier to comply with ethical and legal norms [6].

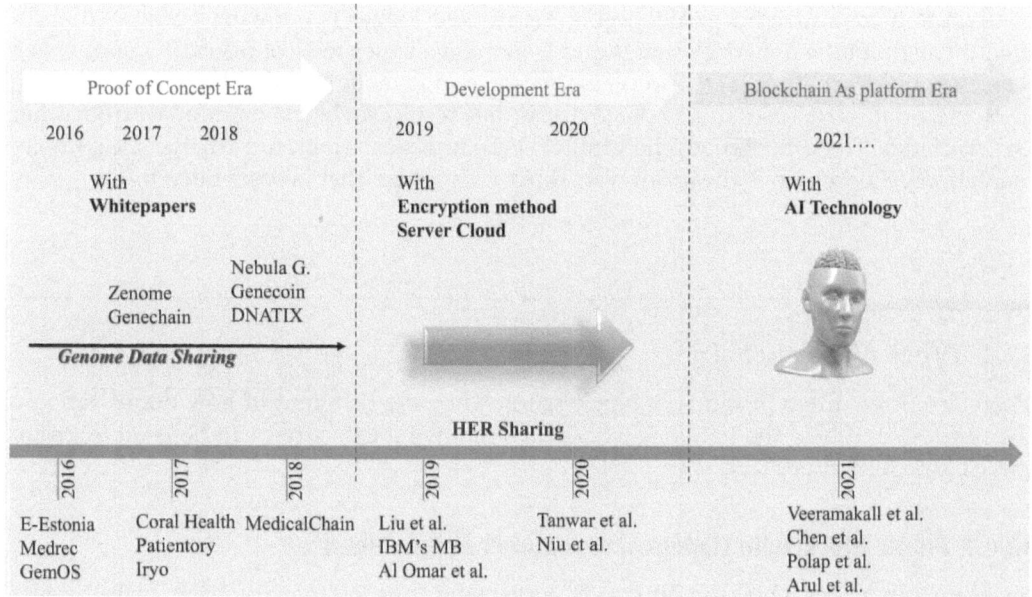

FIGURE 12.1
Timeline of blockchain use in healthcare and genomics.

12.2 What Is Genomics?

Genomics is a field of biology that deals with the structure of the genome and its mapping, editing, function, and evolution. The timeline progress of genomics is depicted in **Figure 12.1**

- A genome is a complete set of genetic information of an organism (also known as DNA) [7].
- DNA, a type of genetic code, is present in every living thing. It controls how an organism develops and interacts with its surroundings, as well as how it performs biological functions. The study of genomics is the art and science of deciphering and applying this DNA code to produce useful outcomes [8].
- Genomics involves the sequencing and the analysis of genomes using bioinformatics and high-throughput DNA sequencing to assemble, function, and structure entire genomes [9].

12.3 Blockchain Technology and Blockchain-Based System

Blockchain that uses hashing algorithms to store data securely aids the business in both ways—data exchange and data security [10]. Despite their close link, there is a slight distinction between distributed ledger technology (DLT) and blockchain technology. In contrast to a centralized organization, a distributed ledger is a database that is distributed throughout the network's nodes and is managed by a group of peers. In contrast to a database, a blockchain is a DLT implementation and is made up of a chain of blocks. The distinctive data structures that make up these data blocks set blockchains apart from other DLT variants. The directed acyclic graph (DAG) and hashgraph are further DLT implementations. Blockchain is the groundbreaking technology that powers Bitcoin [11].

12.4 Types of Blockchain

There are three different kinds of blockchains. They are different in how nodes can join the network and how the network works. The following categories can be used to group these blockchain types [12].

12.4.1 Public Blockchain (Open-Access and Permissionless)

Everyone can access a blockchain that is public (and thus less-trustworthy). Here, anonymous nodes may join the network, and none of the other nodes in the network impose any trust requirements. All nodes receive publicly announced transactions. Any network node can take part in the consensus methods used to verify the blocks. The blockchain of Bitcoin is a prime illustration of this kind of network [13].

12.4.2 Private Blockchain (Private and Permissioned)

As nodes join the network, they are trustworthy because they have been carefully chosen and examined. The blockchain transaction content is more privately protected by the access control mechanism. Also, this kind of blockchain offers improved block confirmation performance. MultiChain is an illustration of this kind of platform [14].

12.4.3 Consortium Blockchain (Public and Permission-Granted)

A hybrid of the first two that makes a balance in between effectiveness and trust, the ledger that a set of nodes has been chosen to administer. Nodes need authorization to join the network, much like private blockchains. Blocks and transactions are validated once a predetermined number of nodes agree. The consensus mechanism's predetermined rules determine the exact process. Hyperledger is an illustration of this kind of platform [15].

Each block in such network stores the hash value of the one before it, creating an immutable chain structure. Also, with blockchain systems, users do not utilize their real identities but rather public and private keys. Public keys are the ones that everyone knows. Private keys are unique to each user and are used to sign transactions. Because of this, the first version of blockchain, which is the Bitcoin network, is called "pseudo-anonymous." The mem-pool is where pending transactions are picked up by miners, who then attempt to properly block-create a block that contains the answer to the given cryptographic. Some of them are listed in Table 12.1 and use hash functions in some way.

The proof-of-work problem in Bitcoin is to find a hash value that starts with certain number of zeros. The created block is broadcast to everyone on the network as soon as one

TABLE 12.1

Different Types of Consensus Algorithms

SI No.	Consensus Algorithms	Explanations
1	PoW	When a user starts a transaction, miners attempt to solve a cryptographic puzzle to prove that they put a lot of effort into it.
2	PoS	For a user to become a validator and build a block, he or she is told to spend more money.
3	PoWeight	Like PoS, but with one key distinction—it is based on a number of additional variables known as weights.
4	PoB	Users will receive incentives based on the amount when they deposit coins back into their wallets that they are unable to reclaim.
5	PoC	The hard disc space of the user can be used by using this protocol.
6	DPoS	Like PoS, but people who own coins will be able to vote and choose witnesses.
7	DBFT	Focuses on a way for expert node controllers to verify blocks that is like a game.
8	PBFT	To ward from malicious users, Byzantium employed a specific procedure.

of the miners achieves the required result. Also, the miner who discovers the new block receives a payout as an inducement to maintain them in the system [16].

12.5 Why Blockchain in Genomics

12.5.1 Genetic Data Security

From a data security standpoint, blockchain delivers great data confidentiality and integrity for genomic data, which is very sensitive and vital. Encryption and other security measures are important for preventing data intrusions, but they do not offer perfect security. Hackers infiltrate several systems of large corporations with the greatest level of protection. Yet blockchain technology benefits enterprises by enhancing data breach security. Blockchain employs hashing algorithms to securely store data, which aids the organization's security and data exchange [17]. The safety and privacy features of the blockchain depend on different kinds of cryptography. Some of these methods were used in the original Bitcoin blockchain design, while others were added to future blockchain implementations to improve privacy. Because the Bitcoin blockchain uses basic security measures, it is guaranteed that the system meets the security standards for online transactions. Blockchain uses the previously mentioned consensus process to make sure that the database is the same on all nodes. Transactions on the blockchain can't be changed by either the miners who confirm them or the outside attackers (threats) who try to change them.

Using cryptographic hashing and a digital signature, if any changes were made to the transaction data, they would be found when the digital signature was checked to make sure it was real. Also, if you want to change a transaction, you have to change the information recorded on all nodes in the blockchain network, since the ledger is kept on all nodes. Because the blockchain network is so decentralized, attacks like distributed denial-of-service (DDoS) are not possible [18].

Though in terms of privacy, blockchain's use of public key infrastructure (PKI) gives it pseudonymity. Instead of their real names, users' public addresses are used to identify their nodes. But this doesn't give complete anonymity, because it's possible to link the public address to the real identities by looking at how people interact with each other. Through the use of public key infrastructure, blockchain provides pseudonymity in terms of privacy. Users' nodes can be identified by their public addresses as opposed to their true identities. However, this does not provide perfect anonymity, because it is feasible to link interactions between parties to the public address in order to determine the real identity of the participants [19]. The fact that transactions and related data can be seen by anyone is another privacy issue with the way blockchain was first made. When transactions and smart contract data are kept private, blockchain can be used for things that deal with sensitive information. To get around the rules, new security methods have been suggested, such as mix, anonymous signatures, and zero-knowledge proofs (ZKP)

The General Data Protection Regulation (GDPR), which was passed by the European Union in 2018, has changed how personal data is handled at all levels and in all fields. Genetic information belongs only to the person who first collected it, so there are rules in place to protect it and keep it private. One example of a blockchain project is the "Genesy Project," in order to determine some broad guidelines for developing a platform for the collaborative exchange of genomic data on the blockchain, with the aim of eventually including all biomedical data [20]. By leveraging blockchain's cryptographic protection and adding additional security measures, Genesy ensures compliance with the General Data Protection Regulation (GDPR). These precautions include requiring secure communication methods to be verified and certified before web-based data access is permitted. They also need to know the name of the server that is providing the service and the name of the client station from which data can be accessed. All private information on the Genesy blockchain is also encrypted with the advanced encryption standard (AES), which is a blocking encryption method that has been used a lot because it is safe and easy to use (AES-256). Because Genesy's business plan calls for a secondary market to form in which data creators sell their data to third parties, it stands to reason that any such data transfers must be regulated to ensure the safety of all parties involved and conform to the guidelines set forth by the General Data Protection Regulation. This is done by having the person who owns the data sign an informed permission document for the data they are ready to release. This is one of the ways the GDPR lets people share personal data. In contrast, the immutability of blockchain data is crucial to its ability to maintain data integrity and inspire confidence in the system [21]. This conflict between blockchain and GDPR might change over time, particularly if more guidance is provided on how to interpret the regulation's application in different kinds of technical settings where data are created and kept [22].

Blockchain data, such as public keys and transaction history, is now the subject of dispute about whether these constitute "personal data" under the regulations of the General Data Protection (GDPR) (European Parliamentary Research Service, 2019) [23].

12.5.2 Genomic Data Sharing

Genomic studies rely heavily on interpretation. Both the individual and the combined effects of several genetic variations on patients may be evaluated. It is depicted in **Figure 12.2**. Combining a patient's genotype with their clinical phenotype may help doctors choose the most effective therapy. The accuracy of these conclusions relies heavily on the data used to draw them.

Benefits and Roles of Blockchain in Genomics

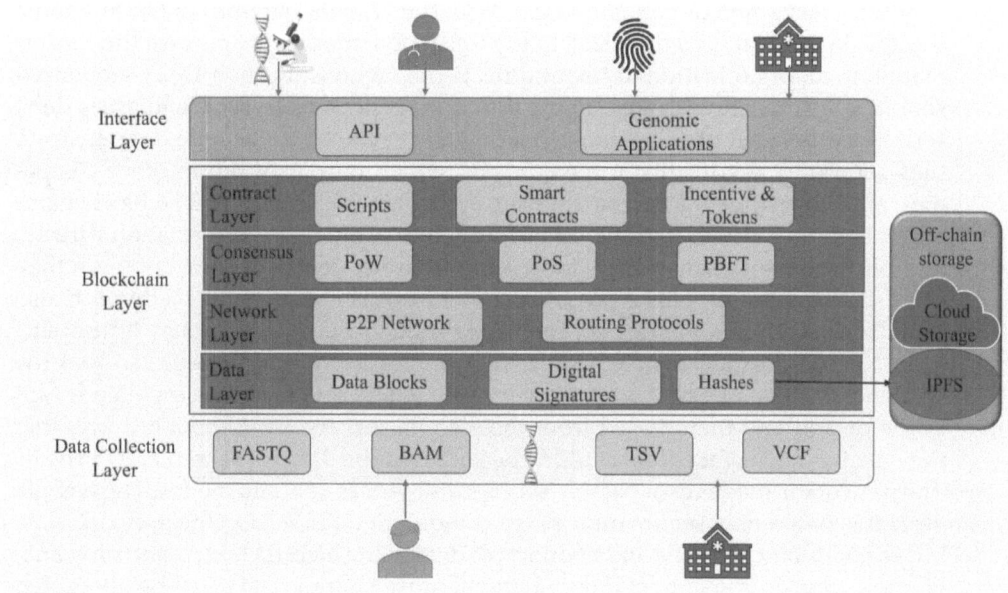

FIGURE 12.2
Generic design for blockchain-based systems for exchanging genetic data.

In order to improve interpretations, it is crucial to share research and clinical expertise. Genomic researchers have firsthand knowledge of how difficult and burdensome the process of exchanging genetic data is. Policies and legislation permit the transmission of genomic data under specific circumstances, but these vary from nation to country. Another problem is the existing limited involvement in genomes research, especially considering the needs in genomics research. Genome-wide association studies (GWAS) typically include thousands of people, but sometimes as many as a million [24]. In order to further study this area, there are a few genomic data exchange platforms that allow scientists to openly share genetic data. Big organizations like Clinical Genome (ClinGen) and the Global Alliance for Genomics and Health (GA4GH), which has a lot of data-sharing projects, have started making reliable tools to fully describe and analyze all changes in the human genome. Beyond 1 Million Genome (B1MG) is one of many large-scale European initiatives designed to facilitate and manage the safe cross-border collecting, storage, and exchange of human genome data. Genomic beacon, a project started by GA4GH, is one of the most visible answers to the problem of widespread genomic data sharing. By responding to inquiries regarding the existence of a given allele in a genome, genomic beacons facilitate data exchange through web services. Beacons may be deployed and linked from inside institutions. Beacons are designed to protect user privacy by giving organizations control over data access and authorization. Nevertheless, subsequent studies have shown that even when data anonymization techniques are applied to the data made accessible by beacons, people may still be recognized [25].

Some of the projects under genomic data sharing are mentioned:

- **Nebula genomics**. It is a network for analyzing genetic data based on Ethereum, but it doesn't have a token yet. They wanted to solve four main problems: how to lower the cost of sequencing, how to protect data, how to gather data, and how to deal with large sets of genomic data. Also, the Nebula network plans to handle the data boom that is coming [26]. In the traditional model, people give their information to an organization in the middle. People who want their DNA sequenced should get in touch with a company that does genetic analysis. Companies don't send the whole set of sequencing data when they analyze genetic data. Instead, they send only the results of the analysis, which they may sell to other companies, since consumers lose control over their data access rights. The blockchain-based Nebula network, on the other hand, lets people give information directly and on their own terms. Users must have their sequences looked at before they can use this network. This is something that Nebula's sequencing facility can also do. It is said that people can get their data sequenced for less money at this site. As a Nebula partner, people send their samples to Veritas Genetics so that the sequences can be put on Nebula servers. The whole set of sequencing data is sent to the person and then erased from the Nebula servers. Even though it says that the data has been erased, we couldn't be sure that the data was completely private. The network is made up of Nebula servers and secure compute nodes. The Nebula system is based on a secure multiparty computation [25,26]. On the network, data buyer nodes buy genomic and phenotypic data using Nebula tokens and only analyze the data on a secure compute node because shared data must be encrypted using the HME format. The bioinformatics platform Arvados is run by secure computing nodes. It works with Intel SGX (software) and, partially, homomorphic encryption. Intel SGX, a set of instruction codes, can be used to make enclaves or private memory spaces. The owner of the data sends data that has been encrypted to a secure computing node. The data is decrypted, and additional calculations are done in the SGX enclave before the results are encrypted and sent to a buyer node. Hence, customers may get the findings without viewing the actual data, partly resolving the privacy issue.

- **Zenome**. The "ZNA coin" stands for the Zenome blockchain ecosystem, which facilitates the sharing of genetic information. Users of Zenome may collaborate on research, control who has access to their data, keep it safely, be paid, recruit new participants, do genetic analysis, and benefit from a variety of additional genetic services [11,25,26]. The technology stores metadata in a completely anonymous fashion across a distributed network. Without the decryption key, it is impossible to have access to an individual's genetic data. There are four different kinds of "nodes" in the system: (1) calculation and storage nodes, which trade computing power and data storage for incentives; (2) user nodes, which trade genetic data and user services; (3) analyst nodes, which analyze genetic data; and (4) service providers, which trade genetic services for payment. Some scientific enterprises, bioinformatics firms, medical facilities, and labs provide genetic services. Zenome is applicable to other creatures and provides users with reports as necessary. The system employs AI techniques and requires all users to use the Zenome software app. The software application from Zenome enables customers to configure their own data privacy (including complete privacy, normal privacy, and public access choices). During raw data preparation, the system is able to identify fraudulent data. To cope with false organisms, the system first searches for coverage according to a threshold and saves them based on fragments. Hence, only a little quantity of data is exchanged over the blockchain. The remaining data might be sent over a secure communication channel [27].

- **Genecoin.** Genecoin, also known as a "GEN token," is a cryptocurrency for the bioeconomy that uses the Ethereum blockchain to ensure the secure transfer of genetic data [27,28]. A user may earn up to one thousand free Genecoin just by inviting their friends to join the global Genecoin network. It takes a DNA sample and stores it on a distributed ledger. DNA samples are distributed to thousands of machines. The business first provides a sample collection kit before coordinating with outside vendors to gather sequencing data. The blockchain may now be read by software that can decipher an individual's DNA. The token distribution is as follows: 10% to the founders, 15% to the community [28].

- **DNATIX.** The goal of this Ethereum-based initiative is to provide a trustworthy, user-friendly, and safe means of exchanging data between businesses, institutions, and individuals. It allows users to submit genetic information anonymously and run genetic tests on that information depending on user-supplied criteria for access. The following is also a major improvement to this system. Tokens may be earned by participants who contribute to the development of applications on next-generation decentralized genetic application (GDApps), which features a virtual machine similar to DNAtixVM and can act as a node. DNATIX's unique approach of condensing long DNA sequences provides a further advantage. The current method can reduce the sequence size by 25%. Like previous initiatives, the platform stores, transfers, and analyses genetic test data via smart contracts. Moreover, the platform may update and cancel access. A reasonable number of nucleotides was identified to calculate the transaction charge [29].

12.5.3 Electronic Health Record–Sharing System

This topic has been the hub of scholarly research between 2019 and the present. Cloud-based and encryption-based sophisticated apps are most frequently offered in the era of blockchain development. At this point, research has focused on creating a healthcare system based on blockchain, like the earlier era. Studies typically focused on how to use various encryption techniques in systems, how to implement modules that support blockchain technology, and how to evaluate performance, while detailed descriptions of the system structure were less common than in the first and third ages, respectively [30].

- **MedRec.** In 2016, it was announced that the first installation of MedRec will take place. The most recent iteration of MedRec, known as MedRec 2.0, does not yet have a token since the MIT Media Lab is currently in the process of developing it using GO-Ethereum and Solidity. It is a platform for exchanging electronic health records that is powered by blockchain technology; it operates in a secure and transparent manner between patients and providers, and it is scalable. Patients are provided with transparency, rapid access, and the ability to amend mistakes made by the authority responsible for their medical information via the use of the MedRec system [31]. The foundation of the system is made up of digital contracts. The MedRec does not directly store the records themselves; it merely stores the metadata associated with the content. The providers themselves are responsible for maintaining the blockchain so that they can protect the confidentiality of their patients and the integrity of the system. There are three distinct kinds of contracts that may be found inside the system. They are: (1) the registrar contract, (2) the patient–provider relationship contract, and (3) the summary contract. IDs of participants are included in the registrar contract so that users may verify their identities [32].

Patients can modify their information, and the registrar will only add this procedure to the contract if the patient verifies that they want it included. The patient–provider relationship contract establishes the connection between the patient node and the provider node and details their relationship. In conclusion, the summary–contract structure is made up of the many connections that exist between the system's members. It contains a reference list of the contracts governing the patient–provider interaction. A status value is assigned to each connection, which indicates when the relationships were first formed and what permissions are associated with them; a request with the patient's ID number is required before a service provider can make changes to a patient's medical file. The contract is examined once the request has been processed on the blockchain network. After the MedRec system has received all confirmations, an update may be applied successfully, and the patient is informed. When a patient wants to see their medical records, they must first make a request to the healthcare provider's database gatekeeper. The database gatekeeper acts as an intermediary between users and the participant-maintained local databases. Following then, the blockchain takes over, and both the summary contracts and the patient–provider contracts are reviewed. The electronic health record (EHR) is made available to the patient upon successful contract validation by the system. It uses delegated contracts to ensure user anonymity, with each provider creating a new Ethereum identity for each patient–provider pairing. Although scalability is one of the most critical difficulties that every blockchain system must confront, the platform does not have a concrete answer to the problem of how it can be scaled [33].

- **IRYO.** It is an EHS sharing and maintaining platform which keeps at least one encrypted live copy of the data in order to protect the data storage system from any potential threats. In this manner, it is possible to ensure the security of all forms of health data. In order to utilize the data that has been saved in ways related to AI, initially the research institution must be validated by IRYO. In order to submit a fresh inquiry, researchers need to make use of the IRYO research software application. A notice will be sent to a patient's phone if the study question that was submitted by a researcher satisfies the patient's requirements. The data are sent to the study organization as soon as the patient gives their consent to the procedure, and the patient is rewarded with some tokens for their participation. After the researcher has completed his study, the patient will get a notice on his phone informing him of the findings of the investigation. Researchers can choose to look at either completely anonymous or partially anonymized datasets within the system. You may access a public blockchain via the IRYO network. Every EOS blockchain storage node must provide patients with cryptographic proof by means of writing hashes. The CHT token, produced by Coral Health, may be used on the Ethereum-based platform that they have built to trade electronic health records and genetic test results for personalized medicine [34]. A precision medicine approach for treatment has the potential to reduce unwanted side effects while increasing efficacy.

- **Coral Health.** This system seeks to overcome issues with genetic data collection and exchange by offering a scalable, interoperable, accessible, and secure healthcare environment. Direct data exchange between patients and their doctors, labs, and other system users is possible. Accounts are used by individuals throughout the process to control who has access to what information. Like Apple Health, Coral Health employs the SMART and Fast Healthcare Interoperability Resource standards. Methodologies for transmitting medical records from one location to another using a patient's mobile device is possible. A notification is delivered to the patient's mobile device once the lab result or prescription is obtained. If a patient verifies the notification, pharmaceutical companies or others may buy sample results. In compliance with the Health Insurance Portability and Accountability Act and the Health Information Trust Alliance (HITRUST), patient data is stored and secured on mobile devices. The data-sharing key is only known to the patient. Also, doctors can have immediate access to a patient's medical history if they arrive at the emergency room while the patient is still unconscious. Doctors can give tailored care based on this patient's unique genetic makeup and other factors. Radiological images, genetic test results, and microbiological test results are all supported by the system [35].

- **Patientory.** Tokenized on the Ethereum blockchain, Patientory (PTOY) is an EHR data-sharing platform. Patients in the traditional system may get copies of their medical records to share with doctors, while physicians can use mobile healthcare apps to keep tabs on their patients' conditions on the go. Yet under the current traditional system, these steps take time, and physicians have access to little information. Also, classical systems are not entirely safe due to the centrality issue. The proposed system makes it simple for users to have access to and manage their own medical records, as well as those of their loved ones and other medical professionals. The Health Insurance Portability and Accountability Act regulation was the major focus throughout system development. The patient-related app is offered at no cost, and each user is given 10 MB of free storage space. Users are required to pay an amount of PTOY once 10 MB of storage space has been used. Via their respective mobile apps, patients are able to construct unique profiles. Patients' records are kept in a blockchain database that is both safe and HIPAA-compliant. Furthermore, individuals may talk to others who are experiencing the same health issues. Similarly to previous initiatives, it employs a smart contract for user data access rights that can be readily modified. This system is global and is not restricted only to the United States [36].

- **Medicalchain.** Medicalchain, represented by the "MTN" token, is an EHR sharing project built on Ethereum and Hyperledger that ensures the secure, instant, and transparent exchange and utilization of private patient health information. It employs a two-blockchain design for its construction. Initiation of the first distributed ledger uses Hyperledger Fabric for its foundation, which allows it to centrally restrict access to medical information. Ethereum, the second blockchain, is what powers all the platform's apps and features. Fabric supports many permission levels, allowing for a variety of control settings. Hence, Hyperledger Fabric may be superior to other options for inspecting health record access. Anybody interested in joining the Hyperledger must first apply to do so, since it is a permission-based network. Hyperledger Fabric is used for applications that demand data confidentiality or that only give select persons access to the data. As an example of one of the benefits of implementing a smart contract in the healthcare system, consider the following. Billing and other insurance-related tasks take up a significant portion of a doctor's day. Smart contracts that are verified by Ethereum may lead to considerable cost reductions if these tasks were completed. The system has teamed up with Civic to safeguard against identity theft. Civic's authentication services are used, wherein identities are safely managed through a decentralized network. Users' identities are confirmed via the use of biometrics. Doctors, patients, and academic institutions all take part. Symmetric key encryption protects patient confidentiality and secures medical records [37]. In the event of an emergency, the Medicalchain also has a secondary access method. Patients participate by wearing a wristband. Scan the bracelet with two different medical devices to unlock and get access to the data so the physicians can quickly access the patient's medical history and provide them the most effective care possible.

- **e-Estonia**. To improve the registration process for multiple government organizations, including the e-healthcare system, Guardtime and the Estonian government have developed e-Estonia, a blockchain-based Health Insurance Portability and Accountability Act and the Health Information Trust Alliance (HITRUST) (www.guardtimefederal.com/ksi/). There is now what's called a "keyless signature infrastructure" (KSI) in Estonia. Its use is widespread because it protects users' privacy and ensures that their networks and data remain unaltered (KSI Blockchain Website). KSI uses hash function cryptography, which is different from other digital signature systems. The integrity of hash functions and the availability of a public ledger are all that is needed to verify KSIs. The term "blockchain" is used to describe this. According to KSI blockchain, traditional methods have problems with scalability and settlement time. Traditional blockchain technology scales linearly in terms of transaction volume. The KSI blockchain, on the other hand, keeps expanding regardless of the number of transactions it processes. The KSI blockchain has limitations due to its distributed consensus design. Agreements may be reached concurrently by reducing the number of participants, eliminating the necessity for proof-of-work, and assuring rapid settlement. Moreover, hash trees are used to store data in KSI blockchain. All the deals done in a certain time period are stored in a hash tree, which can store many different signatures. By linking the trees at their important nodes, we may generate a hash tree. The system has two main applications. Electronic prescriptions follow closely on the heels of electronic medical records. Many different types of medical data are included in the hospital's computerized patient registration system. Access to medical records and other data logs is strictly controlled by the blockchain. Patients who have been given access to their records can do so at any time. Mobile devices can use the system. Every step of the prescription procedure has been handled online. With an e-prescription, the original prescription may be accessed with only the patient's ID card number. A patient who takes a certain drug for a long time may also reduce the frequency of their medical visits. The patient makes a request through the system, and the doctor fulfills it by creating and sending the patient an electronic prescription [38].

12.6 Commercial Scenario of Blockchain

Both academic and industrial communities have become interested in blockchain in genomics, each with a different agenda for applying this technology. We divided the applications in the flowchart into two primary categories: commercial and non-commercial, as shown in Figure 12.3.

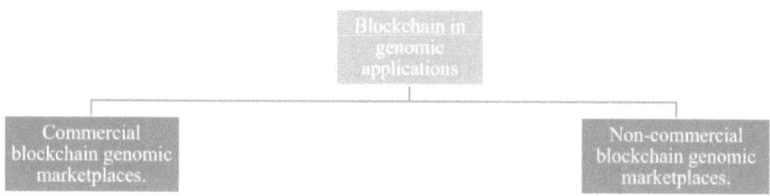

FIGURE 12.3
Commercial blockchain genomic marketplaces.

Commercial genomic customers have become more numerous in recent years as direct-to-consumer (DTC) businesses have begun to commercialize DNA sequencing. This is because technological developments have made genome sequencing considerably more accessible and quicker. Direct-to-consumer enterprises like 23andmMe utilize many strategies to generate cash; one of these is giving pharmaceutical companies access to the DNA sequences that have been gathered. Thoughts about this model's fairness arise when considering the financial benefit from purchasing this genomic data. Some contend that the people should receive the profit, rather than the middlemen [37,38]. Genomic markets built on blockchain technology are designed to eliminate the need for middlemen and offer users access to their data. Those who rent or sell their genetic data receive several kinds of rewards. Bitcoin is the most popular form of incentive in these markets.

The corporation uses outside labs to deliver its sequencing services. The resulting DNA sequence is subsequently encrypted and kept on the Bitcoin blockchain [39]. Several genetic marketplaces highlight traceability and data integrity as essential services they provide. For example, Genomes.io gives consumers the ability to safely manage and save their DNA data throughout the processes of sequencing and blockchain storage. The data is retained exclusively on the users' mobile devices, and access to it is controlled by a private access key provided to them. Another example is Genobank, which examines the use of non-fungible tokens (NFT) for data mobility and traceability. The suggested method comprises assigning a unique NFT to each human sample (such as saliva) and dispersing it on a public blockchain. Only a few applications for the NFT include selecting the lab that will sequence the genome and observing how the generated data are used [40].

12.7 Non-Commercial Blockchain Genomic Marketplaces

The chosen studies on blockchain's non-commercial uses mostly concentrate on sharing genomic data to promote science. Access control, data exchange, and data analysis are a few use scenarios that this research fits within.

The literature is categorized according to the overarching research issue. For instance, one research focused on the exchange of genetic data for the purpose of analysis, while another study focused on blockchain-based storage for the purpose of transferring genomic data that has already been preserved. The Cancer Gene Trust (CGT) is notable because it exemplifies the benefits of utilizing blockchain to exchange genetic data to advance cancer research. To further show the CGT framework's efficacy in a clinical setting, the authors have also initiated a cohort study based on data from actual patients.

TABLE 12.2

Blockchain Applications for Genomics Taxonomy

Main Category	Focus	References
Data sharing	Data exchange platform for securely transferring genetic data	[19,22,24,28,33, 58]
	Sharing and open access to de-identified clinical and genomic data	[26,40]
	A consensus protocol for the exchange of genetic and medical data	[17,48]
Data analysis	Decentralized GWAS with privacy protection	[13]
	Decentralized predictive model learning with privacy protection	[59, 61, 62, 64, 65]
	Using genetic and clinical data, distributed training of machine learning models conducted	[14]
Storage	Raw genomic data storage on-chain	[45]
	DNA sequence data storage and transfer using lossless compression	[69]
	Data storage and retrieval for pharmacogenomics	[46, 60]
Data management and access control	Management of personal genetic data access and consent	[23, 25, 31, 55]
	Management of multi-stakeholder consent	[32]
	Access logs and activities for genomic datasets	[21, 27,44,58,66]
	Dynamic management of consent	[4, 18, 63,]

Cancer patients submitted data for the pilot project, which was subsequently de-identified to protect patient privacy while maintaining the benefits of a distributed, open, cost-effective, and secure interchange of genomic data. De-identification was performed so that the information may be used by other scientists for their own purposes. CrypDist provided a comparable strategy, albeit with additional steps, for disseminating whole-genome data [40]. Finally, a group of articles focused on nontraditional consensus methods with potential genetic and medical implications [41]. To get users to carry out HTS read mapping on their own, Coinami provided incentives for doing so. As compensation, the players receive tokens. This swaps proof-of-work for HTS read mapping to verify blocks before they are included to the chain.

Using blockchain technology for genetic data analysis. One genome-wide association study (GWAS) that took privacy into account was presented. Using a gene fragmentation architecture, they are able to conduct GWAS while protecting users' anonymity. To facilitate storage, sharing, and analysis, this framework partitions enormous genomic datasets and disperses them across a wide variety of service providers in a distributed blockchain environment. As no single provider would therefore have access to all the data, centralization and privacy concerns are mitigated. Numerous articles have promoted blockchain-based decentralized machine learning. Several companies have implemented blockchain technology to train predictive models in a safe, open, and distributed environment [42,43]. Researchers propose using swarm learning (SL) for federated learning on the blockchain. Safely registering members without a coordinator is one way SL decentralizes machine learning. Finally, the model's parameters are integrated once the data are locally learned and the data owner is given control over the enormous store of genetic and medical data.

Dwarna is an online hub that uses blockchain technology to provide real-time approvals. Via the site, researchers may collaborate with study participants. The initiative complies with the General Data Privacy Regulation (GDPR), and participants are guaranteed ongoing control over their data. The suggested architecture makes use of blockchain to document agreement among all parties involved. In other words, when participants' permissions are stored in a blockchain, they become the data's true owners. Only with the explicit consent, the owner may give third parties access to the information. The authors address the master of supply chain management (MSCM) dilemma as applied to the issue of obtaining consent to share individual genetic data. This is because each person's genome may provide light on the person who possesses it and their family tree. That is why it's important to get family members' permission before sharing any personal information about them [44].

12.8 Advantages

- *Incentive (cryptocurrency).* Using blockchain allows us to create an incentive system for sharing genetic data using cryptocurrencies or tokens, which is a huge boon to the field. This is especially important in the context of genetic markets, where a trustworthy system for the trading of personal information is a primary goal. The objective is to streamline data transfers for scientific study and other purposes without compromising the security of the underlying datasets or the rights of real data owners to be compensated financially for sharing their data. In addition, the network's nodes can be rewarded through an incentive system for accomplishing a job, such as mapping sequence (HTS) reads. Anybody may sign up for free and begin performing analysis jobs immediately to earn tokens that can be exchanged for real money [45,46].

- *Decentralization.* Many articles highlighted the importance of blockchain networks' decentralized structure. To a large extent, the consensus process is responsible for the decentralized nature of blockchain. It provides a mechanism for distributed consensus in which no one authority is required for agreement across nodes. Depending on the context, decentralization can have a few advantages. Using blockchain and IPFS, as described in [40], decentralized open access may be realized. In the case of a disease epidemic, such as COVID-19, in order to investigate and create medical therapy, medical resources must be allocated quickly. Another situation in which decentralization works well is for task coordination that involves numerous nodes or locations. To use machine learning and combine the global model, a central server is no longer necessary, as demonstrated in [46]. This eliminates the third party's ability to compromise data privacy by studying aggregated statistics, which is a risk when relying on a third party for coordination due to the single point of failure/control that results. Similarly, it demonstrates a method that uses blockchain to organize GWAS research and ensure that all activity (transactions) inside the network is genuine and confirmed [47].

- *Ownership* is subject to strict regulation. It is preferable for patients or a reliable third party working on their behalf to have access to their genomic data (a doctor, for example). The existing centralized solutions make more work for us by requiring more time-consuming processes for permission and access control. Documents detail the range of control as the primary reason for implementing blockchain technology. Particularly egregious examples of this trend may be seen in genetic markets that promise users agency over who can view their data and for what purposes. There are concepts to promote patient empowerment and uphold their sovereignty over their personal contents; the consent is maintained on the blockchain [48].

- *Invariability.* The selected articles highlight the most desirable feature of blockchains as data storage that cannot be changed or tampered with. Most applications using genetic data rely heavily on the immutability provided by blockchain, which makes it immune to attacks aimed at modifying or erasing information. Blockchain's tamper-proof data structure, which is based on cryptographic hash references, protects against both unintentional and malicious changes to data. Any attempt to tamper with the blockchain's verified blocks will result in inconsistencies that can be easily uncovered by any participating node. This means that even in networks where not all participants can be completely trusted, a stable and consistent shared ledger can be maintained. On-chain storage can be used for data that must be kept indefinitely, such as permission records and audit logs [48], depending on the demands of the underlying application. Because the immutability property applies to on-chain data that is shared by all nodes and is not encrypted, anyone can access it. For this reason, data privacy must be carefully handled [49].

- *Digital agreements.* Token creation and distribution, authorization, and policy enforcement are just some of the many uses for smart contracts. Not all blockchain systems support smart contracts, and not all applications necessitate them. Yet smart contracts have been incorporated into the main parts of some ideas in several articles. Tokens used to motivate individuals to provide genetic data are generated via smart contracts on commercial genomic data exchange platforms. Payment ERC-20 tokens are generated by smart contracts in both Encrypgen and DNAtix. Genomics data may be exchanged for these coins using smart contracts. One further reason to use blockchain is to enforce some kind of access regulation with the help of computerized contracts. For instance, the use of smart contracts to facilitate the transfer of remuneration to the data owners and the provision of access to the data [50].

- *Maintaining trust through openness, accessibility, visibility, and auditability.* Just a few of the publications cited these blockchain features as the primary justification for using the technology. Online model learning, as described, relies heavily on data being readily available across all network nodes, making reliability and availability crucial. Applications that keep data owners apprised of who is accessing their data and how do the best job of emphasizing the significance of transparency and traceability. With these features of blockchain technology, business may win over data owners by putting them in charge of their information. For example, the authors stressed the significance of openness and stated that patients are more likely to provide genetic data for study when they are aware of how their data would be used [51,52].

12.9 Future Direction

Hundreds of gigabytes were generated from a single sequencing run, and it is predicted that 2 billion human genomes will be sequenced in the next decade. Moreover, high-throughput technologies generate several forms of genomics data that require specialized administration, processing, and storage infrastructures. While the possibility to speed up our learning via the reinterpretation of current datasets and gathered datasets is unprecedented, the sharing of these data also poses a number of ethical, legal, and technological concerns. Given these difficulties, it's no surprise that blockchain technology has recently garnered a lot of attention from a wide range of sectors, genomics included. Some blockchain-based initiatives have been established to solve the data-sharing issues in genomics and EHR; nevertheless, only a small number of investigations link the cryptocurrency system with academic studies [53,54].

Off-chain calculations based on the zero-knowledge protocol (ZKP) have made some promising recent advances that could lead to the creation of new blockchain-based applications. One of the nodes performs the calculation off-chain in the off-chain computing paradigm, and the state that results from the computation is preserved on-chain after the confirmation of the computation (verifying the ZKP proof). Arbitrum, on the other hand, employs a reward-based system for confirming off-chain calculations [55]. Given the volume of genomic data and the frequent need for intensive computing in genome analysis activities, we believe that future genomics research employing these off-chain computation approaches is feasible.

Emerging technologies that can be used to create confidence include decentralized identifiers (DIDs) [54,55] and verifiable credentials (VCs); however, they do not receive enough attention. Issues like data integrity and privacy can be resolved by using blockchain to build a decentralized trust architecture. When sharing data for research purposes, it can increase trust in genomic applications to adhere to the trust-over-IP principles [56].

There are many other use cases to research, and the usage of blockchain in genomics is still in its infancy. We believe the present genomic ecosystem will change when blockchain-based solutions are implemented. Patients will play a big part in data sharing because empowering patients to control their data is one of the goals of blockchain technology.

The greater trust and automated operations made possible by blockchain technology and smart contracts will result in a rise in the amount of shared data. Additionally, blockchain enables the creation of incentives that can promote fair genomic data sharing, storing, and analysis, with the ultimate objective of improving our comprehension of the human genome [57,58].

12.10 Limitations of Blockchain

Platforms that are built on blockchain technology are addressing important issues, such as the governance of sharing genetic data, among other issues. The end objective is to make sure that organizations and people may exchange data while maintaining their privacy using algorithms that make it easier to comply with ethical and legal norms. Even though most emerging platforms are still in their infancy, it is reasonable to view them favorably since they offer distinctive strategies to get around governance problems in the sharing of genomic data [10]. Significantly, blockchain is more than just a technological foundation; rather, it represents a fresh approach to managing open networks that harvest the potential of decentralized networks, cater to corporate demands, and consider consumer genomics [59]. Blockchain has the potential to revolutionize the way open networks are governed. So the primary advancement, in this case, is not related to technology but rather is made possible by technology. Blockchain-based networks have the goal of increasing the quantity of data that can be stored while also introducing novel ownership structures and making it easier for users to take an active role while administering the data sharing [60,61]. Opportunities to improve data restriction during collection may arise with blockchain-based solutions. This would improve the openness and honesty of collecting genetic information. As important, smart contracts have the potential to greatly increase the enforceability of access agreements. Assuring all parties involved that future data uses would comply to the T&Cs of data uses is why this initiative is so crucial. This will provide consistency while applying new information [62,63]. Furthermore, if correctly embraced, the blockchain-based solution has the ability to revolutionize the norms and practices around the flow of data. In particular, patients and individuals may play a larger role in the ecology of sharing the data, which might weaken the monopoly that test providers (both commercial and public) presently hold on the administration of the sharing of genetic data. The lack of a private market and the provision of public goods provide an opportunity for blockchain technology to introduce new dimensions. Blockchain-based solutions aim to educate and design around ownership, incentives, and participatory control in order to provide people and patients the power to share and manage their data. [64,65]. Yet blockchain-based solutions still require the backing of legal tools to be effective. Two prominent examples where self-regulation may not be sufficient are the setting of monetary values for genetic databases and the establishment of ownership rights. To provide the best possible rules, it is essential to consider the broader context of biomedical research when doing so [66].

12.11 Conclusions

Research publications that suggest blockchain-based solutions to issues with data processing, data exchange, and storage have recently increased in number. The profusion of blockchain applications, both for-profit and non-profit purposes, created to make the exchange of genetic data easier to do, can be viewed to follow a similar trajectory. In this study, we offered a complete summary of the many efforts that have previously been made in this field.

In the course of our research, we utilized a taxonomy that divides the uses of blockchain technology to genomics into two categories: commercial and non-commercial. The apps that are not for profit have been subdivided even further according to the precise aims they want to achieve, which include data exchange, analysis, safe storage, and restriction of access. The advantages and disadvantages of the suggested strategy were then discussed, along with a comparison of the various suggestions regarding the choice of the blockchain platform and how data is kept, shared, and protected within the proposal, after providing facts about each application.

Some of the most prominent issues are the inconstancy of the software, the inability to interoperate, and the security threats that are related with the rigidity of smart contracts. Another challenge is preserving the information's secrecy and the identity of people who control it.

When implemented in these types of environments, privacy-enhancing technologies like those described previously can be of great use. According to the findings of our investigation, immutability and decentralization appear to be the primary drivers behind the application of blockchain technology in this setting. We found that several of the studies advocated for data owners to be given the ability to exercise control over their own data. Most research articles make use of blockchain technology to provide organizations or people ownership of the data (patients).

Also, we concluded that, even though there is a large opportunity to look into other use cases, the applications or use cases of blockchain technology in genomics are not quite as comprehensive as those in the financial industry. From the vantage point of the many ideas already in place, we compiled a list of outstanding problems and difficulties. We recommend testing distributed analytics based on blockchains, also known as processing, in the field of genomics. In addition, the feasibility of privacy-preserving distributed analytics using blockchain networks can be better understood by comparing the performance of various privacy-enhancing technologies, such as homomorphic encryption, multi-party computation, zero-knowledge proofs, and off-chain computation. Investigating the use of blockchain technology to provide secure and verified access to genetic data is another interesting area for the future. The ideas of trust-over-IP can be applied to facilitate the creation of decentralized identities for researchers and manage such identities.

In conclusion, we believe that blockchain-based genomic applications are still in the research and development stages. Significant societal and technological changes will need to be made for these applications to be deployed. Recent attempts to promote its usage in genomics can help accelerate the adoption of this technology by proving the promise and practicality of utilizing blockchain technology in a range of genomic applications. This might speed up the dissemination of this innovation.

References

[1] Murawa P, Murawa D, Adamczyk B, Połom K. Breast cancer: Actual methods of treatment and future trends. *Reports of Practical Oncology and Radiotherapy*. 19(3) (2014), 165–72.

[2] Thomas C. Precision medicine: Functional advancements. *Annual Review of Medicine*. 69 (2018), 1–18.

[3] Moore C, O'Neill M, O'Sullivan E, Doröz Y, Sunar B. Practical homomorphic encryption: A survey. In *2014 IEEE International Symposium on Circuits and Systems (ISCAS)*, 2014 (pp. 2792–5). IEEE.

[4] Steneck NH. *Introduction to the Responsible Conduct of Research*, 2007. US Government Printing Office.

[5] Shabani M. Blockchain-based platforms for genomic data sharing: A de-centralized approach in response to the governance problems? *Journal of the American Medical Informatics Association*. 26(1) (2019), 76–80.

[6] Baselga J, Tripathy D, Mendelsohn J, et al. Phase II study of weekly intravenous recombinant humanized antip185HER2 monoclonal antibody in patients with HER2/neu-overexpressing metastatic breast cancer. *Journal of Clinical Oncology*. 14 (1996), 737–44.

[7] Gürsoy G, Brannon CM, Gerstein M. Using Ethereum blockchain to store and query pharmacogenomics data via smart contracts. *BMC Medical Genomics*. 13(1) (2020), 1–11.

[8] Worrall D, Ayoubi R, Fotouhi M, Southern K, McPherson PS, Laflamme C, NeuroSGC/YCharOS/EDDU Collaborative Group, ABIF Consortium. The identification of high-performing antibodies for TDP-43 for use in Western Blot, immunoprecipitation and immunofluorescence. *F1000Research*. 12(277) (2023), 277.

[9] Alshafie W, Ayoubi R, Fotouhi M, Southern K, Laflamme C, NeuroSGC/YCharOS Collaborative Group. The identification of high-performing antibodies for Moesin for use in Western Blot, immunoprecipitation, and immunofluorescence. *F1000Research*. 12(172) (2023), 172.

[10] Živi N, Kadušić E, Kadušić K. Directed Acyclic Graph as Tangle: An IoT Alternative to Blockchains. In *2019 27th Telecommunications Forum (TELFOR)*, 2019 (pp. 1–3). IEEE.
[11] Chang V, Baudier P, Zhang H, Xu Q, Zhang J, Arami M. How blockchain can impact financial services – The overview, challenges and recommendations from expert interviewees. *Technological Forecasting and Social Change*. 158 (2020), 120166. https://doi.org/10.1016/j.techfore.2020.120166
[12] Mohammed A, Fatih T, Joeri V D Velde, Karastoyanova D. Blockchain for genomics: A systematic literature review. *Distributed Ledger Technologies*. 1(2) (2022), 1–28. https://doi.org/10.1145/3563044
[13] Zhang Y, Zhao X, Li X, Zhong M, Curtis C, Chen C. Enabling privacy-preserving sharing of genomic data for GWASs in decentralized networks. In *Proceedings of the Twelfth ACM International Conference on Web Search and Data Mining*, 2019 (pp. 204–12). https://doi.org/10.1145/3289600.3290983
[14] Warnat-Herresthal S, Schultze H, Shastry KL, Manamohan S, Mukherjee S, Garg V, Sarveswara R, Händler K, Pickkers P, Aziz AN, et al. Swarm learning for decentralized and confidential clinical machine learning. *Nature*. 594(7862) (2021), 265–70.
[15] Uribe D, Waters G. Privacy laws, genomic data and non fungible tokens. *The Journal of The British Blockchain Association*. 3(2) (2020), 13164.
[16] Talukder AK, Chaitanya M, Arnold D, Sakurai K. Proof of disease: A blockchain consensus protocol for accurate medical decisions and reducing the disease burden. In *2018 IEEE SmartWorld, Ubiquitous Intelligence & Computing, Advanced & Trusted Computing, Scalable Computing & Communications, Cloud & Big Data Computing, Internet of People and Smart City Innovation (Smart- World/SCALCOM/UIC/ATC/CBDCom/IOP/SCI)*, 2018 (pp. 257–62). IEEE.
[17] Silva P, Dahlke DV, Lee Smith M, Charles W, Gomez J, Ory MG, Ramos KS. An idealized clinicogenomic registry to engage underrepresented populations using innovative technology. *Journal of Personalized Medicine*. 12(5) (2022), 713.
[18] Shuaib K, Saleous H, Zaki N, Dankar F. A layered blockchain framework for healthcare and genomics. In *2020 IEEE International Conference on Smart Computing (SMARTCOMP)*, 2020 (pp. 156–63). IEEE.
[19] Shabani M. Blockchain-based platforms for genomic data sharing: A de-centralized approach in response to the governance problems? *Journal of the American Medical Informatics Association*. 26(1) (2019), 76–80.
[20] Pattengale ND, Hudson CM. Decentralized genomics audit logging via permissioned blockchain ledgering. *BMC Medical Genomics*. 13(7) (2020), 1–9.
[21] Nakamoto S, Bitcoin A. *A Peer-to-Peer Electronic Cash System*; 2008. Bitcoin. https://bitcoin.org/bitcoin.pdf.
[22] Dambrot SM. ReGene: Blockchain backup of genome data and restoration of pre-engineered expressed phenotype. In *2018 9th IEEE Annual Ubiquitous Computing, Electronics & Mobile Communication Conference (UEMCON)*, 2018 (pp. 945–50). IEEE.
[23] Park Y-H, Kim Y, Shim J. Blockchain-based privacy preserving system for genomic data management using local differential privacy. *Electronics*. 10(23) (2021), 3019.
[24] Angraal S, Krumholz HM, Schulz WL. Blockchain technology: Applications in health care. *Circulation: Cardiovascular Quality and Outcomes*. 10(9) (2017), e003800.
[25] Pachaury R, Lakshmi CV. Securing genomics data using blockchain technology. In *Advances in Systems Engineering*, 2021 (pp. 473–80). Springer.
[26] Grossman RL. Progress towards cancer data ecosystems. *Cancer Journal (Sudbury, Mass.)*. 24(3) (2018), 122.
[27] Ozercan HI, Ileri AM, Ayday E, Alkan C. Realizing the potential of blockchain technologies in genomics. *Genome Research*. 28(9) (2018), 1255–63.
[28] Ozdayi MS, Kantarcioglu M, Malin B. Leveraging blockchain for immutable logging and querying across multiple sites. *BMC Medical Genomics*. 13(Suppl 7) (2020), 82.
[29] Neto MM, da S Marinho CS, Coutinho EF, Moreira LO, de C Machado J, de Souza JN. Research opportunities for e-health applications with DNA sequence data using blockchain technology. In *2020 IEEE International Conference on Software Architecture Companion (ICSA-C)*, 2020 (pp. 95–102). IEEE.

[30] Arroyo-Mariños JC, Mejia-Valle KM, Ugarte W. Technological model for the protection of genetic information using blockchain technology in the private health sector. In *ICT4AWE*, 2021 (pp. 171–8). https://www.scitepress.org/Papers/2021/104224/104224.pdf

[31] Abul-Husn NS, Kenny EE. Personalized medicine and the power of electronic health records. *Cell*. 177(1) (2019), 58–69.

[32] Beyene M, Thiebes S, Sunyaev A. *Multi-stakeholder consent management in genetic testing: A blockchain-based approach*, 2019. https://publikationen.bibliothek.kit.edu/1000125483

[33] Miyachi K, Mackey TK. hOCBS: A privacy-preserving blockchain framework for healthcare data leveraging an on-chain and off-chain system design. *Information Processing & Management*. 58(3) (2021), 102535.

[34] Sadat MN, Al Aziz MM, Mohammed N, Chen F, Jiang X, Wang S. Safety: Secure gwas in federated environment through a hybrid solution. *IEEE/ACM Transactions on Computational Biology and Bioinformatics*. 16(1) (2018), 93–102.

[35] Glicksberg BS, Burns S, Currie R, Griffin A, Wang ZJ, Haussler D, Goldstein T, Collisson E. Blockchain-authenticated sharing of genomic and clinical outcomes data of patients with cancer: A prospective cohort study. *Journal of Medical Internet Research*. 22(3) (2020), e16810. https://doi.org/10.2196/16810

[36] genecoin.me. 2020. genecoin. Retrieved 01.12.2020 from http://genecoin.me/.

[37] Glicksberg BS, Burns S, Currie R, Griffin A, Wang ZJ, Haussler D, Goldstein T, Collisson E. Blockchain-authenticated sharing of genomic and clinical outcomes data of patients with cancer: A prospective cohort study. *Journal of Medical Internet Research*. 22(3) (2020), e16810. https://doi.org/10.2196/16810

[38] Choi JI, Butler KR. Secure multiparty computation and trusted hardware: Examining adoption challenges and opportunities. *Security and Communication Networks*. 2 (2019).

[39] Sadat MN, Al Aziz MM, Mohammed N, Chen F, Jiang X, Wang S. Safety: Secure gwas in federated environment through a hybrid solution. *IEEE/ACM Transactions on Computational Biology and Bioinformatics*. 16(1) (2018), 93–102.

[40] Drucker N, Gueron S. Combining homomorphic encryption with trusted execution environment: A demonstration with paillier encryption and SGX. In *Proceedings of the 2017 International Workshop on Managing Insider Security Threats*, 2017 (pp. 85–8). https://doi.org/10.1145/3139923.3139933

[41] Kulemin N, Popov S, Gorbachev A. The Zenome Project: Whitepaper blockchain-based genomic ecosystem. *Zenome*, 2017. Available from: https://zenome.io/download/whitepaper.pdf

[42] Schorchit B, Monteiro BA, Gouveia FC, Fischer A, Rebelo MF. Meet Genecoin: The Bioeconomy Currency. *Theoretical White Paper*, 2018. Available from: https://github.com/genecoin-science/genecoin-science.github.io

[43] Gürsoy G, Bjornson R, Green ME, Gerstein M. Using blockchain to log genome dataset access: Efficient storage and query. *BMC Medical Genomics*. 13(7) (2020), 1–9.

[44] Gursoy G, Brannon C, Wagner S, Gerstein M. Storing and analyzing a genome on a blockchain. *Genome Biology*. 23 (2022), 134. https://doi.org/10.1186/s13059-022-02699-7

[45] Dedeturk BA, Soran A, Bakir-Gungor B. Blockchain for genomics and healthcare: A literature review, current status, classification and open issues. *PeerJ*. 9 (2021), e12130.

[46] Lipman A, Ekblaw B, Johnson A, Camaron K, Retzepi NN. *Technical Documentation: MedRec*, 2017 (pp. 1–9). Cambridge.

[47] Park JY, Lee YK, Lee DS, Yoo JE, Shin MS, Yamabe N, Kim SN, Lee S, Kim KH, Lee HJ, Roh SS. Abietic acid isolated from pine resin (Resina Pini) enhances angiogenesis in HUVECs and accelerates cutaneous wound healing in mice. *Journal of Ethnopharmacology*. 203 (2017), 279–87.

[48] Bosworth S, Kabay ME, editors. *Computer Security Handbook*, 2002. John Wiley & Sons.

[49] Alvarez F, Berg PA, Bianchi FB, Bianchi L, Burroughs AK, Cancado EL, Chapman RW, Cooksley WG, Czaja AJ, Desmet VJ, Donaldson PT. International autoimmune hepatitis group report: Review of criteria for diagnosis of autoimmune hepatitis. *Journal of Hepatology*. 31(5) (1999), 929–38.

[50] May A, Ross T. The design of civic technology: Factors that influence public participation and impact. *Ergonomics*. 61(2) (2018), 214–25.

[51] Kumar Y, Munjal R. Comparison of symmetric and asymmetric cryptography with existing vulnerabilities. *International Journal of Computer Science and Management Studies*. 11(3) (2011), 60–63.

[52] Iyer V, Vyshnavi AMH, Iyer S, Namboori PKK. An AI driven genomic profiling system and secure data sharing using DLT for cancer patients. In *2019 IEEE Bombay Section Signature Conference (IBSSC)*, 2019 (pp. 1–5). IEEE.

[53] Kumar R, Tripathi R. Traceability of counterfeit medicine supply chain through Blockchain. In *2019 11th International Conference on Communication Systems & Networks (COMSNETS)*, 2019 (pp. 568–70). IEEE.

[54] Goede M. E-Estonia: The e-government cases of Estonia, Singapore, and Curaçao. *Archives of Business Research*. 7(2) (2019).

[55] Buldas A, Kroonmaa A, Laanoja R. *Secure IT Systems: 18th Nordic Conference*. NordSec.

[56] Kim Y, Park Y-H. Blockchain-based model for gene data management using de-identifying scheme. In *2021 IEEE International Conference on Consumer Electronics-Asia (ICCE-Asia)*, 2021 (pp. 1–4). IEEE.

[57] Mathur G, Pandey A, Goyal S. Immutable DNA sequence data transmission for next generation bioinformatics using blockchain technology. In *2nd International Conference on Data, Engineering and Applications (IDEA)*, 2020 (pp. 1–6). IEEE.

[58] Kuo T-T. The anatomy of a distributed predictive modeling framework: Online learning, blockchain network, and consensus algorithm. *JAMIA Open*. 3(2) (2020), 201–8.

[59] Kuo T-T, Bath T, Ma S, Pattengale N, Yang M, Cao Y, Hudson CM, Kim J, Post K, Xiong L, et al. Benchmarking blockchain-based gene-drug interaction data sharing methods: A case study from the iDASH 2019 secure genome analysis competition blockchain track. *International Journal of Medical Informatics*. 154 (2021), 104559.

[60] Kuo T-T, Gabriel RA, Cidambi KR, Ohno-Machado L. Expectation Propagation Logistic Regression on permissioned block CHAIN (ExplorerChain): Decentralized online healthcare/genomics predictive model learning. *Journal of the American Medical Informatics Association*. 27(5) (2020), 747–56.

[61] Kuo T-T, Gabriel RA, Ohno-Machado L. Fair compute loads enabled by blockchain: Sharing models by alternating client and server roles. *Journal of the American Medical Informatics Association*. 26(5) (2019), 392–403.

[62] Mamo N, Martin GM, Desira M, Ellul B, Ebejer J-P. Dwarna: A blockchain solution for dynamic consent in biobanking. *European Journal of Human Genetics* (2019), 1–18.

[63] Kuo T-T, Kim J, Gabriel RA. Privacy-preserving model learning on a blockchain network-of-networks. *Journal of the American Medical Informatics Association*. 27(3) (2020), 343–54.

[64] Kuo T-T, Pham A. Detecting model misconducts in decentralized healthcare federated learning. *International Journal of Medical Informatics*. 158 (2022), 104658.

[65] Ma S, Cao Y, Xiong L. Efficient logging and querying for blockchain-based cross-site genomic dataset access audit. *BMC Medical Genomics*. 13(7) (2020), 1–13.

[66] Ma L, Liao Y, Fan H, Zheng X, Zhao J, Xiao Z, Zheng G, Xiong Y. PHDMF: A flexible and scalable personal health data management framework based on blockchain technology. *Frontiers in Genetics* (2022), 779.

13

Blockchain for Transaction of Large-Scale Clinical Information

Anusha R., Jayashree J., Vijayashree J., and Mohamed Yousuff

13.1 Introduction

Bitcoin's creation in 2008 introduced the world to a new concept that is now projected to change society. It has the potential to impact every industry, including finance, government, media, law, and the arts, to name a few. Some see blockchain as a revolution, while others believe it will be more evolutionary, with any practical benefits taking several years to materialize [1]. To some extent, this idea is correct, but the revolution, in our opinion, has already begun. Many significant companies throughout the globe are already working on blockchain proofs of concept, recognizing the technology's disruptive potential. Some firms, on the other hand, are still in the early stages of research, though this is likely to change as technology advances. It is a technology that has a significant influence on present technologies and can make a significant difference.

A *blockchain* is a public digital ledger of transactions that a network of computers keeps safe and hard to hack or modify [2]. Courtesy of technological advancements, individuals may interact directly with one another without the need for an intermediary such as a government, bank, or another third party.

Cryptography is employed to connect the ever-growing set of records known as blocks. Through peer-to-peer computer networks, each transaction is verified, time-stamped, and added to a growing data chain. Once data has been captured, it cannot be modified.

Technology has received the greatest attention because of news from the industry and the media about its expansion [3]. The market capitalizations of Ethereum, Bitcoin, Litecoin, Monero, and Dash, for example, are all outstanding. Blockchain, on the other hand, is not only for cryptocurrencies. There are several blockchain-based applications in the commercial and public sectors right now, including crowdfunding, supply chain monitoring, authentication, and voting services, with many more in [4,5]. According to a poll, blockchain is now the most often mentioned technology in financial applications.

13.1.1 How Does Blockchain Work?

Let us look at a more general method of creating blocks. This scheme is presented to provide you with a general overview of how blocks are produced and how transactions and blocks are linked:

1. A node initiates a transaction by producing it and digitally signing it with its private key. A blockchain transaction may be used to represent several different actions [6]. This is frequently a data structure that represents a value transfer between members in a blockchain network. The transaction data format often includes some value transfer logic, suitable rules, source and destination addresses, and other validation data.
2. The Gossip protocol broadcasts (floods) a transaction to peers, who subsequently validate it according to predetermined criteria [7]. In most circumstances, the transaction must be validated by the majority of nodes.
3. The transaction is then placed in a block, which is then sent throughout the network once it has been verified. At this moment, the transaction is deemed finished.
4. The freshly created block has now been added to the ledger, and the next block is cryptographically linked to it. This is a link to a hash pointer. The transaction obtains its second confirmation at this point, while the block receives its first.
5. Transactions are reconfirmed every time a new block is produced. Before a transaction on the Bitcoin network is declared complete, it usually requires six validations.

13.1.2 Consensus

Blockchain innovation in medical care is certainly not an exceptionally basic undertaking. It has some incredible advantages, just as some extreme downsides. Notwithstanding, it is normal that in the coming years, blockchain and AI will dominate in medical services application advancement and hence make it simpler for individuals to seek better therapy. An orderly writing survey was directed fully intent on investigating late writing on blockchain and the medical services space and distinguishing existing difficulties and open inquiries, directed by the bringing up of exploration issues about EHR in a blockchain, to help and work on comprehension of this appropriated record innovation [8]. More than 300 logical examinations distributed over the most recent ten years were inspected, bringing about the advancement of a forward-thinking scientific classification, the distinguishing proof of difficulties and open inquiries, and the assessment and conversation of the main methodologies, information types, guidelines, and structures for the utilization of blockchain in HER [9]. By making electronic well-being records more proficient and secure, this innovation may introduce another period of well-being data trade. Patients who get admittance to their clinical records connect with it in a divided way, which mirrors the way these records are overseen. Blockchain, which considers information trade and trust, could be a future option for telemedicine and accurate medication, considering the collective clinical dynamic [10]. Another utilization case for blockchain in medical care are X-beams performed on the specialist's recommendation on a patient and their stockpiling on the blockchain. This can be refined by securing the patient's protection. The hash of the patient's Aadhar number is utilized to keep up with privacy in the blockchain [11].

13.2 Generations of Blockchain

This section defines the three generations of blockchain technology. Bitcoin's extraordinarily high volatility and many nations' views about its complexity initially impeded its growth, but the benefits of blockchain, Bitcoin's underlying technology, eventually drew global attention. Blockchain's features include a distributed ledger, decentralization, information transparency, tamper-proof architecture, and openness. The evolution of the blockchain has been slow. Blockchains are now categorized as blockchain 1.0, 2.0, 3.0, and X.0, depending on their uses [12].

13.2.1 Blockchain 1.0

This tier was created with the launch of Bitcoin, and it is mostly used for cryptocurrencies. Second, because Bitcoin was the first cryptocurrency, it's only natural to categorize the first generation of blockchain technology as entirely cryptographic currencies. All alternative cryptocurrencies, as well as Bitcoin, are included in this category [13]. It includes important applications, such as payments and apps. With the launch of Bitcoin in 2009, this generation began and terminated in early 2010 [14].

13.2.2 Blockchain 2.0

Financial services and smart contracts are among the applications of the second blockchain generation. Futures, options, swaps, and bonds, among other financial assets, are included in this layer. This layer includes applications that go beyond money, finance, and markets. Ethereum, Hyperledger, and other emerging blockchain technologies are part of blockchain 2.0 [15]. This generation began in 2010 when individuals began to consider how blockchain may be used for numerous purposes.

13.2.3 Blockchain 3.0

Other than banking, this third blockchain generation is utilized to construct applications in government, health, journalism, the arts, and justice. This blockchain technology tier includes Ethereum, Hyperledger, and newer blockchains with the capacity to construct smart contracts, as well as blockchain 2.0. Around the year 2012, multiple applications of blockchain technology in various sectors were investigated, resulting in the formation of this blockchain generation [16].

13.2.4 Hyperledger Fabric

The Linux Foundation hosts an open-source project called Hyperledger Fabric, which is a blockchain system. An arrangement exists that, in a containerized development, incorporates the application thinking known as chain code [17,18]. Transactions that are classified—participants can follow the permeability of exchanges. Permissioned organization—every part has a known personality. Gives validation, access control, and exchange affirmation. Fosters trust, straightforwardness, and responsibility among members [19].

13.2.4.1 Hyperledger Fabric (HLF)

There are a few vital parts in HLF that assume basic parts of the framework. Moreover, it gives three phases of an agreement to approve exchanges before they are transferred to the record. To play out specific favored assignments, HLF gives an assortment of uncommon, assigned chain codes known as framework chain codes [20]. Setup, life cycle, query, endorser, and validator framework chain codes are instances of framework chain codes. A few essential chain codes were planned and executed in our model framework as a feature of our exploration.

Prior to transferring patient information to the EHR framework with the patient's assent, the information is scrambled with a suitable symmetric key [21]. The symmetric key is then unevenly encoded and connected to the scrambled information utilizing the patient's public key [22]. This mixture encryption makes the method more effective as far as both speed and comfort, in light of the fact that symmetric key encryption is quicker than deviated key encryption for enormous information, while the last is more advantageous for little-size cryptographic key encryption [23].

Online applications give electronic UIs and fundamental intuitive capacities for framework members to speak with each other. It is utilized by patients to create key sets to enlist and select their characters in the framework to acquire Eckert's. They can likewise produce intermediary encryption keys and send them to the intermediary [24]. The customer, then again, utilizes this electronic application to produce an exchange proposition and submit it to the blockchain framework for undertakings, for example, deciding a patient's character and making, transferring, and sharing clinical records, metadata, etc.

13.2.5 Blockchain X.0

This generation envisions a blockchain singularity in which, similar to the Google search engine, a public blockchain service would one day be open to anybody and everyone. It will provide services to people from all walks of life [25]. It will be a public and open distributed ledger with general-purpose rational agents (Machina economics) running on it, making choices and interacting with other intelligent autonomous agents on behalf of their owners, and regulated by code rather than legislation or paper contracts. This does not mean that laws and contracts will become outdated; rather, laws and contracts will be programmable [26].

Numerous advantages of blockchain technology have been addressed in a variety of sectors and advocated by thought leaders in the blockchain industry from across the world [27]. Some of the most noteworthy benefits of blockchain technology are as follows:

- **Decentralization.** This is a key principle and advantage of blockchain technology. Validation of transactions does not need the involvement of a trusted third party or intermediary; instead, a consensus mechanism is utilized to agree on the legitimacy of transactions.
- **Transparency and trust.** The system is transparent since blockchains are shared and everyone can see what's on them. As a result, there is an increase in trust. This is especially important in instances when personal discretion in determining recipients is limited, such as the distribution of payments or benefits [28].
- **Immutability.** Once data has been recorded on the blockchain, changing it is extremely difficult. Although it is not completely immutable, keeping an immutable ledger of transactions is seen as a benefit because changing data is so difficult, if not impossible [29].

- **Increased availability.** Because the system is built on thousands of nodes in a peer-to-peer network and the data is duplicated and updated on each node, it is incredibly dependable.
- The network continues to function even if certain nodes depart or become unavailable, making it highly available. There is a high level of availability due to the redundancy.
- **Ironclad security.** On a blockchain, all transactions are cryptographically encrypted, ensuring network integrity.
- **Simplification of existing paradigms.** Many businesses, including banking and health, are now using a disorderly blockchain paradigm. Multiple entities maintain their own databases under this approach, and owing to the different structures of the systems, data exchange might be problematic [30]. However, because a blockchain may act as a single shared ledger for many parties, it can simplify the paradigm by decreasing the burden of administering the several systems that each business maintains.
- **Faster dealings.** The current blockchain approach is unstructured in several areas, including banking and healthcare. In this design, many entities maintain their own databases, and data transfer may be difficult due to the disparate nature of the systems. However, because a blockchain may serve as a single shared ledger for several parties, it has the potential to streamline the process by reducing the administrative burden of each institution's distinct systems [31].
- **Cost saving.** Because the blockchain idea does not necessitate the use of a trusted third party or clearinghouse, it can drastically cut overhead costs associated with fees paid to such institutions.

13.3 A Smart Contracts–Based Blockchain-Based Electronic Medical Health Record

Any healthcare system's most asset is each patient's protected health information. The use of blockchain technology to maintain track of references to distributed patient data is amazing and inventive [32]. An extensive framework that keeps up with individual patient data and well-being records electronically in an advanced configuration is known as an EHR. A patient's personal and medical history is stored in an EHR. The EHR framework attempts to provide a more comprehensive perspective of patient outcomes by going beyond typical clinical data collecting [33].

13.3.1 Smart Contracts for Phases of Clinical Trials

Clinical trials have several phases that can be chained together in blockchain such that every phase is dependent on its predecessor. This ability of blockchain technology to slice and chain different phases is through a process of smart contracts. Smart contracts use cryptographic hash chains to verify and enforce a contract [34]. Smart contracts will only validate a step if the preceding step has been completely validated and verified. Smart contracts can include patients in the database (frozen after data entry) who have consented to the trial, and then each phase of the trial can be chained to ensure a transparent clinical trial with no manipulation of data in any step. Accept that each EHR submits solution, issue, and sensitivity list updates to circulated, decentralized dependable records, guaranteeing that the changes in information are surely known and approved across associations [35]. Thus, EHR shows information from any dataset referenced in the record rather than only one.

13.3.2 EHR Characteristics

- Increases diagnostic accuracy and patient outcomes.
- Enhances the quality of care.
- Streamlines and automates provider workflow.
- Maintained in a digital format that can be shared across multiple organizations.
- Approved suppliers can create and maintain data.

Every block in the blockchain consists of data as well as a digital signature (hash) generated by the encryption of the data. This hash connects two blocks mathematically by chaining them together [36]. The blockchain hash is calculated based on the preceding block's information, and it is used to lock blocks in time and order. It is the idea that binds blockchains together and contributes to the creation of the cryptographic trust. Nodes are the building blocks of the network. Nodes are like machines that run a network security mechanism. Each node holds a complete collection of all transactions recorded in that blockchain [37].

A country with a population of billions and a wide range of diversity undoubtedly demands a healthcare infrastructure that enables each civilian's health records to be handled smoothly and quickly. DeepMind Health, a Google company, is developing a blockchain-like mechanism for monitoring patient information reliably. Unlike conventional blockchain, which requires distributed verification from several participants, DeepMind claims that both changes will improve the system's efficiency.

The fundamental problem with modern healthcare is that organizations' medical records for their patients are numerous and scattered. The EHR framework utilizes blockchain innovation to safely store archives and protect a solitary adaptation of reality. Before submitting a transaction to the distributed ledger, stakeholders will need to obtain authorization to view a patient's history. Enormous scope accessibility, information classification, cost viability, and trust in the data frame may all be accomplished with a blockchain-based arrangement. Hospitals, patients, specialists, doctors, clinical researchers, labs, pharmacies, and drug control agencies, as well as insurance companies, are among the stakeholders.

13.3.3 FHIRChain: Using Blockchain to Share Clinical Data in a Secure and Scalable Way

Safe and versatile information sharing is needed to give patients viable community-oriented treatment and care choices. Patients visit an assortment of care suppliers' workplaces throughout the span of their lives [3]. To guarantee they have the most recent information about persistent medical issues, these suppliers ought to have the option to trade well-being data about their patients in an ideal and secure way.

13.3.4 Clinical Data Sharing Based on Blockchain Requirements

The "Shared Nationwide Interoperability Roadmap" by DeSalvo and Galvez defines technical requirements and guiding principles for developing interoperable health IT systems. Based on our previous experiences, we believe that designing a blockchain architecture to meet these requirements necessitates overcoming significant challenges to effectively use blockchain technology in healthcare. This section examines five key technical requirements fundamental to clinical data–sharing systems before discussing their implications for blockchain-based architectures.

- Storing and exchanging data securely
- Maintaining modularity
- Steady permissioned admittance to information sources
- Applying consistent data formats
- Verifying character and verifying all members

13.3.4.1 Application of Blockchain to Keep Up with Patient Records in Electronic Health Records (EHR)

Electronic health record (EHR) frameworks are progressively being utilized as an effective method for dividing patient records among emergency clinics. In any case, getting to dissipated patient information across various EHRs stays troublesome on the grounds that current EHRs are locally restricted or have a place with partnered medical clinics. As per a report delivered, the main boundary of getting to patient records is the trouble in finding supplier addresses. A channel is made, which is a private subnet of an HLF network where a similar record is divided between emergency clinic individuals. Associations or offices inside them can make autonomous channels with significant records dependent on their necessities. Practically speaking, clinical information is commonly too huge to even think about taking care of straightforwardly in a record; in this manner, information is put away in an EHR, with just the location recorded in the record. Contingent upon if the information is in a record, this kind of capacity is alluded to as on-chain or off-chain stockpiling. A record likewise stores information hash esteems [37]. This guarantees information honesty because once a piece of information is written in a record, it becomes unchanging, permitting the client to decide if the information has been adjusted.

13.3.4.2 A Structure for Secure and Decentralized Sharing of Clinical Imaging Information by Means of Blockchain Agreement

The availability of imaging studies to medical care suppliers and patients is of basic significance. Given the expenses of clinical picture obtaining and the dangers related to deferred admittance to the imaging results, working with the radiological examinations gives us a characteristic objective to further develop medical services proficiency and patient results.

13.3.4.2.1 Medical Picture Sharing
Notwithstanding the inescapable accessibility of advanced imaging and fast organization network, the steady worldview for clinical picture sharing necessitates that an actual duplicate (for example, a CD or DVD) be couriered between suppliers. There is a

clear shortcoming and waste intrinsic in translating a computerized resource onto optical media, which generally is perused just a single time during picture import at the getting site.

13.4 How Blockchain and AI Are Revolutionizing Healthcare Solutions

With the headway of innovation, the quantity of blockchain use cases in medical services is improving. Medical services have some different purposes, separated from making installments. The large issue of the present medical services framework is that it cannot satisfy every one of the necessities of the buyers [38]. Blockchain and AI have concocted an answer for that load of issues.

13.4.1 Blockchain Applications in Medical Care

1. *Admittance to the clinical record.* Blockchain innovation permits putting away every one of the significant patient information in a dataset. Both the specialists and patients can utilize that information adequately.
2. *Following clinical accreditations.* It is vital to really look at the accreditations and confirm the past work insight of the clinical staff. In general, the method involved with recruiting will turn out to be more sensible through blockchain innovation.
3. *Secure installments.* Blockchain innovation is firmly identified with cryptographic money. With cryptographic forms of money, you can follow your installments in a superior manner. Likewise, it lessens the dangers of hacking.
4. *Trial of new medications.* Enormous datasets are assembled and investigated for research purposes. With the assistance of blockchain, that load of information is kept put away so the specialists and patients can profit rapidly.

13.4.2 AI Applications in Medical Services

1. *Simulated intelligence specialists.* Simulated intelligence specialists have made that work as the right hand of the expert specialists.
2. *Man-made intelligence dental specialist.* There are some robot dental specialists that work with AI and capacity consequently. The machine can do a few systems like teeth inserts and so on better than the human dental specialists.
3. *Keeping up with clinical records and remedies.* The primary objective is to distinguish the profile of the patients who are not adhering to the rules. In any case, the AI calculation is not hard to follow those patients and advise them to have meds conveniently.

13.4.3 Drawbacks

1. *Cost.* It is trying to fix a sum for blockchain and AI in the medical services framework.
2. *Approval.* There is no specific system to recognize the proprietor of the information.

3. *Vulnerability.* Because of the absence of mindfulness, there is an absence of new blockchain companies in the medical care industry. It gives a feeling of vulnerability and questions about the eventual fate of blockchain in medical care.
4. *Rules and regulations.* There are no specific standards and guidelines for blockchain in the medical care framework. In addition, it isn't extremely straightforward to anybody how to apply the protection guidelines.

Decentralization, permanence, security, and detectability are totally accomplished by consolidating conveyed records, uneven encryption, and hash calculations in blockchain innovation, which was first known as Bitcoin. It disposes off middle people, shifts certainty from foundations to hard coding, and is viewed as a turning point in the breakdown of the information-restraining infrastructure by re-establishing control of information to individual proprietors. Keen agreements, which are coding programs that independently self-execute the trading of significant worth if explicit arrangements are initiated, gave Ethereum an image of modern advances and their force. A sizeable portion of the applications is accessible to general society [38]. The expression "chain" alludes to the way that everybody locally claims a piece of property. Authorization to see. As the interest in high-security workforce develops, there has been a change in enterprises, like drugstores and medical care. The consortium chain is another kind of blockchain that has developed. It incorporates individuals who have been examined.

Blockchains can be utilized in medical care for a huge scope, where the brought-together structure has made information storehouses for information stockpiling and severe information needs. Data sharing is hampered by security, especially when wearable gadgets make billions of information focuses, with enormous information stockpiling, and use prerequisites man-made reasoning (computer-based intelligence) produces (man-made intelligence). Moreover, blockchains' benefits as far as confirming information possession and expanding the spatial or transient measurement give the blockchain idea a promising future in the medical care industry. Gatekeeper Time cooperated with the Estonian government to dispatch a blockchain-based foundation that would approve patient IDs and secure individuals' well-being records in a patient-driven way across the whole country. Indeed, even with a few partners, this framework guaranteed that patients had responsibility for information and could set admittance freedoms, just as it was impervious to alter [39].

13.4.4 Clinical Trials

At the point when more gatherings and hubs of clinical preliminaries are involved and collaborate a long way from the significant foundations, human-incited botches, regardless of whether accidental or deliberate, are more probable. Wong introduced a blockchain-based clinical preliminary framework that would expect controllers to audit each update to the chain, including various gatherings. Drug production network executives, clinical expert credentialing and licensure, and medical coverage claim organizations are on the whole situation because of changelessness and recognizability. Patients reserve the privilege to both control and participate in the cash produced by their information in the computerized well-being environment.

13.4.5 Gartner Hype Cycle

Blockchain is currently at the "pinnacle of swelled assumptions" and "box of dissatisfaction" stage, as indicated by the Gartner Hype Cycle. Security and protection are two significant difficulties in the medical services area. As a rule, on open chains, where "everybody can see everything," the harmony among transparency and secrecy might be confounded, while different applications might depend on altered arrangements utilizing consortium chains or private chains. Permanence may be a blade that cuts both ways for patients who expect to have the option to erase their information from the chains [40]. Likewise, keeping all clinical information on the blockchain will swell it since it does not change how information is saved but how information is gotten to and shared; subsequently, information is frequently put away outside of the chains with cryptographic location pointers on the chains in many applications. Moreover, specialists should completely investigate and assess the utilization of a blockchain. By taking advantage of shrewd agreement blemishes, programmers had the option to take digital currency esteemed more than 80 million dollars somewhere in the range of 2016 and 2019. Accordingly, before blockchains are broadly utilized in medical care, their value should be assessed on a greater scale.

13.4.6 Evolutions in Technology

As innovation propels, in any case, blockchains might be utilized to scatter information as well as models and handling power, decreasing the risk of setting information on the chain. The AI Record Organization for Medication Disclosure project plans to prepare man-made intelligence models with shifted datasets without modifying information stockpiling or compromising information proprietorship utilizing its fit-for-reason blockchain-based drug application. Quantum processing may likewise prompt crucial changes in the hidden encryption, delivering future scrambled innovation incomprehensible.

13.5 A Blockchain Future for Secure Clinical Data Sharing

In the advanced medical services age, it is basic to bridle clinical information that is spread all through medical services associations to work with inside and outside information examination. Information trade is hampered, notwithstanding, due to the furthest reaches of medical care suppliers' cyberinfrastructure. The issues about clinical information trade and the executives are first brought up in this position paper. We next give a concise outline of the foundation and present status of the craftsmanship. At last, we suggest a couple of potential exploration roads for addressing the current obstacles to clinical information exchange. Because of protection and security concerns, electronic clinical records (EMR) are, much of the time, put away in neighborhood datasets of medical care suppliers as opposed to being divided between clinical examination foundations. Therefore, interoperability of clinical information from assorted sources has turned into a basic hindrance as of late, seriously restricting clinical exploration that requires a tremendous volume of information.

In the time of distributed computing and enormous information, clinical information is quickly being shared across a wide assortment of clinical examination associations to advance better medical services benefits and make clinical arrangements. At the point when clinical information and clinical preliminaries from all through the nation are converged in a comprehensive manner, it opens unparalleled possibilities for exact therapy plans and clinical conclusions, just as bringing down the expenses of rehash clinical testing. As per security and security guidelines, for example, the healthcare coverage Convenience and Responsibility Act and Well-Being Data Innovation for Monetary and Clinical Well-Being in the United States, and the Overall Information Insurance Guideline in Europe, information should be put away and partaken in a solid and protection-saving way [41].

13.5.1 Blockchain to Improve the Quality of Clinical Research

The traditional field of biomedical research has several problems, like scientific misconduct, from errors due to human carelessness to even fraud; small mistakes have the potential to undermine the research quality of a clinical study. In the context of clinical records, the violation and chronological history of data is protected by the feature of blockchain, which ensures that each event in the clinical trial is tracked in the correct chronological order. The integrity of the data in the clinical trials is preserved through using validation using cryptography principles. This feature can help prevent the falsification of data or even the invention of data that was not uncovered in the clinical trial. Blockchain can help keep the data free from manipulation but also maintain confidentiality.

13.5.2 Sharing Data in Community-Driven Medicine

As blockchain is a trustless system, that is, trust is built into the system; therefore, clinical researchers can allow people to be enrolled into protocols using community management. In Estonia, researchers have been successful in implementing a blockchain-based storage system where millions of patients are able to store and access their medical health records through a system of "keyless signature infrastructure." On the researcher side, blockchain can be used to share anonymized raw data and can also be distributed to enable secure cloud sharing. Therefore, researchers can analyze datasets and share information among many users—investigators, publishers, and even patients [42].

13.5.3 Sharing Key Information on a Blockchain

Before the trial even begins, the required consent forms, the field of the study, and the research outcomes can be stored in data structures stored on the blockchain. As blockchain is decentralized and information can never be deleted, only when most users vote for an event will it get added to the chain.

13.5.4 Cloud-Based Methodologies

Secure information partaking in a circulated setting has been a hot and hard point since the beginning of distributed computing. Since clients and cloud suppliers are habitually in particular authoritative or security areas, the intricacy of cloud-based information sharing is dictated by the degree of trust clients have in cloud specialist organizations [43]. The test turns out to be more tangled with regard to cloud-based clinical information organization. Permitting clients to oversee keys would further develop information security; however, it would be an expense for themselves and limit the versatility of information dividing between an enormous number of examination associations. Mentioning responsibility for keys from cloud suppliers, then again, may raise the danger of information spillage, since cloud heads can alter the keys and even interpret the information.

13.6 Solutions with Blockchain Technology

Each clinical data trade of the patient has related costs, like affirmation, security, assurance, interoperability, and institutional course of action. High upkeep costs can impact the medical results and treatment.

1. *Interoperability with blockchain.* Interoperability can be avoided; blockchain enables a centralized distributed mechanism for the management of authentication. Gordon et al. suggested a method for interoperability by establishing an API connection to the systems. They suggested another method using patient identity. As per that method, if two systems want to exchange the patient's data, the patient identity should be resolved initially.
2. *Cost of maintenance.* Blockchain-circulated nature, open-source innovation, and different properties can diminish the asset's expense fundamentally. The huge figuring measure is fundamental for blockchain-based applications. The expense of registering power depends on the volume and size of the exchanges associated with that application. Be that as it may, it is hard to foresee the expense of working a blockchain at the big business level. In this manner, to anticipate the expense of a completely scaled framework dependent on blockchain innovation client need, target examinations and normal rules are vital.

13.7 Blockchain to Establish IoT-Based Healthcare

IoT has tremendous uses in the field of healthcare—it can provide real-time healthcare data with the use of different sensors. However, the data collected is stored in a "centralized" database, and from here, it is analyzed and processed. The problem with this kind of centralized system is that if there is a small error that causes failure, all the healthcare data will be lost; also, a centralized system poses security threats, such as tampering with the stored data and manipulating it. To solve this issue, we can combine the IoT system with blockchain technology, which can decentralize the system and use the popular consensus algorithms in blockchain to validate the information in healthcare.

13.7.1 Useful Features of Blockchain That Can Be Used in e-Health

- *Decentralizing the information stored.* In the status quo, all the information stored is under the control of a single entity, which gives the owner the power to transfer or manipulate the data. With decentralization, every user can safely secure their contracts or healthcare documents directly via the Internet with no middleman.
- *Transparency.* Since each transaction on the blockchain has to be validated by every user on the network, all the holdings are in public view.
- *Immutability.* Blockchain is immutable, so regardless of how powerful a user is, they cannot change a transaction; in case of an error, a new transaction can be initiated that can reverse the error. Both transactions will be visible, however, in the records.

13.8 IoT Blockchain-Based e-Healthcare

In traditional IoT networks, the model generally followed is the server–client model, where the devices are connected via cloud servers. The server–client model does not fare well when the networks are scaled up because of the increase in cost and increased susceptibility to a single-point failure. IoT networks are also susceptible to information attacks. Blockchain can correct these drawbacks by establishing a peer-to-peer network which will immediately reduce the cost of installation and maintenance. Since every device on the network is able to communicate, it reduces the problem of single-point failure. Blockchain, along with cryptography, can help solve information security issues.

The blockchain-based IoT systems architecture comprises four layers—IoT healthcare, a blockchain platform, connectivity to the Internet, and lastly, IoT devices. Using two-factor authentication schemes will allow the user to communicate with other nodes in the network, thus ensuring authenticity and security. IoT healthcare will comprise sensors, actuators, signals, and wearables. This will transfer information to the blockchain platform that will use different modes of authentication and, finally, using Internet connectivity will relay that information to decentralized apps.

13.8.1 Blockchain to Enable Secure Medical Record Access

Electronic health records can be shared between multiple organizations upon the authorization of the patients with the use of smart contracts. The information for the health records can be collected via IOT devices, such as wearables or sensors. The blockchain layer can then permanently and publicly store the patient's authorization, the public keys of patients, and the organizations who have attempted to access the patient's data.

13.8.2 Assessing Claims and Billings

In e-healthcare, fraudulent claims and bills cause huge losses to the industry—if a claim is made regarding medical procedures that have not even been performed, overcharging of the provided service, and unnecessary usage of medical services to extract more money from a patient, etc. By using blockchain, the entire process can be automated by a decentralized system such that all parties can share a copy of their transaction and contract while making a claim so that the whole process can be more effective and fraudulent-free.

13.8.3 Medicinal Drug Supply Chain Management

Counterfeit pharmaceutical drugs cause two major problems—the fake drugs can have severe repercussions on the health of an individual and, in some cases, even result in death; secondly, pharmaceutical companies can also incur huge losses due to the presence of cheap fake drugs in the market. The processes involved in drug manufacturing to supply to the patient are primarily comprised of the following stages: transportation of the drugs, handling of the medications, appropriate storage (as some medications may need to be maintained at a particular temperature), and finally, selling the medications. Now, due to the system being heavily dependent on human intervention, it opens up the possibility of human error or intentional malicious activity. With the help of blockchain, the records of the medicine, right from manufacture to sale, can be entered into the blockchain; due to its permanent, decentralized, and immutable nature, it can make the process of medicine supply more transparent.

13.9 Challenges and Solutions of Integrating Blockchain in Healthcare

There is a very close link that exists between healthcare data mining and big data (complex large set of data that is evaluated for patterns). Several diseases can be identified in their early stages by simply analyzing the patterns in a person's characteristics of walking (as an example) using machine learning techniques. The patient data can be recorded by an IoT wearable that contains sensors that can record body temperature, sweating, sleep quality, blood pressure, and breathing pattern.

13.9.1 Privacy Concerns Over Healthcare Data

Every person's online identity carries information or attributes that directly relate to themselves or their organizations. While digital identity helps authenticate an individual on the World Wide Web, it can also result in all their personal information and activities online being visible to certain entities. This kind of revealing or sensitive information is known as *personally identifiable information (PII)*, which can be used to distinguish a particular person. Login information, user's living address, and full legal name are classified as PII, while race, sex, height, and weight can be classified as potential PII. A combination of the two kinds of information can be very effective in exactly identifying a person. There are several methods to anonymize this kind of big healthcare data:

- Aggregate the data such that no one can detect the source of information and mining any useful information or patterns will be impossible.
- Remove or censor certain fields of the data such that it becomes difficult to guess the missing values.
- Deliberately add falsifications or irrelevancies to the data.
- Approximate all numerical values in such a way that any machine learning techniques will fail to make predictions

There are certain countries that are now passing policies or regulations for the privacy of information.

13.9.2 Blockchain Applied to Secure Clinical Big Data

- *Trust.* Since blockchain is a trustless system (trust is built into the protocol), patients don't need to rely on data handlers or worry about breaches and private information leaking out.
- *Data mining.* Through decentralization and consensus, the privacy of healthcare data is ensured, and any interested stakeholders, like researchers, scientists, politicians, and doctors, can just join the network as a miner and then study the information. This can lead to better research quality.

- *Interoperability.* IoT wearables data and feedback, the lab results of a patient, and the medicine consumption status can be shared among the patients, businesses, doctors, and labs, which can enable healthcare workers and insurance companies to create policies on the blockchain using smart contracts.
- *Counterfeit medicines.* By making the cycle of drug manufacture and sale transparent and immutable, the sale of fake drugs will significantly reduce, which can save lives and prevent pharmaceutical companies from losing money [44].

13.9.3 Challenges of Blockchain

- *Storage.* Since IoT wearables produce huge amounts of data, it becomes very costly to scale up and store the information on the decentralized and hashed architecture of blockchain. Therefore, as data size increases, the cost of the blockchain application increases.
- *Modification capability.* Due to its immutability, it's impossible to delete or change data, which means that when these applications are developed, it must be conscious that the data modification required must be kept to a minimum.
- *Scalability.* This is not such a critical issue because of the decentralized nature of blockchain; however, there is large computational power required that will, in turn, consume lots of electricity, which can have environmental concerns.

13.10 Conclusion

This chapter defines blockchain in clinical information sharing securely in healthcare systems. IoT and blockchain support the healthcare system. It also defines the fundamentals of blockchain and IoT. In this article chapter we examine the past, present, and future of blockchain in clinical information sharing using blockchain.

References

[1] Pandey P, Litoriya R. Implementing healthcare services on a large scale: challenges and remedies based on blockchain technology. *Health Policy and Technology.* 2020 Mar 1;9(1):69–78.
[2] Vardhini B, Dass SN, Sahana R, Chinnaiyan R. A blockchain based electronic medical health records framework using smart contracts. In *2021 International Conference on Computer Communication and Informatics (ICCCI),* 2021 Jan 27 (pp. 1–4). IEEE.
[3] Zhang P, White J, Schmidt DC, Lenz G, Rosenbloom ST. FHIRChain: applying blockchain to securely and scalably share clinical data. *Computational and Structural Biotechnology Journal.* 2018 Jan 1;16:267–78.
[4] Tith D, Lee JS, Suzuki H, Wijesundara WM, Taira N, Obi T, Ohyama N. Application of blockchain to maintaining patient records in electronic health record for enhanced privacy, scalability, and availability. *Healthcare Informatics Research.* 2020 Jan 31;26(1):3–12.
[5] Patel V. A framework for secure and decentralized sharing of medical imaging data via blockchain consensus. *Health Informatics Journal.* 2019 Dec;25(4):1398–411.

[6] Adithya K, Girimurugan R. Benefits of IoT in automated systems. *Integration of Mechanical and Manufacturing Engineering with IoT: A Digital Transformation*. 2023 Jan 23:235–70.

[7] Mayer AH, da Costa CA, Righi RD. Electronic health records in a blockchain: a systematic review. *Health Informatics Journal*. 2020 Jun;26(2):1273–88.

[8] Yun D, Chen W, Wu X, Ting DS, Lin H. Blockchain: chaining digital health to a new era. *Annals of Translational Medicine*. 2020 Jun;8(11).

[9] Luo Y, Jin H, Li P. A blockchain future for secure clinical data sharing: a position paper. In *Proceedings of the ACM International Workshop on Security in Software Defined Networks & Network Function Virtualization*, 2019 Mar 19 (pp. 23–7). https://doi.org/10.1145/3309194.3309198

[10] Zhuang Y, Sheets LR, Chen YW, Shae ZY, Tsai JJ, Shyu CR. A patient-centric health information exchange framework using blockchain technology. *IEEE Journal of Biomedical and Health Informatics*. 2020 May 8;24(8):2169–76.

[11] Sharma A, Bahl S, Bagha AK, Javaid M, Shukla DK, Haleem A. Blockchain technology and its applications to combat COVID-19 pandemic. *Research on Biomedical Engineering*. 2020 Oct 22:1–8.

[12] Hemalatha K, Hema K, Deepika V. Utilization of blockchain technology to overthrow the challenges in healthcare industry. In *Emerging Research in Data Engineering Systems and Computer Communications: Proceedings of CCODE 2019*, 2020 Feb 11 (pp. 199–208). Springer.

[13] Benchoufi M, Ravaud P. Blockchain technology for improving clinical research quality. *Trials*. 2017 Dec;18(1):1–5.

[14] Yu G, Zha X, Wang X, Ni W, Yu K, Yu P, Zhang JA, Liu RP, Guo YJ. Enabling attribute revocation for fine-grained access control in blockchain-IoT systems. *IEEE Transactions on Engineering Management*. 2020 Feb 10;67(4):1213–30.

[15] Onik MM, Aich S, Yang J, Kim CS, Kim HC. Blockchain in healthcare: challenges and solutions. In *Big Data Analytics for Intelligent Healthcare Management*, 2019 Jan 1 (pp. 197–226). Academic Press.

[16] Zhang P, Walker MA, White J, Schmidt DC, Lenz G. Metrics for assessing blockchain-based healthcare decentralized apps. In *2017 IEEE 19th International Conference on E-Health Networking, Applications and Services (Healthcom)*, 2017 Oct 12 (pp. 1–4). IEEE.

[17] Mahmood Z. Impact of blockchain technology in healthcare sector during COVID-19 pandemic. In *Computer Science & Information Technology: International Conference on AI, Machine Learning and Applications (AIMLA 2021), August 28~ 29, 2021, Dubai, UAE*, 2021 (Vol. 11, No. 13, pp. 75–88). AIRCC Publishing Corporation.

[18] Kaur H, Alam MA, Jameel R, Mourya AK, Chang V. A proposed solution and future direction for blockchain-based heterogeneous medicare data in cloud environment. *Journal of Medical Systems*. 2018 Aug;42:1.

[19] Chowdhury D, Anni LT, Hasan MM, Bhuiyan NA, Islam N, Pervez R. Cryptographic ledger of blockchain technology in healthcare. *GSC Advanced Research and Reviews*. 2021;7(3):28–37.

[20] Rani M, Verma P, Kumar S, Tayal N, Pant S. *Transforming healthcare system with blockchain*, 2021. https://doi.org/10.32628/CSEIT217434

[21] Maslove DM, Klein J, Brohman K, Martin P. Using blockchain technology to manage clinical trials data: a proof-of-concept study. *JMIR Medical Informatics*. 2018 Dec 21;6(4):e11949.

[22] Kuo TT, Bath T, Ma S, Pattengale N, Yang M, Cao Y, Hudson CM, Kim J, Post K, Xiong L, Ohno-Machado L. Benchmarking blockchain-based gene-drug interaction data sharing methods: a case study from the iDASH 2019 secure genome analysis competition blockchain track. *International Journal of Medical Informatics*. 2021 Oct 1;154:104559.

[23] Vazirani AA, O'Donoghue O, Brindley D, Meinert E. Implementing blockchains for efficient health care: systematic review. *Journal of Medical Internet Research*. 2019 Feb 12;21(2):e12439.

[24] Mamoshina P, Ojomoko L, Yanovich Y, Ostrovski A, Botezatu A, Prikhodko P, Izumchenko E, Aliper A, Romantsov K, Zhebrak A, Ogu IO. Converging blockchain and next-generation artificial intelligence technologies to decentralize and accelerate biomedical research and healthcare. *Oncotarget*. 2018 Jan 1;9(5):5665.

[25] Siyal AA, Junejo AZ, Zawish M, Ahmed K, Khalil A, Soursou G. Applications of blockchain technology in medicine and healthcare: challenges and future perspectives. *Cryptography*. 2019 Jan 2;3(1):3.

[26] Hussein AF, Alzubaidi AK, Habash QA, Jaber MM. An adaptive biomedical data managing scheme based on the blockchain technique. *Applied Sciences*. 2019 Jun 19;9(12):2494.
[27] Kleinaki AS, Mytis-Gkometh P, Drosatos G, Efraimidis PS, Kaldoudi E. A blockchain-based notarization service for biomedical knowledge retrieval. *Computational and Structural Biotechnology Journal*. 2018 Jan 1;16:288–97.
[28] Mytis-Gkometh P, Drosatos G, Efraimidis PS, Kaldoudi E. Notarization of knowledge retrieval from biomedical repositories using blockchain technology. In *Precision Medicine Powered by pHealth and Connected Health: ICBHI 2017, Thessaloniki, Greece, 18–21 November 2017*, 2018 (pp. 69–73). Springer.
[29] Sharma A, Bahl S, Bagha AK, Javaid M, Shukla DK, Haleem A. Blockchain technology and its applications to combat COVID-19 pandemic. *Research on Biomedical Engineering*. 2020 Oct 22:1–8.
[30] Pandey P, Litoriya R. Securing and authenticating healthcare records through blockchain technology. *Cryptologia*. 2020 Jul 3;44(4):341–56.
[31] Liu H, Crespo RG, Martínez OS. Enhancing privacy and data security across healthcare applications using blockchain and distributed ledger concepts. In *Healthcare*, 2020 Jul 29 (Vol. 8, No. 3, p. 243). MDPI.
[32] Liang X, Zhao J, Shetty S, Liu J, Li D. Integrating blockchain for data sharing and collaboration in mobile healthcare applications. In *2017 IEEE 28th Annual International Symposium on Personal, Indoor, and Mobile Radio Communications (PIMRC)*, 2017 Oct 8 (pp. 1–5). IEEE.
[33] Dwivedi AD, Malina L, Dzurenda P, Srivastava G. Optimized blockchain model for internet of things based healthcare applications. In *2019 42nd International Conference on Telecommunications and Signal Processing (TSP)*, 2019 Jul 1 (pp. 135–9). IEEE.
[34] Sammeta N, Parthiban L. Hyperledger blockchain enabled secure medical record management with deep learning-based diagnosis model. *Complex & Intelligent Systems*. 2022 Feb;8(1):625–40.
[35] Sravanthi C, Chowdary S. Deep learning and blockchain for electronic health record in healthcare system. In *Intelligent System Design: Proceedings of INDIA 2022*, 2022 Oct 28 (pp. 429–36). Springer.
[36] Farouk A, Alahmadi A, Ghose S, Mashatan A. Blockchain platform for industrial healthcare: vision and future opportunities. *Computer Communications*. 2020 Mar 15;154:223–35.
[37] Wang K, Dong J, Wang Y, Yin H. Securing data with blockchain and AI. *IEEE Access*. 2019 Jun 7;7:77981–9.
[38] Drosatos G, Kaldoudi E. Blockchain applications in the biomedical domain: a scoping review. *Computational and Structural Biotechnology Journal*. 2019 Jan 1;17:229–40.
[39] Mettler M. Blockchain technology in healthcare: the revolution starts here. In *2016 IEEE 18th International Conference on E-Health Networking, Applications and Services (Healthcom)*, 2016 Sep 14 (pp. 1–3). IEEE.
[40] Azaria A, Ekblaw A, Vieira T, Lippman A. Medrec: using blockchain for medical data access and permission management. In *2016 2nd International Conference on Open and Big Data (OBD)*, 2016 Aug 22 (pp. 25–30). IEEE.
[41] Esposito C, De Santis A, Tortora G, Chang H, Choo KK. Blockchain: a panacea for healthcare cloud-based data security and privacy? *IEEE Cloud Computing*. 2018 Mar 28;5(1):31–7.
[42] Zhang J, Xue N, Huang X. A secure system for pervasive social network-based healthcare. *IEEE Access*. 2016 Dec 29;4:9239–50.
[43] Al Omar A, Rahman MS, Basu A, Kiyomoto S. Medibchain: a blockchain based privacy preserving platform for healthcare data. In *Security, Privacy, and Anonymity in Computation, Communication, and Storage: SpaCCS 2017 International Workshops, Guangzhou, China, December 12–15, 2017, Proceedings 10*, 2017 (pp. 534–43). Springer International Publishing.
[44] Dwivedi AD, Srivastava G, Dhar S, Singh R. A decentralized privacy-preserving healthcare blockchain for IoT. *Sensors*. 2019 Jan 15;19(2):326.

14

Sharing and Interpretation of Genomic Datasets using Blockchain

Mohamed Yousuff, Jayashree J., Vijayashree J., and Anusha R.

14.1 Introduction

Blockchain is a distributed ledger system that allows for the safe, transparent, and tamper-resistant recording of transactions. A *blockchain* is a digital ledger of transactions that is spread across a network of computers. Each block in the chain contains a set of transactions that have been verified and added to the ledger. The concept of blockchain was first introduced in 2008 by a pseudonymous person or group known as Satoshi Nakamoto, who created the blockchain-based cryptocurrency Bitcoin [1]. However, blockchain technology has been utilized for various purposes other than cryptocurrency, such as managing supply chains, developing voting systems, and handling digital identities. The fundamental aspect of a blockchain is that it comprises a distributed network of computers or nodes that collaborate to confirm transactions and preserve the accuracy of the record. All nodes retain a copy of the ledger, which is continually revised as new transactions are appended. When a transaction is initiated on the blockchain, it is broadcast to the network and verified by multiple nodes through a process known as consensus. This ensures that the transaction is valid and has not been tampered with. Once the transaction is verified, it is added to a new block in the chain, along with other transactions that have been validated by the network [2].

Every block in the blockchain includes a distinct cryptographic hash that connects it to the preceding block, forming an unchangeable account of all the transactions that have transpired on the blockchain. Because each of the blocks is linked to the preceding block, any attempt to alter or delete a transaction in one block would require altering all subsequent blocks in the chain, which is virtually impossible due to the computational power required to do so [3]. This makes blockchain a highly secure and transparent technology for record-keeping, as all transactions are stored in a tamper-proof and publicly accessible ledger. Additionally, because the ledger is decentralized, there is no need for a centralized authority to manage and validate transactions, which can reduce the potential for fraud or corruption [4]. Blockchain is a distributed ledger technology that provides a secure, transparent, and tamper-proof way to contain and manage transactions. It has the potential to transform many industries by improving transparency, reducing fraud, and increasing efficiency in record-keeping and other processes.

Genomics is a field that incorporates multiple disciplines and is focused on comprehensively researching the structure, function, and evolution of genomes. A *genome* constitutes an organism's complete genetic material, including its genes, non-coding deoxyribonucleic acid (DNA), and regulatory components [5]. The field of genomics encompasses a range of techniques, including DNA sequencing, bioinformatics, and functional genomics, which are employed to investigate and evaluate the extensive genomic data. DNA sequencing is the procedure in which the practitioner determines the precise order of nucleotides in a DNA molecule, which enables researchers to identify and study the genes and other functional elements in the genome. The development of high-throughput sequencing (HTS) technologies has made it possible to sequence entire genomes quickly and efficiently, which has led to a tremendous increase in the availability of genomic data [6,7].

Bioinformatics is a computational approach to analyze and interpret large amounts of data generated by DNA sequencing. It involves the use of algorithms and statistical models to identify patterns and relationships within the genomic data, as well as to predict the function of genes and other genomic elements. Functional genomics is another important area of genomics that involves studying the function of genes and other genomic elements in living organisms. This includes transcriptomics, which focuses on the study of gene expression, and proteomics, which focuses on the study of proteins [8]. In agriculture, genomics has been used to improve the quality and yield of crops and livestock. It has enabled the development of genetically modified organisms that are resistant to pests, diseases, and environmental stresses. In environmental science, genomics has been used to study the microbial communities in various ecosystems, which has provided insights into the roles of microorganisms in the environment [9]. Genomics is a rapidly evolving field that has the potential to revolutionize our understanding of the genome and its role in health, agriculture, and the environment. Its multidisciplinary nature and the vast amount of data it generates make it an exciting and challenging field for researchers [10].

14.2 Genomics

Genomics is the study of a human's entire genome, including how their genes interact with one another and their surroundings. A genome is an organism's entire collection of hereditary data, also referred to as DNA. Genomics also requires the chronology and examination of genomes by utilizing bioinformatics and high-throughput DNA sequencing. All the information required for an individual to develop and grow is contained in their genome. Understanding how genes interact with one another, the environment, and other illnesses like cancer, diabetes, and heart disease may be improved by studying the genome. The study of genomes has a lot of potential to improve healthcare. The field of precision medicine is being propelled forward by the genomic data obtained through advanced techniques such as HTS. This method enables the acquisition of distinct health-related data for everyone without the need for invasive procedures [11,12].

Genomic studies provide scientists with methods to rapidly analyze genes and their products en masse. Sequencing methods were the first high-throughput tools to be created. Thus, the genomes of numerous diverse species have been sequenced. Presently, genomics is primarily concerned with investigating the expression and functionality of genes. Over the past 5–10 years, the utilization of genomic, proteomic, and high-throughput microarray technologies has significantly enhanced our capacity to examine the molecular mechanisms of cells and tissues in various states of health and disease. This has resulted in a comprehensive and novel outlook on the subject matter. For instance, analysis of diagnostic possibilities for tumor classification and prognostication has emerged in cancer research. Metabolomics and lab-on-a-chip methodologies for metabolic research are recent and exciting development. However, significant computational development is needed in order to interpret the vast quantity of data [1,13].

The whole collection of genetic instructions for an organism is contained in its genome. Each genome is equipped with all the data necessary to create the specific organism, support its development, and enable growth. Every cell in the body contains a full copy of the roughly 3 billion DNA base pairs or letters that comprise the human genome. The term *genomic information* pertains to the genome and DNA information of an organism. *Bioinformatics* is the field that encompasses the gathering, storage, and analysis of genomes of living organisms. Typically, the processing of genomic data requires the use of specialized software and significant storage and analysis capacity. Big data processing and analysis techniques mainly use genomic data. A bioinformatics system or program for processing genomic data collects such data [9,11]. Genomic data is typically processed using a variety of data analytical and management techniques to discover and analyze genome parameters like genome structures and various others. Genomic data are frequently subjected to processes like variation analysis and data sequencing analysis methods. The purpose of genetic data analysis is to ascertain the roles played by particular genes [3].

14.2.1 Challenges in Genomics

- Genetic data collection has increased, which has led to some problems with data access, security, and privacy. Sometimes, other research companies purchase the individual's genetic data.
- To broaden the participation of racially and ethnically diverse groups in human genomics studies.
- Haplotype phasing and methods that produce long sequencing reads are used to create more diverse reference genomes in order to take into consideration the substantial structural variation that is probably present both within and between populations.
- The instruction of a more diverse group of scientists conducting a genomic study.
- The creation of improved techniques for correctly predicting phenotypes and genetic risk across racial and ethnically diverse groups, as well as for separating the effects of genes.
- Without people's genetic data consent, businesses are making enormous profits by selling this genetic material.
- It is more difficult to identify, monitor, and treat diseases when genomics data is incorrectly combined with other types of available data.
- The extension of human genome sequencing is significantly hampered by the ability to keep genomic data securely and with high integrity.

14.2.2 Applications of Genomics

- *Predicting disease risk at the individual level.* Individual-level genome analysis is utilized for the purpose of screening asymptomatic individuals for potential disease susceptibility. Despite the increasing accessibility of genetic sequencing and the growing reliability of analytical tools, unresolved ethical issues persist with regard to population-level genomic analysis. The genomic data was scrutinized by the researchers through the utilization of databases and various methodologies that have been previously established by other scholars. Despite the increasing accessibility of genetic sequencing and the growing reliability of analytical tools, unresolved ethical issues remain regarding population-level genomic analysis [14].

- *Pharmacogenomics and toxicogenomics.* Pharmacogenomics, alternatively referred to as toxicogenomics, involves the evaluation of the effectiveness and potential adverse effects of pharmaceuticals through the analysis of an individual's genetic information. Prior to commencing research involving human subjects, it is common practice to investigate the genomic reactions to pharmaceuticals in laboratory settings or through experimentation on animal models, such as rodents. This approach has been documented in literature. The investigation of alterations in gene expression can yield insights into the transcription profile in the presence of a drug, which may serve as an early indicator of the likelihood of toxicological consequences [15].

- *Microbial genomics.* The conventional approach to teaching microbiology emphasizes on the use of pure culture conditions, where a single type of cells is isolated and grown in the laboratory, as the most effective way to study microorganisms. On the other hand, the examination of the combined genomes of multiple organisms that coexist and interact within a specific environmental setting is referred to as metagenomics. Metagenomics can aid in analyzing the influence of contaminants on the environment and in expediting the discovery of new species [10,16].

- *Genomics in agriculture.* Genomics has the potential to mitigate the experimentation and errors that are inherent in scientific research, thereby augmenting the caliber and quantity of agricultural crop production. Genomic data is utilized by scientists to identify favorable characteristics and subsequently transfer them to an alternate organism. Scholars are currently investigating the potential of genomics to enhance the quantity and quality of agricultural yield. As an illustration, researchers may employ advantageous characteristics to enhance an extant commodity or create a novel one, such as enhancing the drought resistance of a crop that is vulnerable to aridity [17].

- *Mitochondrial genomics.* Since mitochondrial DNA mutates quickly, it is frequently used to investigate evolutionary connections. Because of this, lineage research frequently makes use of mitochondrial genomics. Forensic examination has utilized genetic markers, and evidence and indications obtained from DNA samples found at crime locations have been admitted as evidence in legal proceedings. Genomic analysis has also been advantageous in this field, as seen in the case of anthrax sent through the US Mail Service. Microbial genomics analysis was able to identify that the same strain of anthrax was used in all the shipments [17].

14.3 Blockchain

A blockchain is a decentralized database that maintains an ever-growing collection of sequenced records, known as blocks, that are interconnected through cryptographic techniques. Every individual block comprises of transaction details, a specific date, and a cryptographic hash value of the preceding block. The blockchain is a digital ledger that is decentralized, distributed, and open. It is utilized for recording activities across multiple computers in a manner that precludes retroactive alteration of the record without modifying all subsequent blocks and achieving network consensus. Blockchains can be categorized into four distinct classifications based on the network's operational mechanisms and the methods by which users can participate in the network, as shown in Figure 14.1.

1. *Public blockchain*. A public database is accessible to everyone. There is no requirement for trust among network participants, and any anonymous node may participate. All the nodes receive a public broadcast of the events. The consensus methods used to validate the blocks can be utilized by any node in the network. The Bitcoin blockchain is an illustration of this kind of network. It is public and permissionless [18].

2. *Private blockchain*. Nodes are pre-selected and screened before joining the network, and once they do, they are trusted. Blockchain transaction information is more privately protected by the access control mechanism. Additionally, this kind of blockchain offers improved block confirmation speed. MultiChain is an illustration of this kind of network. It is private and permissioned [19].

3. *Consortium blockchain*. A hybrid of the first two that offers a balance between effectiveness and confidence. The ledger that a set of nodes has been chosen to handle.

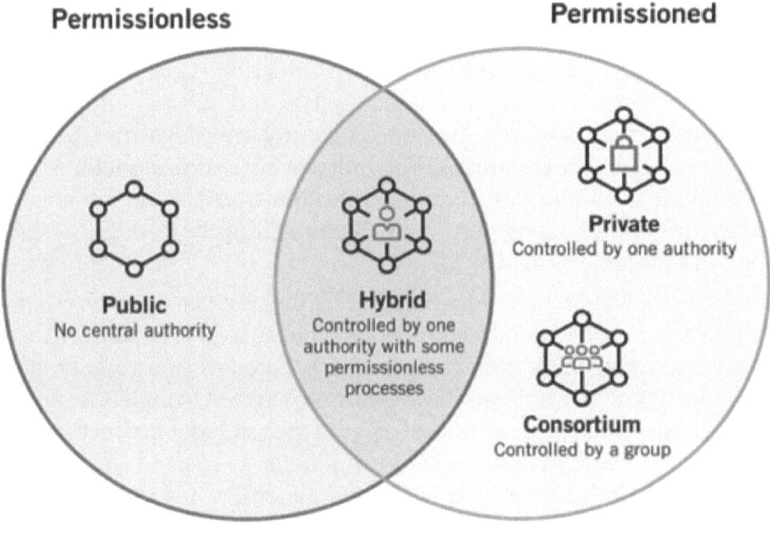

FIGURE 14.1
Different categories of blockchains.

Nodes need to be authorized to join the network, just like on private blockchains. Blocks and transactions are validated once a predetermined number of peers agree. The consensus mechanism's predetermined rules determine the exact procedure. Hyperledger is an illustration of this kind of application. It is public and permissioned [9].

4. *Hybrid blockchain.* Hybrid blockchains are a type of blockchain technology combining the greatest characteristics of public and private blockchains. They provide a more adaptable approach to blockchain implementation, enabling enterprises to adjust their blockchain solutions to their particular requirements [20].

The four foundational ideas of blockchain:

- *Shared ledger.* A shared ledger refers to a decentralized system of records that is distributed across a company's network and operates on a "append-only" basis. The utilization of a shared ledger ensures that transactions are recorded singularly, thereby eliminating the redundant efforts that are commonly associated with traditional business networks [21].
- *Permissions.* Permissions ensure that actions are safeguarded, validated, and authorized. By imposing restrictions on network participation, entities can effectively comply with data security regulations, such as the European General Data Protection Regulation (EU GDPR) and the Health Insurance Portability and Accountability Act [22].
- *Smart contracts.* Smart contracts refer to a predetermined agreement or a set of regulations that oversee a commercial transaction. These contracts are stored on the blockchain and are executed automatically as an integral part of a transaction [8].
- *Consensus.* The network-verified transaction is universally accepted by all participants through a process of consensus. Various consensus methods are employed by blockchains, such as multi-signature, practical Byzantine fault tolerance, and proof-of-stake [23].

14.4 Blockchain in Genomics

Bitcoin technology holds great promise for creating the systems of the future and reshaping the medical industry. The goal of a blockchain is to store all the data on its network in a digital, decentralized public database. Blockchain is widely used in many industries, including banking, education, healthcare, and others. Despite being relatively new, blockchain technology is already having a significant impact on healthcare, particularly in genetic medicine [4]. Scientists will be able to comprehend disease mechanisms better as the technology is applied more frequently in genomics and can treat patients and treat diseases while maintaining privacy and security with the aid of this knowledge [3]. Blockchain realizes the psychological empowerment of users within the platform and provides new ways to address data ownership, data sharing, and data security problems in genomic big data platforms [17].

Blockchain technology has been observed to play a crucial role in the field of bioinformatics and health applications due to its ability to reduce the cost of analysis. Data transactions made using blockchain systems are quicker and more effective than those made using conventional methods. The greatest benefit of the blockchain is that unlike data stored in the central system, which can be altered, the data stored in the blockchain cannot be modified. Every data exchange with the blockchain is more transparent and traceable because it is a distributed system. Compared to other systems, blockchain is superior at preventing fraud and unauthorized activity. Genomics can potentially benefit from blockchain technology in various ways, such as secure storage and sharing of genomic data, monitoring and administration of laboratory procedures and samples, and motivating people to participate in research studies [3].

Shivom is a blockchain-based platform for the secure storage and sharing of genomic data. Users can select whether to share their genomic data with researchers, pharmaceutical companies, and other interested parties after uploading it to the portal. The platform makes use of smart contracts to guarantee data confidentiality and privacy [24]. Zenome is a decentralized platform that allows users to store, share, and monetize their genomic data. By engaging in clinical trials or providing their genomic data to research projects, users can earn tokens. The platform also includes tools for genetic analysis and personalized medicine [25]. EncrypGen is a blockchain-based platform that allows users to securely store and sell their genomic data. Users of the platform have complete control over their data and may decide with whom to share it, thanks to the usage of smart contracts. Researchers and pharmaceutical companies can purchase data directly from users on the platform [22].

Nebula Genomics is a blockchain-based platform that allows users to securely store and share their genomic data. By taking part in studies and providing their data to researchers, users can earn tokens. Tools for genetic analysis and tailored therapy are also included in it. Users can gather and exchange their health data, including genomic data, via the blockchain-based platform Seqster. Users of the platform have complete control over their data and may decide with whom to share it, thanks to the usage of smart contracts [22]. Seqster also has resources for clinical trial matching and tailored medicine [26]. Based on the Ethereum network, Genecoin, also known as the GEN token, is a bioeconomy currency that enables the secure sharing of genomic data. The system will provide rewards, up to 1,000 Genecoin, without charge, to a user who successfully brings another user into the Genecoin network. DNA from a person is sampled, and it is stored on the blockchain network [1]. Some blockchain-based firms, such as EncrypGen [27], Nebula Genomics, and Shivom aspire to develop a safe and decentralized platform for individuals to store, control, and share their genomic data. With blockchain technology, these platforms ensure that data is secure, anonymous, and tamper-proof. People retain sovereignty over their genomic data while having the option to share it with researchers, healthcare providers, or other parties on a case-by-case basis.

Numerous blockchain-based platforms, like Luna DNA, Genomes.io, and Genomic Data Commons, aim to offer a secure and decentralized platform for researchers and institutions to share genetic data. These systems employ blockchain technology to assure the security, transparency, and traceability of data [13]. Researchers can access and use the data on the platform for research purposes, but people retain ownership of their data and control who gets access. Consent management is a crucial part of genomics research since it guarantees that individuals are aware of how their data will be used and can provide informed consent for its application. Genomes.io and MyBitBlock are blockchain-based platforms that attempt to build a safe and decentralized platform for managing consent in genomics research. These platforms use smart contracts to ensure that individuals are aware of how their data will be used and can consent to its use [28].

The storage and management of massive volumes of genetic data represent a substantial problem for genomics research. Blockchain-based technologies, such as Shivom and

Genomes.io, seek to develop a decentralized and secure platform for storing and managing genomic data. With blockchain technology, these platforms ensure that data is secure, tamper-proof, and transparent [29]. In addition, these systems can also provide a uniform format for genetic data, allowing for interoperability between various data sources. Blockchain-based platforms, such as Zenome, aim to establish a decentralized and secure platform for handling intellectual property and royalties in genomics research. These platforms leverage smart contracts to recompense individuals and organizations for their contributions to research. Overall, blockchain-based methods and approaches in genomics are still in their infancy, but they have the potential to offer substantial advantages in terms of secure and efficient data sharing, consent management, data storage and management, intellectual property and royalty management, and patient empowerment. As blockchain technology continues to evolve and improve, creative blockchain-based solutions in the field of genomics are likely to increase [25][21].

14.5 The Genesy Model for a Blockchain-Based Fair Ecosystem of Genomic Data

The Genesy model presents a blockchain-oriented approach toward establishing an ecosystem that is impartial and just for genomic data. The objective of the model is to tackle the obstacles pertaining to data privacy, data ownership, and data sharing that are encountered in the domain of genomics research. The model has been constructed utilizing blockchain technology, thereby guaranteeing the integrity and immutability of the data that is shared. The implementation of security measures serves to mitigate the risk of unauthorized alterations to the data, thereby safeguarding its integrity and confidentiality. Genesy aims to promote collaboration among users and external entities to facilitate the development of a sophisticated genomics ecosystem, which can efficiently gather and handle the vast quantities of data produced by sequencing endeavors [30].

The Genesy architecture, in its present state of development, comprises a private blockchain consisting of peer nodes that are exclusively owned and operated by Genesy Project SRL. This blockchain is responsible for storing user personal information, user phenotype data, and biometric information [14]. The Genesy model is depicted in Figure 14.2. The system works by allowing individuals to upload their genomic data to the blockchain, where it is encrypted and stored securely. Participants can choose to share their data with researchers, pharmaceutical companies, or other interested parties and set the terms and conditions of data use through smart contracts. The Genesy model is designed to promote fairness and openness in the sharing of genomic data. It provides a secure and transparent platform for sharing genomic data, which can help advance research in the field. By facilitating the sharing of data, the Genesy model can help accelerate the development of new treatments and cures for diseases [16,31].

14.5.1 Features, Benefits, and Potential Impact of the Genesy Model

The Genesy model is built on blockchain technology, which ensures the integrity and immutability of the shared data. This helps prevent any unauthorized changes to the data and ensures that it remains secure. The model is designed to promote fairness and openness in the sharing of genomic data, with an emphasis on ensuring that all

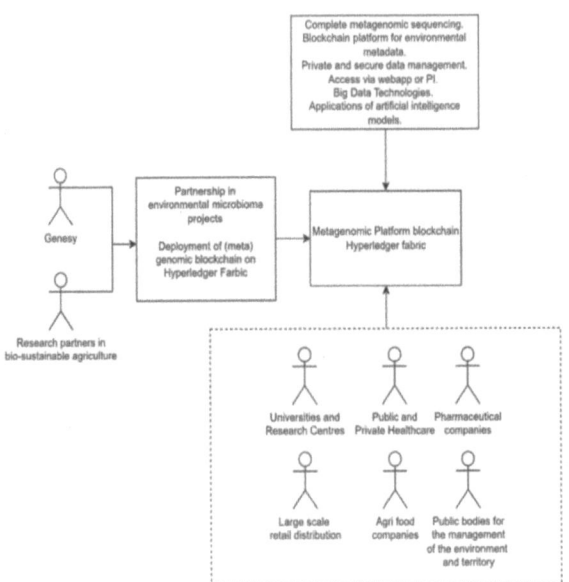

FIGURE 14.2
Genesy model.

participants in the ecosystem are treated fairly and that the benefits of sharing genomic data are distributed equitably. This is achieved through the use of smart contracts, which can automatically enforce the terms of the sharing agreement and ensure that all parties receive the appropriate compensation. The Genesy model offers several benefits over traditional models of sharing genomic data. Firstly, it provides a secure and transparent platform for sharing genomic data, which can help advance research in the field. By facilitating the sharing of data, the Genesy model can help accelerate the development of new treatments and cures for diseases. Secondly, the Genesy model ensures that participants are treated fairly and that the benefits of sharing genomic data are distributed equitably. This can help address some of the existing inequities in the field of medical research and ensure that all participants are able to benefit from the sharing of data [14].

The Genesy model has the potential to significantly impact medical research and treatment. By providing a more secure and equitable way of sharing genomic data, the model can help accelerate the development of new treatments and cures for diseases. This can lead to improved health outcomes for patients and a reduction in healthcare costs. Additionally, the Genesy model can help address some of the existing inequities in the field of medical research, ensuring that all participants are able to benefit from the sharing of data. This can help promote greater collaboration and innovation in the field, leading to further breakthroughs in medical research and treatment. The model represents a promising new approach to sharing genomic data. By leveraging the power of blockchain technology, the model can help create a more secure and equitable system for sharing data, which can ultimately lead to new breakthroughs in medical research and treatment. The Genesy model has the potential to significantly impact the field of medical research and treatment, and it is an exciting development that warrants further exploration and discussion [14].

14.6 Blockchain in Genomics Applications

Customers have become more numerous in recent years as direct-to-consumer businesses have begun to commercialize DNA sequencing. This is because technological developments have made genome sequencing considerably more accessible and quicker. Concerns about this model's fairness arise when considering the financial benefit of purchasing this genomic data. Some contend that the public should receive the benefit, rather than the middlemen. As a result, a new breed of businesses has emerged that employ blockchain to enable an open market for the exchange of genetic data [12].

14.6.1 Commercial Genomics Marketplace

Genomic markets built on blockchain technology are designed to eliminate the need for middlemen and offer users access to their data. Several kinds of rewards are given to those who rent or sell their genetic data. In these markets, Bitcoin is the most typical incentive. A summary of the utilized incentives as well as the blockchain platform that is being used and the services that platform offers are explored in this chapter. Genecoin represented the first attempt to use blockchain in genomics. The corporation uses outside labs to deliver its sequencing services. The resulting DNA sequence is subsequently encrypted and kept on the Bitcoin blockchain. The emergence of numerous markets has facilitated the exchange of genomic data for cryptocurrencies (tokens), which can subsequently be traded on cryptocurrency exchanges, thereby enabling genomic data owners to participate in this novel economic activity [27].

The Genecoin model has been widely adopted by most marketplaces, with the aim of endowing patients with agency over their data and expediting genomic research by increasing the accessibility of data. Shivom and Zenome are two distinct marketplaces that differentiate themselves by providing supplementary services, such as pipelines and computational resources, for the examination of genomic data that is transacted on their respective platforms. Researchers have the option to utilize provided pipelines for their research by remitting fees in the form of cryptocurrencies or tokens. The significance of traceability and data integrity is underscored as pivotal services provided by numerous genomic marketplaces. Genomes provide a secure means for customers to store and manage their DNA data from the point of sequencing until its deposition on the blockchain. Users are provided with a confidential access key that is utilized to limit data access and is exclusively stored on their mobile devices. The investigation of non-fungible tokens (NFT) for data tracing and mobility is exemplified by Genobank. The proposed methodology involves assigning a unique NFT to every individual sample of human bodily fluid, such as saliva, and subsequently disseminating it on a publicly accessible blockchain. The NFT serves various functions, such as determining the laboratory authorized to sequence the genome and monitoring the utilization of the resultant data [27].

14.6.2 Non-Commercial Applications

Several studies investigated the work of blockchain to speed up processing or analysis of genetic data. A novel approach for conducting genome-wide association studies (GWAS) with a pivot on privacy was presented. GWAS is carried out utilizing a sharing protocol that protects anonymity and has a gene fragmentation framework at its core. Large genomic files are divided up into smaller pieces in this architecture, which are then given to various service providers to build a decentralized blockchain network for storage, sharing, and analysis [32]. This resolves the centralization and privacy issues by removing the prospect of one source possessing all the data. Some studies suggested merging blockchain technology with machine learning to accomplish decentralized machine learning. Predictive models were trained across various businesses, with blockchain facilitating the process in a safe, open, and decentralized manner. Swarm learning (SL), a blockchain approach for federated learning, was also suggested. By first securely enrolling users without the need for a central coordinator, SL accomplishes decentralized machine learning. The huge amount of medical and genetic data is then kept in the possession and control of the data owner once the data are trained locally and the model parameters are combined [3][23].

Secure storage. Blockchain was used to reserve and search pharmacogenetics data. Each piece of data is added to the smart contract and given a special ID that serves as a mapping key. It is a good idea to have a backup plan in case something goes wrong. Comparing the magnitude of the pharmacogenomics data used in this work to other popular genomic data formats, it is fairly tiny. Sequence alignment map files, which can be in the range of 10s of gigabytes in size, were the focus of the investigation into alternatives for storing larger data files. This was accomplished using a brand-new data format that was created by fusing data compression methods with a private blockchain network [12].

Data management and access control. Many studies focused on the application of blockchain for managing permission to grant and deny access to genomic data that may be stored elsewhere. A website called Dwarna uses blockchain to enable dynamic consent. Participants and researchers in a research partnership are connected by the portal. The initiative complies with GDPR and seeks to guarantee that participants retain control of the data. The suggested architecture records participant permission on a blockchain. By storing consent in a blockchain, participants can take ownership of the data; as a result, third parties can only access the data with the owner's permission in the multi-stakeholder consent management dilemma as it relates to an agreement for the data-sharing. This is because each genome has the potential to provide details about the owner as well as relatives of the owner of the genomic data. Hence, obtaining their permission is necessary to protect the relatives of a person's privacy, using blockchain to address this consensus issue and win the approval of various parties. The application of blockchain as a universal logging system was examined in task 1 of the 2018 IDASH competition; such a system can deliver an access log that records individual access to all data in all the genomic data repositories of the system [33].

A decentralized cross-site logging system has many benefits over the traditional, centralized internal logs that are presently used in practice. Most importantly, the problem of one specific point of failure and malicious changes to the logs has been solved. There were multiple competitors, and the submissions were judged according to predetermined standards, including accuracy and speed. This is so that the competition may assess the effectiveness and performance of blockchain as a cross-site logging system in addition to its viability as such. The competition demonstrated that using blockchain to create a cross-site genomic data access record is, in fact, practical. Given the solution's promising performance, it is fair to assume that with additional improvements, a system of this caliber can be configured for use in practical applications [13][2].

14.7 Motives for Blockchain Application in Genomics

The blockchain technology is a decentralized and transparent digital ledger that has attracted considerable interest in recent years because of its promise to provide a safe and tamper-resistant mechanism for recording and distributing data. The discipline of genomics, which is concerned with the study of genetic information, is one that could profit from how blockchain technology is used. The rationale will be discussed for implementing blockchain technology in genomics.

Safe and confidential data sharing. Genomics data contain sensitive information that should be protected from unauthorized access, given the potential for discriminatory exploitation of this data. Blockchain technology can provide a decentralized and secure platform for exchanging genetic data while ensuring that only authorized parties have access to the data. Because blockchain employs cryptographic techniques to establish a safe and transparent network, this is the case. A hash can be found in each block of the chain; it serves as a distinct digital fingerprint of the data in the block's contents. It is a tamper-proof system because once a block is put to the chain, it cannot be changed or removed without the consent of all other nodes on the network. Individuals are able to exchange their data without revealing their identity; hence, blockchain can also guarantee anonymity for data sharing [3].

Interoperability. Data from different sources, including hospitals, research institutes, and genomic testing corporations, are utilized in genomics research. Nevertheless, these data sources frequently employ disparate formats and standards, making it challenging to combine and evaluate data from several sources. Blockchain technology can provide a common format for genetic data, allowing for the interoperability of disparate data sources. This can assist in streamlining the research process and facilitating collaboration between institutions [16].

Traceability of data. In genomics research, it is essential to assure data integrity and prevent data manipulation. This includes the creation, sharing, and analysis of genetic data. Each transaction is recorded on the blockchain with a time stamp and a hash of the transaction data, which prevents the data from being altered or erased. In addition, blockchain can assist researchers in tracing the provenance of genomic data, which is crucial for quality control and the reproducibility of research [17].

Incentivizing data sharing. Sharing genetic data might be difficult due to privacy and ownership considerations. Individuals can keep ownership of their genomic data while still being able to securely and anonymously share it with researchers via blockchain technology, thereby incentivizing data sharing. With smart contracts, it is possible to construct a system that rewards individuals for sharing their genomic data. For instance, researchers could give Bitcoin compensation to individuals who contribute genetic data to a research project. Smart contracts can be created to guarantee that individuals retain ownership of their data and are compensated for its use [21].

Patient empowering. Patients can have greater control over their genomic data through the use of blockchain technology. Patients can opt to share their data with healthcare professionals, researchers, and other organizations on an individual basis. This can inspire more individuals to participate in genetic research by fostering trust between patients and scientists. The usage of a patient's data can be made more transparent and accountable thanks to blockchain technology. Patients may monitor the transactions on the blockchain and understand how their data is being utilized, which can assist in guaranteeing that it is being used ethically and for the intended purpose. The application of blockchain technology to genomics has the potential to yield many advantages, including safe and private data sharing, interoperability, data traceability, data sharing incentives, and patient empowerment. These advantages can promote the secure and effective sharing of genomic data, which is crucial for advancing genomics research and enhancing patient outcomes [23][17].

14.8 Current Problems, Difficulties, and Future Scope

The list of current issues and restrictions with blockchain and genomics is provided here.

Standardization. Lack of standardization in the display of genomic data on the blockchain is a significant barrier to the application of blockchain technology in genomics. Without a generally established standard, it can be challenging to assure the integrity and quality of data across many platforms and applications. This lack of standards can also impede interoperability between blockchain-based platforms and conventional databases [7].

Scalability. The amount of genetic data collected is growing at a rapid rate, and typical blockchain systems may not be able to accommodate the vast volume of data. This may result in sluggish transaction speeds and hefty transaction costs, which may hinder the adoption of blockchain-based solutions in genomics. To overcome this issue, sharding, off-chain storage, and side chains are being considered as potential solutions [34].

Privacy. Despite the fact that blockchain technology can enable safe and tamper-proof storage for genomic data, privacy concerns remain. Since the blockchain is decentralized, anyone can access its data, which could result in the accidental revelation of sensitive information. Therefore, it may be able to identify individuals based on their genomic data even if the data on the blockchain is encrypted. To deal with this issue, methods including differential privacy, homomorphic encryption, and zero-knowledge proofs are being researched [3].

Regulation. Another barrier to the blockchain technology's use in genomics is the lack of clear standards. Despite the fact that the technology is still in its early stages, there are no set guidelines for its application in genomics research. Confusion and regulatory challenges may come from this, making it more difficult for the genomics industry to use blockchain-based solutions. To solve this issue, clear rules and regulations controlling the application of blockchain technology in genomics are needed [35].

Interoperability. Due to differences in data formats and architectures, achieving interoperability between multiple blockchain-based platforms and traditional databases can be challenging. Without interoperability, it might be difficult for multiple platforms and applications to communicate data, which can reduce the utility of blockchain-based solutions in genomics. To address this issue, standards such as the genomic data commons and the global alliance for genomics and health are being established [17].

Technical complexity. The technical intricacy of blockchain technology can be a problem for uninitiated researchers and healthcare practitioners. This can impede the adoption and deployment of blockchain-based solutions in genomics. User-friendly interfaces and educational resources are required to address this difficulty. Despite the fact that blockchain technology has the potential to deliver considerable benefits to genomics research, there are still a number of unanswered questions and obstacles to be resolved. Standardization, scalability, privacy, regulation, interoperability, and technological complexity are just some of the obstacles that must be solved before blockchain-based solutions in genomics may be extensively implemented [21][3].

Blockchain technology might transform the genomics business by providing a safe and efficient way to organize and exchange genetic data. The biggest challenge in the genomics industry is data privacy and security. Blockchain offers a solution to this problem by providing a decentralized and tamper-proof system for storing and sharing data. This implies that data of each patient can be encrypted and stored safely, and only individuals with authorization can access it. The benefits of blockchain in genomics are significant and cannot be ignored. Researchers can securely access and analyze data from multiple sources without the need for intermediaries or complex data-sharing agreements. This can lead to faster and more accurate results, ultimately improving patient outcomes. Additionally, blockchain can facilitate the development of personalized medicine by providing a secure and efficient way to store and share genetic information [3][4].

One potential application of blockchain in genomics is in the sharing of genomic data for research purposes. Currently, there are many challenges with sharing genomic data, including concerns around data privacy and ownership. However, by using blockchain technology, individuals can control who can access their data and under what conditions, while also being incentivized to share their data through token-based reward systems. This can encourage greater collaboration and data sharing in genomics research, leading to more significant breakthroughs in disease diagnosis, treatment, and prevention. Another potential application of blockchain in genomics is in the management of clinical trials. Blockchain technology can make certain the integrity of trial data, from the collection of patient data to the analysis of results. By using smart contracts to automate the management of clinical trial data, blockchain can reduce the risk of errors, fraud, and data tampering. In addition to these applications, blockchain technology can also provide new opportunities for personalized medicine [8].

The utilization of blockchain technology can facilitate the creation of tailored treatment strategies that are based on an individual's genomic data, through secure storage and sharing of data. This can lead to more precise and effective treatment options for a range of diseases. However, there are still some challenges that need to be addressed before blockchain technology can be widely adopted in genomics. One of the biggest challenges is the lack of standardization in the industry. There is a need for clear guidelines and regulations to ensure that data is being collected, stored, and shared in a consistent and secure manner. Other challenges include technical issues, such as scalability and interoperability, as well as regulatory and ethical concerns around data privacy and ownership [7].

14.9 Conclusion

The number of case studies offering blockchain-based solutions for storing, sharing, and analyzing genomic data, as well as the number of commercial and non-commercial blockchain apps aiming to facilitate exchange of genomic data, is increasing. Using a taxonomy that organizes genomic blockchain applications into commercial and non-commercial groups, with further subcategories depending on specific aims, such as data exchange, analysis, safe storage, and access control. The benefits and drawbacks of each application include comparing proposals regarding blockchain platform selection and data storage, sharing, and protection methods and identifying obstacles, including software instability, interoperability, security risks, and the protection of data privacy and owner identities. The key drivers for blockchain in genomics are immutability (or consistency) and decentralization. There is always a need for data owners to have control over their data. Compared to financial applications, genomics blockchain applications are now restricted, but there is room for expansion. Future research areas include exploring blockchain-driven distributed analytics and assessing the effectiveness of techniques that boost privacy, such as homomorphic encryption, multi-party computation, zero-knowledge proofs, and off-chain computation. Furthermore, investigating trustworthy and verifiable access to genetic data using blockchain and adopting trust-over-IP principles to sustain decentralized identities for researchers are captivating avenues for future research. Genomic blockchain applications are currently in the initial stages of research and are still being developed, and additional societal and technological revolution is required for widespread use, which suggests that efforts be made to promote the usage of blockchain in genomics in order to demonstrate its ability and viability for many genomic applications.

References

1. Adanur Dedeturk B, Soran A, Bakir-Gungor B. Blockchain for genomics and healthcare: a literature review, current status, classification and open issues. *PeerJ*. 2021;9:e12130.
2. Dagher GG, Mohler J, Milojkovic M, Marella PB. Ancile: privacy-preserving framework for access control and interoperability of electronic health records using blockchain technology. *Sustain Cities Soc*. 2018;39:283–97.
3. Ozercan HI, Mollah MNH, Ozdogan M, Kantarcioglu M, Malin B. Realizing the potential of blockchain technologies in genomics. *Genome Res*. 2018;28(9):1255–63.
4. Malin B, Benitez K. Standardizing data sharing consent for genomics research. *Genet Med*. 2018;20(8):730–2.
5. Hang L, Chen C, Zhang L, Yang J. Blockchain for applications of clinical trials: taxonomy, challenges, and future directions. *IET Commun*. 2022;16(20):2371–93.
6. Shabani M. Blockchain-based platforms for genomic data sharing: a de-centralized approach in response to the governance problems? *J Am Med Informatics Assoc*. 2019;26(1):76–80.
7. Botta A, De Donno M, Persico V, Pescapé A. Integration of blockchain and IPFS for secure and privacy-preserving sharing of genomic data. *Futur Gener Comput Syst*. 2019;97:583–96.
8. Zhang P, White J, Schmidt DC, Lenz G, Rosenbloom ST. FHIRChain: applying blockchain to securely and scalably share clinical data. *Comput Struct Biotechnol J*. 2018;16:267–78.
9. Institute NHGR. *A Brief Guide to Genomics* [Internet]. 2021. Available from: www.genome.gov/about-genomics/fact-sheets/a-brief-guide-to-genomics
10. Crouch J, Turnbull A. The legal implications of blockchain in healthcare and life sciences. *Blockchain Healthc Today*. 2018;1:1–7.
11. GeeksforGeeks. *Blockchain in genomics* [Internet]. 2022. Available from: www.geeksforgeeks.org/blockchain-in-genomics/
12. Shendure J, Balasubramanian S, Church GM, Gilbert W, Rogers J, Schloss JA, et al. DNA sequencing at 40: past, present and future. *Nature*. 2017;550(7676):345–53.
13. Shabani M. Blockchain-based platforms for genomic data sharing: a de-centralized approach in response to the governance problems? *J Am Med Informatics Assoc*. 2018;26(1):76–80.
14. Carlini F, Carlini R, Dalla Palma S, Pareschi R, Zappone F. The genesy model for a blockchain-based fair ecosystem of genomic data. *Front Blockchain*. 2020;3:483227.
15. Sultan K, Ruhi U, Lakhani R. Conceptualizing blockchains: Characteristics and applications. *arXiv*. 2018.

16. Das M, Patel A, Pandya A. Genomics in the era of blockchain and distributed ledger technologies. In: *Advances in Computers*. Elsevier. 2019, pp. 75–91.
17. Iyer V, Vyshnavi AMH, Iyer S, Namboori PKK. An AI driven genomic profiling system and secure data sharing using DLT for cancer patients. In: *2019 IEEE Bombay Section Signature Conference (IBSSC)*. 2019, pp. 1–5. https://doi.org/10.1109/IBSSC47189.2019.8973020
18. Nakamoto S. Bitcoin: *A Peer-to-Peer Electronic Cash System*. 2008. Available from: https://www.ussc.gov/sites/default/files/pdf/training/annual-national-training-seminar/2018/Emerging_Tech_Bitcoin_Crypto.pdf
19. Greenspan G. *Multichain Private Blockchain-White Paper*. 2015, p. 85. Available from: www.multichain.com
20. Cachin C, others. Architecture of the hyperledger blockchain fabric. In: *Workshop on Distributed Cryptocurrencies and Consensus Ledgers*. 2016, pp. 1–4. https://efaidnbmnnnibpcajpcglclefindmkaj/https://www.zurich.ibm.com/dccl/papers/cachin_dccl.pdf
21. Lee JH, Choi JY, Lee JE, Kim JH. A blockchain-based platform for trustworthy data sharing and storage in the genomic domain. *J Biomed Inform*. 2018;88:67–73.
22. Grishin D, Obbad K, Estep P, Cifric M, Zhao Y, Church G. *Nebula Genomics: Blockchain-Enabled Genomic Data Sharing and Analysis Platform*. 2022. Available from: https://nebula.org/whole-genome-sequencing-dna-test/
23. Bernasconi M, Stranieri A, Spagnuolo C. Towards blockchain interoperability: reference architecture and use cases. *IEEE Access*. 2019;7:63911–28.
24. Healtheuropa. *Shivom: A Precision Medicine Data Secure-Sharing and Analysis Ecosystem* [Internet]. 2021. Available from: www.healtheuropa.com/shivom-precision-medicine/90476/
25. Kulemin N, Popov S, Gorbachev A. *The Zenome Project: Whitepaper Blockchain-Based Genomic Ecosystem*. 2017. Available from: https://zenome.io/
26. Philippidis A. *Seqster Platform to Integrate Genomic, EHR, and Wearable Health Data* [Internet]. 2018. Available from: www.seqster.com/seqster-platform-to-integrate-genomic-ehr-and-wearable-health-data/
27. EncrypGen. *Gene-Chain: A Blockchain-Based Genomic Data Platform* [Internet]. 2022. Available from: https://encrypgen.com
28. Albalwy F, Brass A, Davies A, others. A blockchain-based dynamic consent architecture to support clinical genomic data sharing (ConsentChain): proof-of-concept study. *JMIR Med Inform*. 2021;9(11):e27816.
29. Kim Y, Park Y-H. Blockchain-based model for gene data management using de-identifying scheme. In: *2021 IEEE International Conference on Consumer Electronics-Asia (ICCE-Asia)*. 2021, pp. 1–4. https://doi.org/10.1109/ICCE-Asia53811.2021.9641994
30. Yuan X, Tong J. Blockchain for genomics: opportunities and challenges. *Theor Biol Med Model*. 2020;17(1):4.
31. Zheng Z, Xie S, Dai H, Chen X, Wang H. An overview of blockchain technology: architecture, consensus, and future trends. In: *2017 IEEE International Congress on Big Data (BigData Congress)*. 2017, pp. 557–64. https://doi.org/10.1109/BigDataCongress.2017.85
32. Zhang Y, Zhao X, Li X, Zhong M, Curtis C, Chen C. Enabling privacy-preserving sharing of genomic data for GWASs in decentralized networks. In: *Proceedings of the Twelfth ACM International Conference on Web Search and Data Mining*. 2019, pp. 204–12. https://doi.org/10.1145/3289600.3290983
33. Beyene M, Thiebes S, Sunyaev A. Multi-stakeholder consent management in genetic testing: a blockchain-based approach. In: *Pre-ICIS SIGBPS 2019 Workshop on Blockchain and Smart Contracts Munich*. 2019. https://publikationen.bibliothek.kit.edu/1000125483
34. Alghazwi M, Turkmen F, van der Velde J, Karastoyanova D. Blockchain for genomics: A systematic literature review. *arxiv* [Internet]. 2021; abs/2111.10153. Available from: https://arxiv.org/abs/2111.10153
35. Samani F, Pahl C. Blockchain for secure and efficient sharing of medical data: a systematic review. *Electron Mark*. 2018;28(2):161–84.

15

Improved Data Transmission Technique for Healthcare Emergency Vehicle Using Blockchain in VANET

R. M. Rajeshwari and S. Rajesh

15.1 Introduction

Vehicular ad hoc network (VANET) facilitates an intelligent transport system (ITS) that enhances improved and safe driving experience. It provides a harmless and effective traffic management system. The life support emergency vehicles that travel on the road act as mobile nodes, and they communicate with each other. The messages exchanged among the nodes intimate the drivers to take the necessary action in case of any emergency, thereby preventing unnecessary deaths [1]. VANETs facilitates in optimizing the traffic, generating warning message for collisions and tracking location services [2]. VANET supports three types of communication, including vehicle-to-vehicle communication, vehicle-to-infrastructure communication, and infrastructure-to-infrastructure communication. The VANET architecture has three important entities, namely, trusted authority (TA), on-board units (OBU), and roadside units (RSU), for real-time traffic management [3]. The TA maintains the real identity of OBU of each life support emergency vehicle and RSU on the road of each zone. The RSU tracks the attacker vehicles and facilitates information sharing between the TA and OBUs. OBUs are responsible for getting registered with the RSUs for enhancing their safety while driving. The fake vehicles are distinguished from original vehicles by the information transmitted between the source ID and the destination ID. The authentication mechanism authenticates both the RSU and the life support emergency vehicles in the network, which also tracks the same. Any network communication should support CIA parameters (confidentiality, integrity, and availability) throughout the entire data transmission for the security constraint. Here, the life support emergency vehicles should be called by its pseudoID every time, which is obtained by periodically updating the links [4] [5].

15.2 Motivation

Achieving secure data transmission in VANET is always a big matter of deal. The life support emergency vehicles in the network exchange messages to take immediate action for maintaining a secure and safe driving scenario. The broadcast is done frequently in a time period of 100 to 300 milliseconds [6]. The actions have to be taken within the expiry of the message to prevent road crash. Despite several advantages, the vehicle ad hoc network is vulnerable to various security attacks, such as blackhole attack, distributed denial-of-service (DDoS), playback attack, and so on. Hence, the messages exchanged between the life support emergency vehicles have to be cross-checked for authentication and non-repudiation. The message modified by fraudulent vehicles may cause serious effects to the driver as well as the passenger's life. It is also important that life support emergency vehicles not reveal its original identity, for the driver's safety purpose. Sometimes, due to network fault and time delay, life support emergency vehicles may not receive messages on time. These factors catalyze us to implement novel security features to the vehicles.

Previously, VANETs managed the data transmission process by mobile crowd sensing (MCS) to track vehicles in case of emergency. This chapter achieves a model for better data communication by differentiating emergency and normal messages. The messages are set with an expiry time stamp to avoid unnecessary congestion in case of delay in the delivery of messages. Furthermore, the privacy-preserving data transmission in vehicles is achieved by implementing one-way blockchain-based cryptography hash chain mode (7).

15.3 Objectives of the Proposed Work

The contributions of the proposed model are as follows:

- To create packet classification and fusion model for efficient data communication.
- To achieve secure data and privacy preservation in mobile nodes by one-way hash blockchain cryptography model.

For ease of users, the chapter is organized as follows:

Section 15.3.1 deals with the literature survey, which discusses how previous technologies were used to achieve secure data transmission in vehicles and their limitations of the models.

Section 15.3.2 discusses how the proposed one-way hash blockchain cryptograph model is used to achieve privacy preservation of data in vehicles.

Section 15.4 deals with the performance analysis of the proposed model with the existing models. Section 15.5 ends the chapter with the scope of future work.

15.3.1 Related Works

Here, various relevant works and research of different authors related with the achievement of secure data transmission using blockchain technology in mobile vehicles, along with the difficulties faced by them while implementing the concepts in reality, are discussed.

Privacy preservation is achieved in VANET by keeping information about the location and identity of the vehicle as confidential. [8] discusses about the two entities of self-organizing VANET, namely, trust authority and the vehicles, which play a vital role. The system is initialized by a fully trusted entity so-called a TA and is responsible for generating keys. The traffic data are shared between vehicles with the help of shared secret keys. PPTMS ensures the privacy preservation of location, identity, and data. It also promises data integrity and efficiency of self-organizing VANET. On the other hand, computational cost and communication overhead show linear exponentiation with the number of vehicles. [9] deals with how a VANET-based privacy-preserving mutual authentication scheme without bilinear pairing addresses security limitation and achieves QoS. The paper also discusses the elimination of several security attacks, such as impersonation attack, modification, and side channel attack [10]. To generate a signature for each transaction in blockchain, a private key is used. Each transaction is authenticated, and it is free from malicious behavior, as confirmed by the generated signature, and is used to derive the public key mathematically. Public keys are practically irreversible, that is, we can easily derive public key from the private key, but it would take millions of years to do vice versa. The paper also discusses the hierarchical deterministic cryptocurrency wallet derived from a known seed, which allows for the generation of child keys from the parent key. There is a hidden relationship that exists between the child and parent keys, unaware to the seed. [11] deals with how the messages are delivered to the desired vehicles in a social network region with dynamic privacy-preserving authentication protocol DPPAP, a combination of AES and ECC cryptographic mechanism. In this paper, the Lahore City map is taken as instance, and it is segregated into various minor regions using NS3 simulation. Each region is identified by latitude and longitude coordinates stored in the OBU. Social networks create a cluster of smart vehicles based on a region ID using haversine formulae. The selection of vehicles and the data transmission are based on region ID. This paper guarantees that the functioning of the proposed protocol can withstand a high load factor. Cloud computing technology is adopted to disseminate messages, which are encrypted, using the attribute-based encryption for warning the vehicles in the network. The encryption and decryption processes are outsourced to attain computational efficiency. The anonymous vehicles are authenticated using the identity-based signature technique that has the ability to track the malicious vehicles. This scheme helps in reducing computational overhead and improves integrity checking [12]. A fully aggregated privacy preservation mechanism is utilized along with pseudonym to reduce the computation overhead caused in tamper-proof devices. The vehicles in the communication network communicate by a certificateless aggregate signature that reduces resources, such as bandwidth consumption. The tracing authority generates pseudonym to track the vehicles' identity [13]. The public key infrastructure-based symmetric key encryption algorithm lacks high-end privacy preservation values. Hence, the appropriate features of symmetric key encryption are extracted to combine with asymmetric cryptographic techniques, which ensure integrity, privacy, and non-repudiation in services [14]. A privacy preservation mechanism is proposed to help the communication of vehicles with the infrastructure using signature-based bilinear mapping. The signature generation and its verification are effectively done at the RSUs using one-way hash functions. The scheme is highly suitable for large-traffic-density areas as it supports batch signature verification to reduce computational overhead

[15]. A non-Diffie-Hellman-based algorithm, namely, lattice-based privacy preservation, is proposed to ensure mutual authentication and privacy. Since the Diffie-Hellman-based algorithms require polynomial time to solve the problem, the complexity is reduced using lattice-based algorithms [16]. The certificate revocation list that facilitates identity-less authentication results in computational overhead. This issue is resolved by the generation of temporary secret key of a group of vehicles. The communication overhead is increased due to periodically changing pseudonyms; hence, the lightweight privacy preservation system generates a permanent pseudonym ID [17]. The delay in message recovery signature may affect the traffic of VANETs; hence, the validity of the signature is verified in a rapid manner. The process supports batch verification to reduce time complexity by verifying more than one signature at the same time. This scheme also resists reply attacks and provides data confidentiality [18]. The fully homomorphic encryption is integrated with pseudonym to reduce the overhead and ensure security. The logical and physical address that varies based on the location of the emergency vehicle decides the pseudonym; hence, it tends to vary over time and prevent vehicles from being traced by an adversary [19]. The process of multi-hop message dissemination and security is achieved using an intelligent transport system of smartphones in VANET. The location-based protocol that chooses the sender and receiver node is incorporated along with a certificateless cryptographic technique. It verifies authenticity of nodes and data integrity [20]. An RSU cooperation detection mechanism is proposed to eliminate selfish message propagation and to check whether the propagated messages reach the destination on time. The mechanism identifies a Sybil attack using triangulation and fake propagation. The nodes are designed in such a way that they receive the digitally signed message from valid source nodes (21).

15.3.2 Proposed Work

This portion deals with what happens when any type of vehicle enters into the communication zone and how data are transmitted between vehicles via CA and RSU.

Figure 15.1 shows from very first step, that is, vehicle entry, participation, data transmission, and exit.

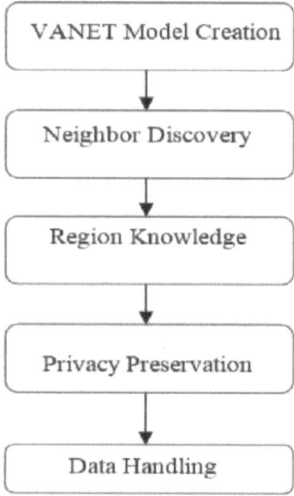

FIGURE 15.1
General steps in the VANET model.

15.3.2.1 System Model

The VANET system consists of on-road vehicles (both normal and emergency), roadside units (RSUs), certificate authority (CA), regions, and law enforcement authority (LEA). The life support emergency vehicles in the network are assigned a unique digital identity from the motor vehicles department of the government. These identities are registered in the database of the CA to make the emergency vehicle an authorized unit in the network. The security-related activities are dealt by the LEA to prevent and recover the emergency vehicle from serious concern. Any emergency vehicle acts as a transceiver of the messages from its neighboring vehicles. The sender can broadcast the messages, which in turn will be verified by the receiver. The CA and the emergency vehicle are communicated via the RSUs, which act as a gateway. The RSUs register the life support emergency vehicles that come in contact with the corresponding region. The CA generates the credentials and verifies them accordingly. The CA is responsible for maintaining the cryptographic credentials of the life support emergency vehicles for security reason. When an emergency vehicle moves from one region to another, its credentials have to be matched with the region credentials in accordance with certificates and time of expiry. The malicious activities in broadcasting the messages are monitored by the LEA, which in turn intimates the CA to block the malicious vehicle ID. The flow of the proposed model is given in Figure 15.2.

15.3.2.2 Blockchain Technology–Based Cryptography

A *block* is a container data structure of blockchain which contains a set of confirmed transactions. A block could contain different information, and a chain of these blocks evolves into a blockchain as long as it links one and the other. All blocks in blockchain

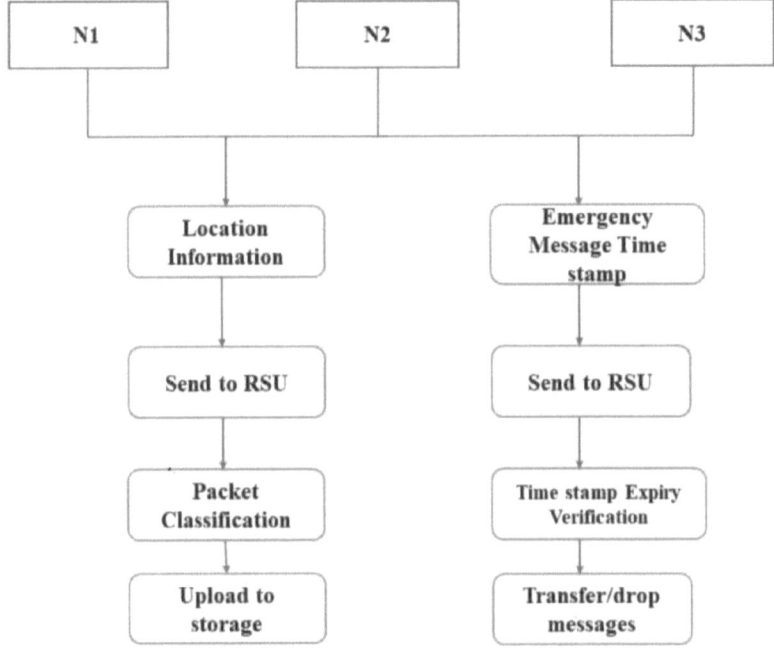

FIGURE 15.2
Overall flow of the proposed model.

are composed of a header, identifiers, and a long list of transactions. To identify a block, we need to have a cryptographic hash, a digital signature. This is created by hashing the block header twice with the SHA256 algorithm. The fundamental backbone of blockchain is Bitcoin, which is one of the cryptocurrencies that help in achieving privacy and security in the networks. This concept has been applied in VANET to ensure the privacy of broadcast beacons and its integrity. The messages from emergency vehicle nodes are mapped with public blockchain to verify the reliability of the emergency vehicle. The basic Bitcoin technology has become insufficient in VANET application due to the lack of assurance in the case of disseminating critical information. In addition to the hashing sequences in the block, a new block in accordance with event messages is also incorporated in VANET. Each region in the VANET has independent local blockchains for transmission in the particular region. The information about all the nodes is maintained in a public blockchain in that region. The consensus mechanisms are adopted to secure and scale the blockchain to the required level.

15.3.3 Algorithms Used

Let us say life support emergency vehicles as emergency vehicles in the following algorithms.

15.3.3.1 Emergency Vehicle Registration Algorithm

Step 1: Emergency vehicle obtains real ID from the Road Transport Office (RTO) and creates a secure path between the CA and itself, then sends its original ID and other details to the CA.

Step 2: The CA first checks the originality of the registered emergency vehicle; if it exists, it then generates a valid document containing the pseudoID, a pair of public and private keys (PKi, Ski) generated by ECC.

Step 3: From those credentials, the CA evaluates two hash functions needed for the authentication of the life support vehicle, and its identity is stored in the CA for future communication.

Where hash values are defined as follows:

$$H0 = (P\ IDi\ ||Pki)\ \text{and}\ H1 = (V\ IDi\ ||cert)$$

Step 4: The RSU holds the hash value H0 sent by the CA.

Step 5: The registered emergency vehicle obtains a pseudoID, certificate, H1, and a pair of public–private keys from the CA and stores these in the on-board unit (OBU).

15.3.3.2 Certificate Validation and Revocation Algorithm

Step 1: The emergency vehicle requests for an authentication to the RSU by submitting its pseudoID and public key Pki.

Step 2: Now, the RSU evaluates the hash value based on the H0 algorithm and yields the actual result. To check the originality of the emergency vehicle, the RSU, in turn, maps the values with the CA. If the actual result coincides with the stored result, the CA returns "True" to the RSU, which means the emergency vehicle is justified. Otherwise, authentication is not approved.

Step 3: After determining the authenticity of the emergency vehicle identity, the RSU initiates the random integer negotiation process, which sends a random integer RN_1 encrypted by the emergency vehicle's public key Pki.

Step 4: The emergency vehicle decrypts the cipher text by its Ski and stores random number (RN_1) in the on-board unit for the forthcoming communication between vehicles.

Step 5: To check the integrity of the received random number, the emergency vehicle in turn selects another random number (RN_2) from the RSU and recalculates the hash values of both. If the hash values are the same, the integrity of the random number is preserved. Otherwise, there is an error in data transmission. Additionally, in order to prevent the CA from malicious activity, the emergency vehicle evaluates the signature based on the H1 algorithm. Then the resultant values are mapped with the values stored in the blockchain network. Finally, the emergency vehicle sends SigSki (H1) ||H2(RN_1 ||RN_2)||RN_2 to the RSU.

Step 6: Hash function H1, along with its random integer (RN_2) and its signature, evaluates the hash value. Likewise, the hash function H2, along with a random integer (RN_1) and its corresponding signature, evaluates the hash value. While comparing if both values are the same, settlement of random number is successful.

Step 7: The RSU behaves as a peer node BC network, binds up a transaction Tx1 (sigSki (H1) ||P IDi ||Pki), and stores it in the BC network, where all RSUs are able to handle transaction Tx1.

15.3.3.3 Emergency Vehicle Advertisement (Neighbor Discovery and Message Forwarding) Algorithm

Step 1: To maintain the integrity constraint of the particular event D, the emergency vehicle uses RN_1 given by the RSU. The emergency vehicle delivers the message, which contains the traffic conditions, emergency vehicle identity, and hash value H3 (RN_1 ||D||PIDi), to the RSUs.

Step 2: Now the RSU, in turn, checks the integrity of the event D.

Step 3: If the result is okay, the RSU initiates a new transaction (Tx2).

Step 4: The RSU generates the traffic event to initiate a new transaction, whose content is Tx2 (H3||D||P IDi||timestamp).

Step 5: The contents of the transaction Tx2 are split into several parts, which are stored in different CAs.

Step 6: After hashing the Tx2 about event D, the RSU stores H4 (Tx2) in blockchain and broadcasts this transaction to all mobile nodes.

Step 7: Each emergency vehicle evaluates the time stamp of alarm message and calculates the message expiration time.

Step 8: Any emergency vehicle that participated in the data transmission can forward the message to its neighboring vehicles before the timer expires.

Step 9: After the timer expires, vehicles stop transmitting the data. If any new data communication arrives, then the emergency vehicle starts generating a random number from step 1.

15.4 Results and Discussion

The model is implemented using Simulation of Urban Mobility (SUMO), which is efficient in simulating road traffic. The parameters for the SUMO are shown in Table 15.1. The proposed one-way hash-based blockchain model is evaluated by comparing with the existing models, namely, bSPECs, Xiaoyan, BLS, and ECPP. The metrics used for comparisons are data collection per user, message delivery ratio, total amount of data collected, end-to-end delay, and energy consumption.

15.4.1 Data Collected per User

Figure 15.3 shows the amount of data collected in terms of bytes by the receiver. The existing models, like bSPECS, Xiaoyan, BLS, can only transmit data less than or slightly equal

TABLE 15.1

Simulation Parameters

Parameter	Values
No. of nodes	100
Speed	40 m/s
Acceleration	3.6 m/s^2
Length of the emergency vehicle	~6.77 m
Width of the emergency vehicle	~2.3 m
No. of RSUs	15
RSU coverage	1,000 m

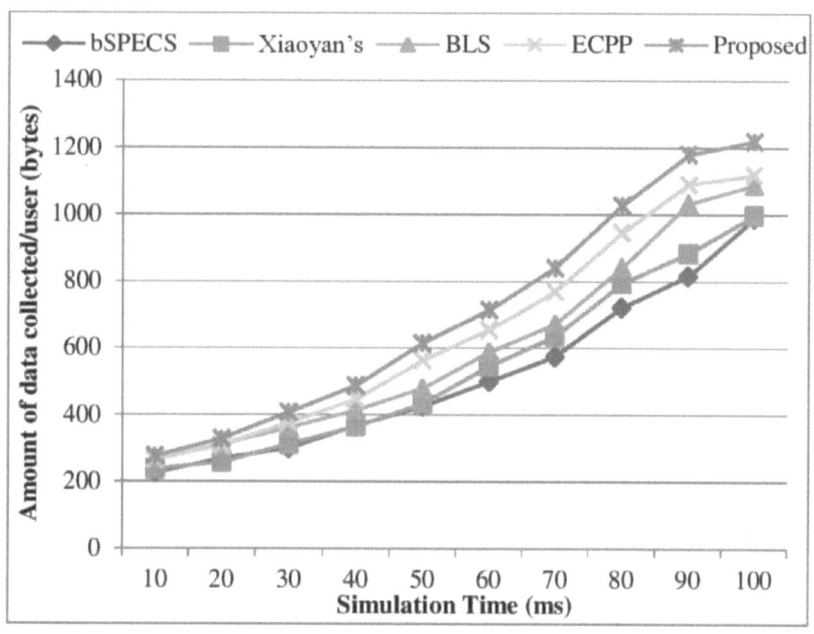

FIGURE 15.3
Comparison of amount of data collected per user in VANET.

to 1 packet length, whereas our proposed model can transmit more than 1,024 bytes in the prescribed time limit. This reveals that our model has the better data collection ability compared to the existing methods.

15.4.2 Message Delivery Ratio

The number of successful messages to the total number of messages delivered is the message delivery ratio. Its calculation is shown in equation 1.

$$Message\,Delivery\,Ratio = \frac{No.\,of\,Successful\,packets}{Total\,No.\,of\,packets} \quad (1)$$

Figure 15.4 shows that there is detrimental change in the delivery of messages when the number of malicious node increases. Even though our proposed model could withstand in the simulation environment while delivering the messages compared with the existing system.

15.4.3 Total Amount of Data Collected

The data collected by all the life support emergency vehicles in a network during a particular simulation period is termed as the total amount of data collected. Figure 15.5 shows that the proposed model can recollect 8,000 bytes of data, where other existing models are

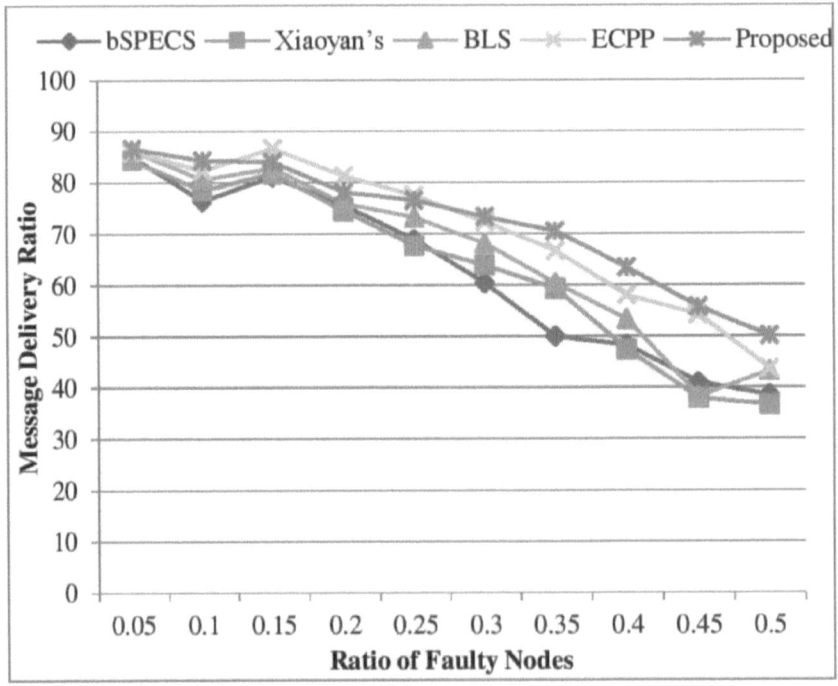

FIGURE 15.4
Comparison of message delivery ratio of the proposed VANET model.

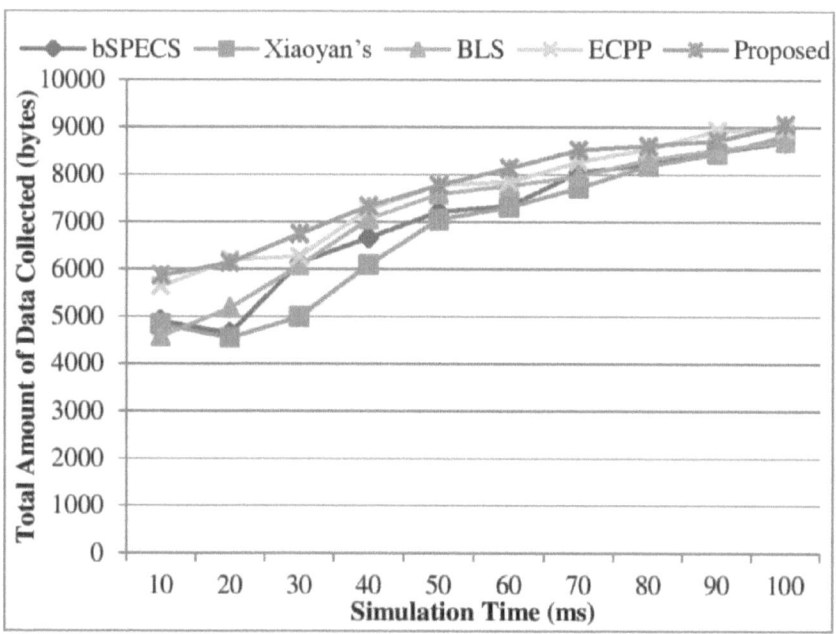

FIGURE 15.5
Comparison of total amount of data collected by all the users in the network.

struggling to collect 6,000 bytes of data. This depicts that the resilience of the proposed model is good compared to the existing models.

15.4.4 End-to-End Delay

The difference in time between the departure and arrival of the message in the network is the end-to-end delay. Indirectly, EED speaks with the speed of data. Our proposed model takes a maximum of 1 ms for delivering the message, where other models take the same as the minimum time constraint of delivering the message.

15.4.5 Energy Consumption

The efficiency of the model is calculated by the energy consumed by each node in the network. The energy consumption of nodes is highly fluctuating in other models, whereas our proposed model shows linear and gradual increase with the amount of time.

This characteristic is observed as one of the qualities of the standard system. Our proposed model comes under the aforementioned category too.

15.5 Conclusion

The potential of VANETs in broadcasting beacons to enhance safety measures has made VANET a popular research topic. Still, VANET is open to several network attacks, such as

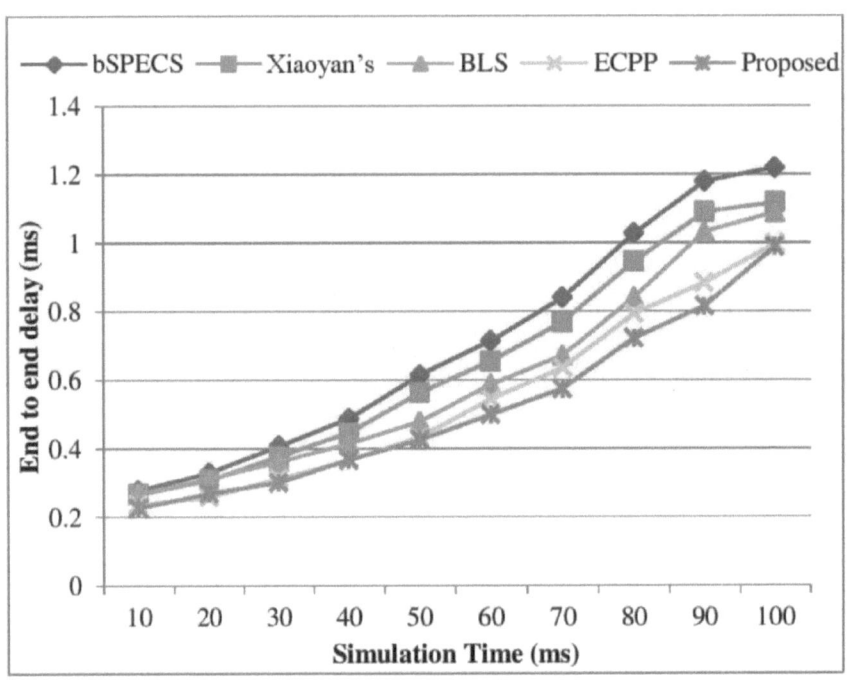

FIGURE 15.6
Comparison of end-to-end delay of the VANET models.

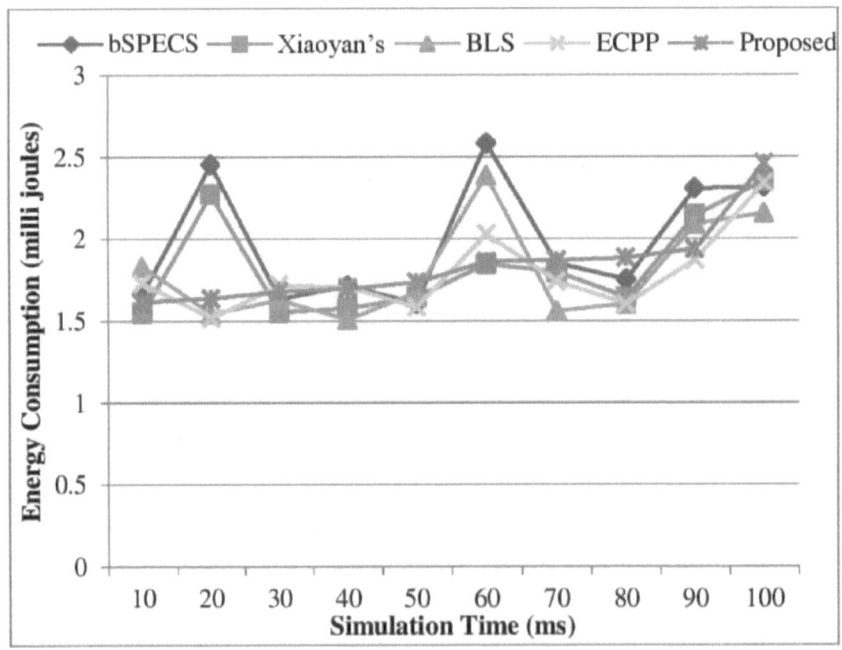

FIGURE 15.7
Plot for energy consumption of the VANET models.

DoS attack, Sybil attack, impersonation attack, and so on. In this chapter, our proposed model ensures the reception of actual messages about road conditions in order to support life supporting vehicles like ambulances in a timely manner, saving one's life by taking the exact route. In addition, privacy and data integrity are also ensured by setting time stamps to the message sent by each node. The proposed model is simulated using SUMO by setting parameters, as shown in Table 15.1. The results show that the blockchain-based one-way hash model outperformed other existing models considered for comparison, namely, bSPECs, Xiaoyan, BLS, and ECPP. The message delivery ratio is high, which in turn reduced the end-to-end delay of the model. The model resulted in standardized energy consumption; hence, the overall efficiency of the model is enhanced.

References

1. S.S. Tangade and S.S. Manvi, "A Survey on Attacks, Security and Trust Management Solutions in VANETs." In *4th IEEE international Conference on Computing, Communications and Networking Technologies*; 2013, pp. 1–6. https://doi.org/10.1109/ICCCNT.2013.6726668
2. B. Parno and A. Perrig, "Challenges in Securing Vehicular Networks." In *Workshop on Hot Topics in Neworks*; 2005. https://efaidnbmnnnibpcajpcglclefindmkaj/https://netsec.ethz.ch/publications/papers/cars.pdf
3. R.G. Engoulou, M. Bellache, S. Pierre and A. Quintero, "VANET Security Surveys." *Computer Communications*. 2014; 44: 1–13.
4. M. Raya, P. Papadimitratos and J. Hubaux, "Securing Vehicular Communications." *IEEE Wireless Communication*. 2006; 13(1): 8–15.
5. X. Hou, Y. Li, M. Chen, D. Wu, D. Jin and S. Chen, "Vehicular Fog Computing: A View Point of Vehicles as Infrastructures." *IEEE Transactions on Vehicular Technology*. 2016; 65(6): 3860–73.
6. Y. Zhang, X. Lin and C. Xu, "Blockchain Based Secure Data Provenanace for Cloud Storage." In *International Conference on Information and Communications Security*; 2018. Springer, pp. 3–19.
7. F. Tschorsch and B. Scheruermann, "Bitcoin and Beyond: A Techncal Survey on Decentralied Digital Currencies." *IEEE Comunication Surveys & Tutorials*. 2016; 3(18): 2084–123.
8. L. Zhu, et al., "Traffic Monitoring in Self Organizing VANETs: A Privacy Preserving Mechanism for Speed Collection and Analysis." *IEEE Wireless Communications*. 2019; 6(26): 18–23.
9. J. Cui, et al., "Secure Mutual Authentication with Privacy Preservation in Vehicular Adhoc Networks." *Vehicular Communications*. 2020; 21: 100–200.
10. M. Crosy, P. Pattanayak, S. Verma and V. Kalyanaraman, "Block Chain Technology: Beyound Bicoin." *Applied Innovation*. 2016; 2: 6–10.
11. S.A. Shah, et al., "A Dynamic Privacy Preserving Authentication Protocols in VANET Using Social Network." In *International Conference on Software Engineering, Artificial Intelligence, Networking and Parallel Distributed Computing*; 2019. Springer.
12. S. Wang and N. Yao, "A RSU Aided Distributed Trust Framework for Pseudonym Enabled Privacy Preservation in VANET." *Wireless Networks*. 2019; 25(3): 1099–115.
13. Q. Huang, et al., "Secure and Privacy PreservingWarning Message Dissemination in Cloudasssisted Internet of Vehicles." In *IEEE Confrence on Communications and Network Security*; 2019, pp. 1–8. https://doi.org/10.1109/CNS.2019.8802649
14. H. Zhong, et al., "Privacy Preserving Authentication Scheme with Full Aggregation in VANET." *Information Sciences*. 2019; 47(6): 211–21.
15. F. Tahir, S. Nasir and Z. Khalid, "Privacy Preserving Authentication Protocol Based on Hybrid Cryptography for VANET." In *International Conference on Applied and Engineering Mathematics*; 2019, pp. 80–85. https://doi.org/10.1109/ICAEM.2019.8853808
16. I. Ali and F. Li, "An Efficient Conditional Privacy Preserving Authentication Scheme for Emergency Vehicles to Infrastructure Communication in VANET." *Vehicular Communication*. 2019:100–228.

17. S. Mukherjee, D.S. Gupta and G.P. Biswas, "An Efficient and Batch Verifiable Conditional Privacy Preservingauthentication Scheme for VANETs Using Lattice." *Soft Computing*. 2019; 12(101): 1763–88.
18. S.A. Alfadhli, et al., "An Efficient Light Weight Condiional Privacy Preserving Authenticaion Scheme Based on Hash Function and Local Group Secret Key for VANET." In *The World Symposium on Software Engineering*; 2019. Association for Computing Machinery, pp. 32–36. https://doi.org/10.1145/3362125.3362128
19. S. Jian, et al., "Secure Real Time Traffic Data Aggregation with Batch Verification for Vehicularcloud in VANETs." *IEEE Transactions on Vehicular Technology*. 2020; 69(1): 807–17. https://doi.org/10.1109/TVT.2019.2946935
20. N.K. Prema, "Efficient Secure Aggregation in VANETs Using Fully Homomorphic Encryption." *Mobile Networks and Applications*. 2019; 24(2): 434–42.
21. H. Galeana-Zapien, et al., "Smartphone Based Platform for Secure Multihop Message Dissemination in VANETS." *Sensors*. 2020; 20(2).

16

Blockchain-Based Digital Twin to Predict Heart Attacks

Venkatesh Upadrista, Sajid Nazir, and Huaglory Tianfield

16.1 Introduction

Remote health monitoring (RHM) is a research area that is gaining a lot of interest within the research community due to the nature of personalization it allows by providing targeted treatments and preventive care for each patient using the person's past medical history, genetic factors, in combination with real-time health indicators. The digital twin for remote health monitoring is a virtual representation (digital twin) of a human and can bring in a lot of value to RHM use cases, where the human body parameters are replicated virtually and then proactively monitored for a disease occurrence. The digital twin (DT) for a human can use sensors, actuators, and other sources of data to create a virtual representation of health data [1].

Several papers have discussed DT by focusing on specific body organs. As an example, DT of heart was derived from echo scans [2], computerized tomographic scans [3], or other imaging techniques [4], including electrocardiogram databases and mathematical techniques [5–8]. Few other papers have discussed about models that would be helpful to build a DT for ischemic diseases and hypertension [9], [10], [8]. There were some other interesting papers which have described the models that can be enhanced to create a full-blown heart prediction DT model [11–13]. These research papers can be best described as preliminary work that can be used as guidance to build either an active or semi-active fully functional and real-time digital twin model. Data privacy and security are other areas which were not discussed in these papers, which can be considered as a research gap.

Some other papers have discussed about remote health monitoring for elderly care [14–16]. In [13], [17], authors have discussed about detecting the severity of carotid stenosis, and [11] describes a model for heart rate monitoring. However, all these dealt with basic RHM use cases, which can only perform reactive treatments and, at the same time, have not focused on security and privacy aspects, which are few of the biggest challenge with RHM use cases [18–20], as RHM use cases deal with sensitive patient data. Therefore, we need a secure mode that can proactively detect a disease for serious health conditions.

In this chapter, we have proposed a blockchain-based digital twin application (referred as **BDT app**) to predict heart attacks using Optimized XGBoost–based heart attack machine learning model. The health readings of patients (data feeds), which are currently simulated data, are fed as inputs into this heart attack machine learning model to predict heart attacks. Headless architecture has been used to ensure that we minimize any changes to our **BDT app** code even when the source of the data feed changes in future (for example, wearable devices to send patient health readings).

Security and privacy concerns tend to be the biggest challenge in healthcare [18–22], and not many digital twin architectures in literatures have sufficiently covered this aspect. Our model uses blockchain to overcome security and privacy issues, thereby making the model foolproof [20], [22–25]. The reasons for using the blockchain for digital twin use cases are its prominent features to enhance security and privacy of data generated by patients. In our model, only the patient metadata is being stored on the blockchain, thereby making the blockchain very light. This is in contrast to other literatures, where all data is stored on the blockchain.

We have used chaos engineering to test **BDT app** security. *Chaos engineering* is a technique in which chaos experiments are conducted to identify problems in a live production system. These tests are conducted to build confidence in the capability of the system to ensure that it can withstand turbulent conditions in production [26]. Chaos engineering has been applied since we wanted to test the application's reliability in real time with full datasets in production, in contrast to testing with limited data in a test environment. The chaos engineering tests are important for the **BDT app** because data tampering can happen during cyberattacks. Since our application deals with critical and high-health-risk patients, it is important that we perform security testing on a full production system and test the reliability in real time thoroughly rather than testing it in a constrained environment and leaving chances for errors.

We have organized the rest of this chapter as follows: Section 16.2 covers the literature review, Section 16.3 shares the **BDT app** architecture, and in Section 16.4 we describe the experiments, evaluations, and results. Finally, Section 16.5 shares a discussion, and Section 16.6 provides a conclusion.

16.2 Literature Review

We performed a literature review to understand the implementation of digital twins for proactive disease detection, specifically to understand the models that address cardiovascular diseases. Based on these reviews [2–13], [27–31], it can be inferred that there is lot of attention focused on the DT models for cardiovascular diseases. The conceptual models that are defined as part of these papers can be treated as precursors to creating a full-fledged DT model to proactively and reactively detect cardiovascular diseases. There was no specific mention of security and privacy in these papers.

16.2.1 Abdominal Aortic Aneurysm (AAA)

An AAA is a bulge that is formed in the wall of the large artery just below the heart [27]. The large artery is referred to as the aorta. The bulge is caused at the weakest section in the artery wall, which is at a risk of tearing. There are different treatments for AAA, out of which endovascular repair is the most prominent one.

Auricchio et al. [5] performed a comparison between preoperative simulation of the DT implant using a specially made endograft prediction with postoperative outcomes of a specific patient. The experimental results demonstrated a high level of quantitative and qualitative agreement between the postoperative analysis and the simulation prediction. Based on the results, which were considered encouraging, it was inferred that there are high potential benefits to investigate aortic endografting by using patient-specific simulations using DT. The proof-of-concept was developed as part of the paper, but only limited details on endograft prediction were shared.

Hemmler et al. [6] had proposed to mitigate complications related to infrarenal endovascular repair (as against open-surgical abdominal aortic aneurysm repair) by creating a digital twin for stent-graft size and material during preoperative selection. They used a morphing algorithm and patient-specific preoperative data that can help predict configuration of wall stress and postoperative graft, which includes geometry of aneurysms and mechanical modelling of graft. A theoretical model was also shared as part of the paper.

There are several techniques to treat intracranial aneurysms, but minimally invasive treatment approaches, such as percutaneous stent implants, are becoming quite popular these days. The results of such treatments are due to factors such as aneurysm and vessel geometry, including conditions related to hemodynamic and device design. Because of this reason, Larrabide et al. [7] developed a tool that can assist in finding alternatives for stenting. As part of the experiments, authors had used a phantom (virtual human) to perform in vitro experiments, where a contrast injection was given to the phantom. After these experiments, computational fluid dynamics analysis was performed on the "virtual/digital twin of the phantom" using the virtually released stent. In vitro experiments and computational fluid dynamics analysis were then compared using virtual angiographies. Comparison was then performed by generating data from contrast time–density curves for in vitro and computational fluid dynamics. When comparing the contrast–density curves specifically, the results demonstrated that both experiments (phantom vs. digital twin of the phantom) were comparable, indicating that digital twins can be used to perform experiments related to stenting.

Biancolini et al. [28] discussed about the reduced order model framework. The framework was developed to reduce the computing costs that are needed for blood flow prediction in computational fluid dynamics techniques. The effect of form parameter changes on the entire flow field can be seen in real time using the inspection tool the authors have created. The tool provides patient-specific data that can be used for surgery planning, treatment, and prevention. A proof-of-concept was developed and shared as part of the paper.

Chakshu et al. [29] use a virtual patient database and share a model to detect AAA and severity classification. The authors applied recurrent neural networks and an inverse analysis system for the prediction of blood flow to classify the severity of AAA. A proof-of-concept was developed using inverse analysis with neural networks and deep learning techniques for waveform calculation and vessel dynamics.

16.2.2 Occlusive (Ischemic) Heart Disease and Hypertension

The narrowing of the arteries cause inadequate blood flows to the heart, which leads to occlusive arterial disease. Though these symptoms are most often seen in the legs and arms, there are chances that it can occur directly in the heart or the brain [32].

Parr et al. [8] used machine learning models to detect stenoses and aneurysms. They used an algorithm that can use patterns and biomarkers from an already-existing dataset and presented a model to quantify classification accuracy of arterial disease by using flow rate measurements and pressure in the arterial network at specific body locations. Multiple machine learning models were discussed, such as gradient boosting, Naive Bayes, random forests, and multilayer perceptron, for proof-of-concept.

Martinez-Velazquez et al. [9] created an edge computing–based application using body sensors connected via a Bluetooth connection and a 5G network to detect ischemic heart disease. Convolutional neural networks were used to classify non-myocardial and myocardial conditions. The results of the implementation had shown an accuracy of 85.77%, and each sample classification was performed in 4.8 sec. These results prove that the developed proof-of-concept is capable of supporting demand processing by creating digital twins using edge.

A digital twin was developed using two-chambered heart and baroreflex blood pressure control as part of [10] that can produce synthetic physiological data under atherosclerotic and healthy settings. A methodology for creating synthetic PhotoPlethysmoGraphy signals using a digital twin created specifically for the cardiovascular system was also proposed. A successful initial validation was performed by clustering coronary artery disease and data from non–coronary artery disease PhotoPlethysmoGraphy and by bringing forward features from the synthetically generated PhotoPlethysmoGraphy and finally comparing it with PhotoPlethysmoGraphy that was generated from Physionet data.

16.2.3 Arrhythmia

Cardiac arrhythmia is a disease that causes irregular heartbeats. Electrophysiology tests are performed to check if a person is suffering from arrhythmia. It is a test where the heart's electrical system or activity is monitored for abnormal heartbeats, or arrhythmia. Catheters and wire electrodes are inserted to measure the electrical activity, through blood vessels that enter the heart [30].

Peirlinck et al. [2] researched a new computational model that utilizes cardiac magnetic resonance imaging–based modelling, simulation, and non-invasive electrocardiographic data for efficient quantification of properties related to subject-specific ventricular activation. Sequential Monte Carlo approximation Bayesian approach was used to simultaneously estimate the root nodes, the endocardial, and the myocardial conduction speeds. The authors also quantified the accuracy of recovering these activation properties using a cohort of 20 virtual subjects. The concept was explained using a statistical methodology.

Generating high-fidelity digital twins of heart (cardiac) encompasses two stages [3]. One stage is related to anatomical generated from tomographic data, and the second one is functional twinning, which is derived from electrocardiogram. A study [3] brings forward limitations of both these stages that impede accuracy and efficiency for clinical utility. Further, in order to address these challenges, authors had presented a proof-of-concept that can help increase the value of a biophysically detailed digital twin that replicates ventricular electrophysiology, utilizing techniques like parameter vector and fast-forward electrocardiogram model.

Pagani et al. [4] have discussed about several promising mathematical models that have emerged to predict unforeseen health events in addition to reproducing patient-specific clinical indicators. Once specific patient information is fed into these models, these provide predictions of diseases specific to the model code. The authors also noted a number of issues with combining clinical information from cardiac electrophysiology (such as rhythm and imaging) to develop numerical models for patient-specific prediction. They emphasized these issues as research gaps for further investigation.

To mimic the natural behavior of the heart, a framework with mechano-electric feedback and bidirectional coupling is required [31]. Adapting this framework allows ion channels personalization to the organ level that can be used to model digital twins. A fully coupled multi-scale model of human heart with parameterizations for electrophysiology and a closed-loop circulation model was presented. The authors also showcased validity of the model by performing a simulation on customized heart geometry that was developed using magnetic resonance imaging data of a healthy person.

16.2.4 Heart Failure

A heart failure can be caused if the blood supply to the heart is suddenly blocked due to a blood clot [33].

Winokur et al. [11] discussed using a heart monitoring wearable device to proactively detect cardiovascular diseases. They developed a proof-of-concept using a wearable heart monitoring device that can be plugged in the ear just like a hearing aid. The device was wirelessly connected to a laptop for recording the data and then to perform analytics. The heart monitor used a triaxial microelectromechanical system accelerometer to measure the ballistocardiograph motion of the head.

In Chakshu et al. [12], an inverse analysis method was proposed to create a cardiovascular digital twin. For nonlinear systems—as an example, blood flow in the circulatory system (which generally involves a significant degree of nonlinearity)—the inverse analysis approaches frequently fail or were proven ineffective. In order to solve this problem, a virtual patient database was used, and a methodology was developed for inverse analysis by employing recurrent neural networks for the cardiovascular system. Inverse analysis was performed using the method described in this study with high degree of accuracy. It was able to accurately identify issues like AAA and determined the severity with an accuracy rate of 97.79%.

Using a coupled blood flow and head vibration, a digital twin model for RHM was created to assess the severity of carotid stenosis (narrowing of heart arteries) from a video of a human face [13]. The digital twin was developed as a proof-of-concept, in a partially active mode which uses patients' face image to detect the percentage of blockage to the carotid arteries.

16.3 Blockchain-Based Digital Twin Architecture

The architecture of the BDT app is depicted in Figure 16.1.

We have created a data feeds interface to simulate the communication of the DT actors, such as creating new twins (adding new patients) or updating existing twins (updating existing patients' data). We used headless architecture, where the data feeds are separated from backend services. Figure 16.1 depicts the technical architecture of our digital twin application.

Data feeds refer to individual patient's real-time data, such as body mass index, hypertension levels, electrocardiogram, or ST slope. Data feeds entered using the data feeds interface (Figure 16.2) are written to an *XML file*. The advantage of using headless architecture is that, in the future, data feeds interface can be replaced with wearable devices that send patient data, and our **BDT app** will work seamlessly without any changes to the

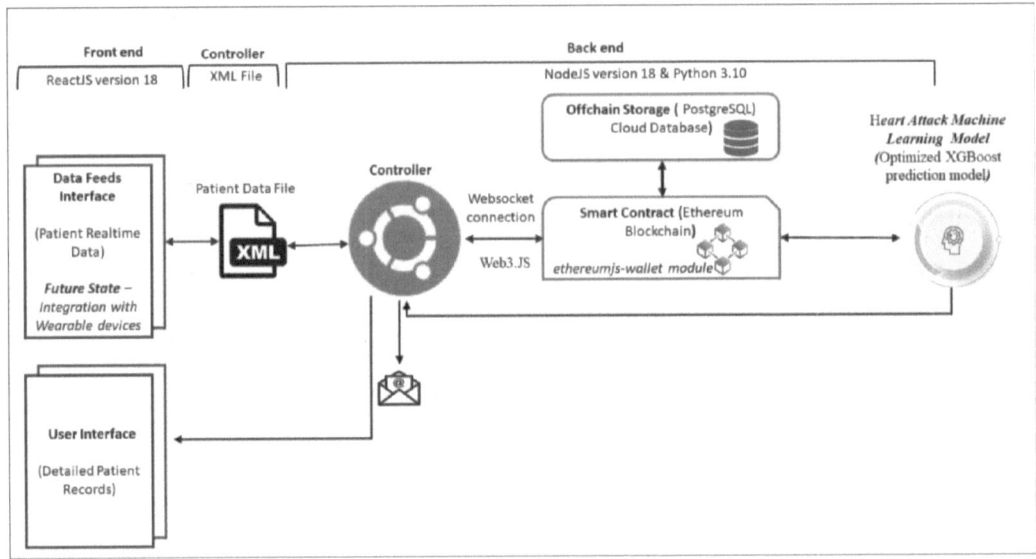

FIGURE 16.1
Blockchain-based digital twin architecture.

application code. The only configuration that will need to change for the wearable devices will be to write data directly to the *XML file* and our **BDT app** will run as is.

Controller continuously monitors the *XML file*, and as soon as a change is detected, the smart contract on the Ethereum Ganache private blockchain is invoked. To manage the blockchain account, we have used an **ethereumjswallet** module.

The blockchain account provides access to the private and public keys. During first access, key pairs are generated dynamically and kept in the BDT app cache for later use. Sending signed transactions, including the private key, to the smart contract on the Ganache blockchain was accomplished by using Web3.JS library. The *controller* is connected to a Ganache blockchain node using a WebSocket connection. WebSocket connections perform better than HTTP connections because they offer a two-way communication channel between the Ethereum node and the client. As a result, there is no need to create separate HTTP connections for every request. The device agent uses WebSockets to subscribe to smart contract events, which typically uses publish–subscribe method and is another feature that is useful for synchronization. During development, we achieved a noticeably faster data load time by switching to a remote procedure call connection based on WebSockets.

We propose an off-chain solution to store patients' data, as storing the entire health record of a patient on the blockchain would increase the size of the entire chain and storage at each node. Therefore, we are only recording the events using the blockchain technology as a ledger, whereas the patient data (i.e., linked transactions) are stored in an off-chain data store (i.e., PostgreSQL database on cloud).

We have created an **upload module** that uses the blockchain account to upload off-chain data to PostgreSQL database. PostgreSQL has been modified so that its identification system uses Ethereum accounts. For dynamic content, we have used Chainlink data feeds. Chainlink data feeds have a fixed address determined by the user (Ethereum account) and topic (any SHA3 hash) and can only be modified with a public key signature, which makes

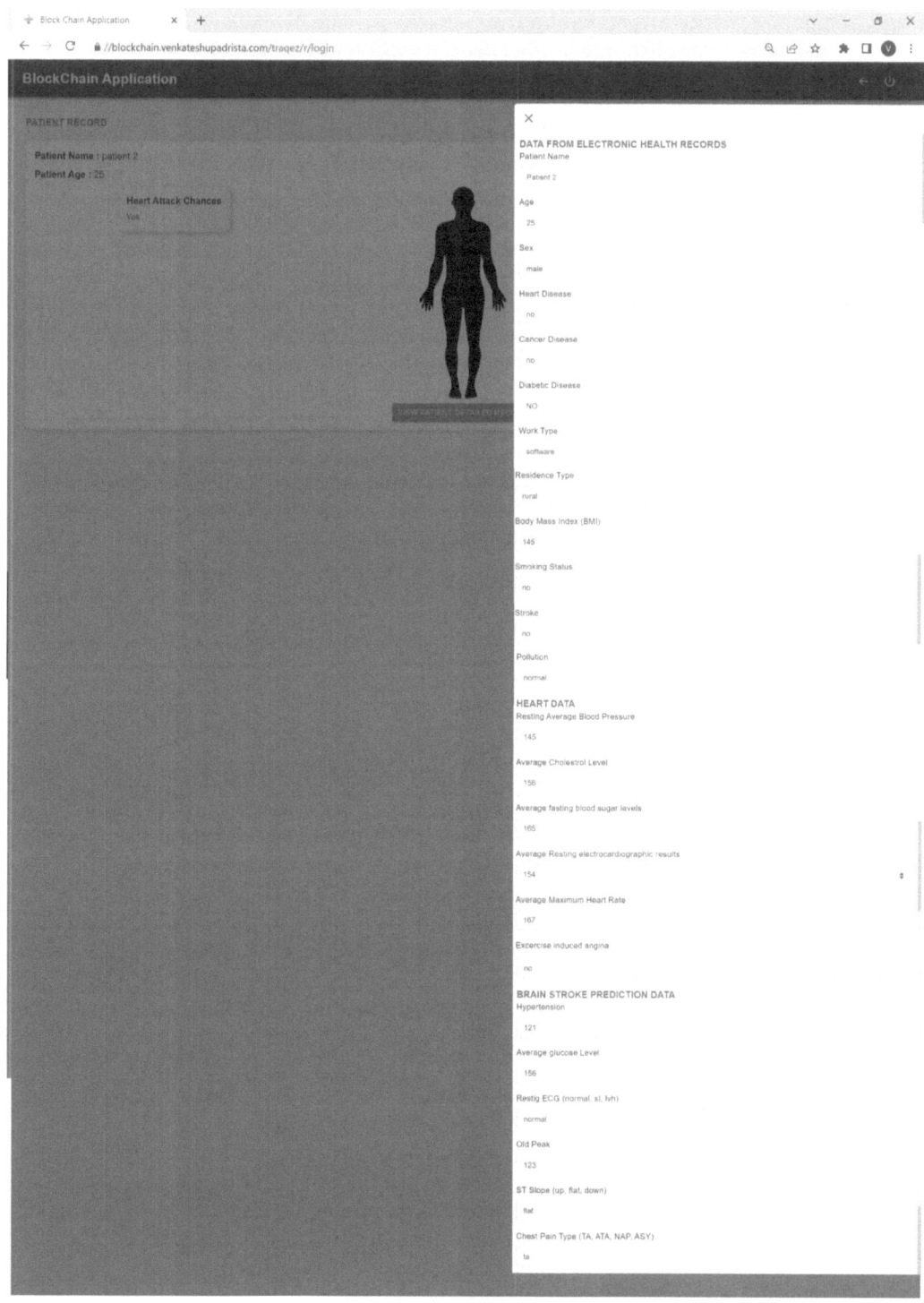

FIGURE 16.2
Data feeds interface to enter patient data.

it fully secured. After data is stored on the Ganache private blockchain and PostgreSQL, the smart contract next invokes the trained *heart attack machine learning model*. We have initially used the basic version of random forest classifier to predict heart attacks. In order to develop our model, we first divided the data into the training and test set. The dependent variables were then trained to anticipate the outcomes. The accuracy of the outcome predicted by the random forest classifier was roughly at 71.4%. Since we required higher accuracy, we then used the enhancement technique to increase the prediction accuracy. A *random forest* is a set of multiple decision trees which has different accuracy rate for each decision tree. We selected the decision tree model which had the highest prediction rate, and then hyperparameter tuning was applied. While splitting a node, a hyperparameter can either choose multiple decision trees in the random forest or can choose multiple features in each tree. In our model, we have proposed the use of automated data visualization to find discrepancies in data, and then the best tree features were selected using feature selection. After this process, the model was used for classification. We finally achieved the best random state *heart attack machine learning model*, increasing the accuracy of predictions from 71.4% to 97.1%.

For each patient, the *heart attack machine learning model* is invoked, and results are sent to the digital twin utility, which in turn sends an email to the registered doctor's email ID if the machine learning model determines a heart attack risk.

16.4 Experimental Evaluation

16.4.1 Systems Setup

We have used Linux server which uses x86-based Elastic Compute Cloud instance with Mac instances hosted on Amazon Web Services. The server is based on Intel's eighth generation with 3.2 gigahertz core i7 processors using 32 gigabytes of memory.

ReactJS version 18, NodeJS version 18, and Python 3.10 were used to develop the application, and PostgreSQL version 12 was used as the relational database.

The *heart attack machine learning model* that we created to detect heart attack uses Optimized XGBoost, which is tuned to predict heart diseases. Categorical features were encoded using the one-hot encoding technique during the data pre-processing stage, followed by Bayesian optimization technique, which further improved the prediction results. XGboost is a package that is owned by the distributed machine learning community [34]). The *heart attack machine learning model* was trained using the Heart Failure Prediction Dataset Kaggle [35]. This is one of the largest datasets available for research purposes, created by combining five heart datasets with 11 shared features [35].

Ganache private blockchain has been used to guarantee data security. Ganache is simpler to configure and is lightweight, hence can be run on laptops or desktops.

We used Solidity object-oriented programming language for implementing the smart contract. Clique proof-of-authority [36] has been used as the consensus algorithm. Clique is an Ethereum implementation of the proof-of-authority which is based on the Go language. Proof-of-authority is one of the most popular consensus algorithms that is widely used across permissioned blockchain environments to safeguard the network. The algorithm is well-known to accelerate the consensus process, and hence, we were able to achieve faster data storage in our case, which is an essential requirement of our application, since we preform real-time processing of patient data. On the other hand, Clique does not need huge computing power and resources, thereby making it energy-efficient. In contrast to the proof-of-work algorithm, only predefined authority known as validators are permitted to take part in the consensus process in proof-of-authority algorithm. This is achieved by first validating the transactions, after which blocks are created and appended to the blockchain. The hospital serves as the validator in our scenario.

16.4.2 Prediction Accuracy

We calculated the accuracy of the machine learning algorithm using Sklearn's accuracy_score() function after fitting the random forest model in scikit-learn. The true labels of the sample are accepted by the accuracy_score() method, and the proposed *heart attack machine learning model* accuracy was 97.1%.

After we fitted the random forest model, we were able to see each individual decision tree from the random forest. The sample source code, as shown in code listing 16.1, first fits the random forest model and then shows all the estimators (i.e., decision trees) from the random forest.

We chose the estimators (decision trees) that gave the maximum accuracy at 97.1%. One of the key challenges while plotting the single decision tree from the random forest is that the decision tree can grow quite deep (large) when it is fully grown (default hyperparameters), and generally, any tree with depth greater than 6 is very hard to read. Since we wanted to have the tree visualization in a readable format, we built the random forest with max_depth <7 and selected the best estimator that gave us the maximum accuracy, that is, 97.1%.

```
Code Listing. 16.1 : Sample Random Forest source code
fn=data.feature _ names
cn=data.target _ names
fig, axes = plt.subplots(nrows = 1,ncols = 5,figsize = (10,2), dpi=900)
for index in range(0, 5):
    tree.plot _ tree(rf.estimators _ [index],
         feature _ names = fn,
         class _ names=cn,
         filled = True,
         ax = axes[index]);
axes[index].set _ title('Estimator: ' + str(index), fontsize = 11)
fig.savefig('rf _ 5trees.png')
```

16.4.3 Data Analysis and Notifications

As soon as a new patient data is added to the *XML file*, the *controller* invokes the *smart contract* and patient data is stored on the Ganache blockchain and PostgreSQL. Subsequently, the smart contract invokes the *heart attack machine learning model*, and results are sent to the *controller*. If the risk of heart attack is predicted, the *controller* will send an email notification (Figure 16.3) to the doctor indicating the risk of heart attack. In case the doctor needs additional readings, fresh data from the patient can be requested and entered using data feeds interface. Once data is entered using data feeds interface, the *XML file* will be updated, the *controller* will be invoked, the heart attack risk will be reevaluated on the new data, and notifications will be sent appropriately.

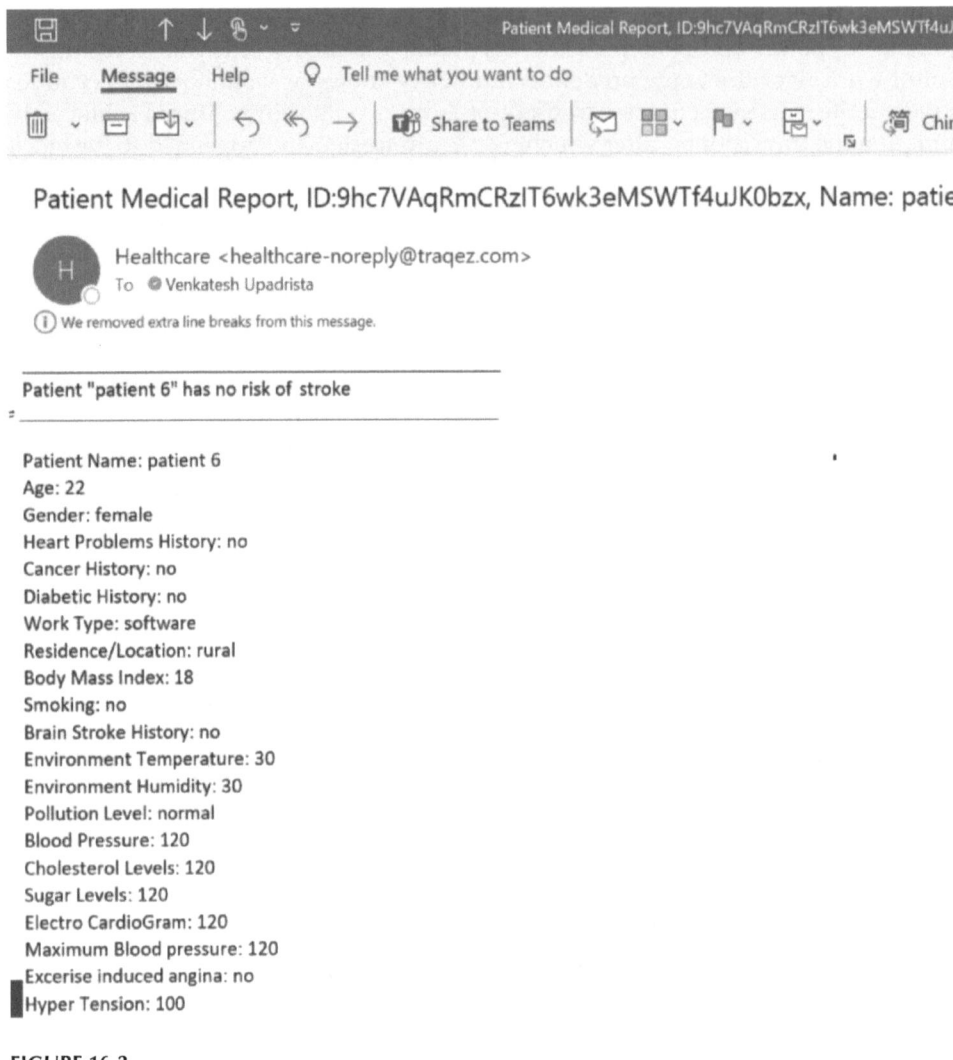

FIGURE 16.3
Email notification.

16.4.4 Data Visualization

The doctors can get email notifications for a patient's heart attack risk as the main application flow for our **BDT app**.

Alternatively, in some cases, doctors may want to review patients' detailed real-time health data, including their past medical history, from electronic health records. To facilitate this, we have created an alternate flow (user interface) which the doctors can use to view detailed patients' medical reports. The doctor can view all his patients' records along with any associated heart attack risks by logging to the user interface as shown in Figure 16.4. The details of each patient's data can be viewed by the doctor by clicking on the individual patient's name hyperlink.

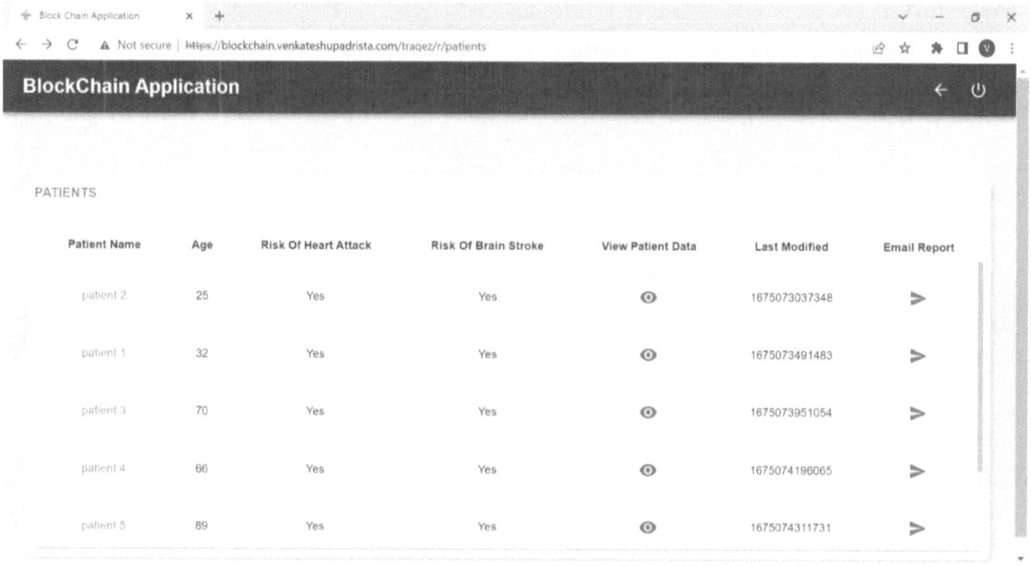

FIGURE 16.4
User interface (patient summary screen).

16.4.4.1 The Chaos Engineering Experiment to Test Reliability

Chaos engineering experiments purposefully try to create turbulent conditions in real production environment to test the system and find weaknesses in real time. We conducted chaos engineering experiment to prove the reliability of the **BDT app** by simulating the tampering of patient data from the backend for a specific patient, and then compared the "before tampering" results with results "after tampering."

First, we ran the steps as described in Section 3.1 by adding data for a new patient, that is, Patient 6. As soon as the new Patient 6 record was added, the **controller** was invoked, and steps, as discussed in Section 3.1, were executed. Finally, an email was sent to the doctor with the readings as shown in Scenario A column of Table 16.1.

We then tampered the values for Patient 6, from the backend on PostgreSQL database to invalid values. The tampered values are shown in the Tampered Values column of Table 16.1, where we have modified the body mass index value to 100, and blood pressure and cholesterol level values to 190 and 190, respectively. Maximum blood pressure was tampered to 101, and hypertension was changed to 250.

After these values were changed from the backend, we ran the **BDT app** again. The *controller* was invoked, and steps as disused in Section 3.1 were executed. An email was sent to the doctor with the readings as shown in Scenario B of Table 16.1.

Based on the comparison between Scenario A values and Scenario B values, it is clear that our blockchain system was able to detect the tampering and revert the records back to the original values, thereby ensuring data reliability against malicious tampering. This is accomplished through the inherent nature of the blockchain, as the application will be able to identify and retrieve correct data values from other blockchain nodes in the network.

TABLE 16.1

Patient 6 Data (Before and After Tampering)

Patient Data	Scenario A	Tampered Values	Scenario B
Patient Name	Patient 6		Patient 6
Age	22		22
Gender	Female		Female
Heart Problem History	No		No
Cancer History	No		No
Diabetic History	no		no
Work Type	Software		Software
Residence/Location	Rural		Rural
Body Mass Index	18	*100*	18
Smoking	No		No
Brain Stroke History	no		no
Environment Temperature	30		30
Environment Humidity	30		30
Pollution Level	Normal		Normal
Blood Pressure	120	*190*	120
Cholesterol Levels	120	*190*	120
Sugar Levels	120		120
Electrocardiogram	120		120
Maximum Blood Pressure	120	*101*	120
Exercise-Induced Angina	No		No
Hypertension	100	*250*	100
Glucose Levels	60		60

Blockchain is a technology that can be used together with digital twin to eradicate several security and privacy concerns for healthcare uses cases [23], [37], [38], [21–23], which we have proved using this experiment.

16.5 Discussion

The concept of digital twin has been applied in many domains, including healthcare, which extends the digital twin concept to combine system models and analysis with real-time personal data that can be used to enhance health and life expectancy [39].

The digital twin of a human has been investigated for specific use cases, such as elderly care [14], [40], detecting the severity of carotid stenosis [41], and diagnosis of heart diseases [42]. Few other papers have discussed models that would be helpful to build a DT for ischemic diseases and hypertension [9], [10], [8]. In addition, we find some interesting papers about DT concepts for cardiovascular diseases [11–13] which can be enhanced to create a full-blown heart prediction DT model. Based on these reviews, it can be inferred that there is a lot of ongoing research to create digital twins. However, most of the methods discussed so far [4], [5], [9], [10], [12], [28], [29], [31], [35] can be treated as simulations and modelling techniques and are best described as initial basic models that need to be enhanced to build something meaningful, as none were fully integrated into real-time implementations or have considered privacy and security of patient data. In summary, these can be considered as preliminary investigations to build either an active or semi-active digital twin.

Security and privacy concerns tend to be the biggest challenge in healthcare [18–22], and not many digital twin architectures in literatures have sufficiently covered this aspect.

In contrast to the applications developed, we have created a fully functional digital twin app that can be used to predict heart attacks. We have built the app using a loosely coupled architecture to enable future enhancements without changing the existing functionality or source code. Our model uses blockchain-based solutions to overcome security and privacy issues, thereby making the model foolproof. We used Ganache private blockchain–based smart contract to store and retrieve data from blockchain, as well as PostgreSQL. Secondly, we are not storing all data on the blockchain but are using a combination of PostgreSQL database and blockchain to distributed patient data. In our model, only patient metadata is being stored on the blockchain, thereby making the blockchain very light. This is in contrast to other literatures, where all data is stored on the blockchain. The app delivers a high degree of accuracy and was tested from patient data security and privacy perspective using the relevant technique from chaos engineering.

16.6 Conclusion

Digital twin usage in cardiology is creating a profound impact for both patients and medical professionals alike. The digital twin technology has the potential to help patients and healthcare professionals proactively detect worsening health conditions, thereby helping in saving lives. This chapter proposes a digital twin application called **BDT app** which is integrated with machine learning model to predict heart attacks. To ensure that in the future any type of wearable devices can also be integrated easily without any code changes to our application, we have used a headless architecture where the patient data (data feeds) are kept loosely coupled from the **BDT app** backend code. Blockchain was used as part of the architecture, which can significantly increase security and privacy of medical data to meet administrative and regulatory requirements.

The results show that the **BDT app** can predict heart attacks with a 97.1% accuracy. Further, high reliability was achieved with the **BDT app**, which was demonstrated with the chaos experiments by simulating tampering of the data from the backend. It was shown that the **BDT app** can intelligently predict, alert, and revert back to the correct data for any malicious or unauthorized data updates.

It can be concluded that the proposed **BDT app** is highly accurate and secure, and the headless architecture facilitates ease of integration with any future wearable devices without requiring any changes to the application code. As future work, we plan to enhance the application security with advanced encryption standard across device layer and the cloud platform.

References

[1] S. Abdulmotaleb, "Digital twins: The convergence of multimedia technologies," *IEEE MultiMedia*, vol. 25, no. 2, pp. 87–92, Apr.–Jun 2018.

[2] M. Peirlinck, S. Costabal, J. Yao, J. M. Guccione, S. Tripathy, Y. Wang, D. Ozturk, P. Segars, T. M. Morrison, S. Levine and E. Kuhl, "Precision medicine in human heart modeling," *Biomechanics and Modeling in Mechanobiology*, pp. 803–31, 2021.

[3] K. Gillette, M. A. Gsell, A. J. Prassl, E. Karabelas, U. Reiter, G. Reiter, T. Grandits, C. Payer, D. Štern, M. Urschler, J. D. Bayer, C. M. Augustin, A. Neic, T. Pock and E. J. Vigmond, "A framework for the generation of digital twins of cardiac electrophysiology from clinical 12-leads ECGs," *Medical Image Analysis*, vol. 71, p. 102080, Jul 2021.

[4] S. Pagani, L. Dede, A. Manzoni and A. Quarteroni, "Data integration for the numerical simulation of cardiac electrophysiology," *Pacing Clin Electrophysiol*, vol. 44, no. 4, pp. 726–36, Apr 2021.

[5] F. Auricchio, M. Conti, S. Marconi and S. T. Trimarchi, "Patient-specific aortic endografting simulation: From diagnosis to prediction," *Computers in Biology and Medicine*, vol. 43, no. 4, pp. 386–94, Feb 2013.

[6] A. Hemmler, B. Lutz, G. Kalender, C. Reeps and M. W. Gee, "Patient-specific in silico endovascular repair of abdominal aortic aneurysms: Application and validation," *Biomechanics and Modeling in Mechanobiology*, vol. 18, pp. 983–1004, Mar 2019.

[7] I. Larrabide, M. Kim, L. Augsburger, M. C. Villa-Uriol, D. Rüfenacht and A. F. Frangi, "Fast virtual deployment of self-expandable stents: Method and in vitro evaluation for intracranial aneurysmal stenting," *Medical Image Analysis*, vol. 16, no. 3, pp. 721–30, Apr 2012.

[8] J. Parr, P. Nithiarasu and S. Pant, "Machine learning for detection of stenoses and aneurysms: Application in a physiologically realistic virtual patient database," *Biomechanics and Modeling in Mechanobiology*, vol. 20, pp. 2097–146, Jul 2021.

[9] R. Martinez-Velazquez, R. Gamez and A. E. Saddik, "Cardio twin: A digital twin of the human heart running on the edge," in *IEEE International Symposium on Medical Measurements and Applications (MeMeA)*, pp. 1–6, 2019. https://doi.org/10.1109/MeMeA.2019.8802162

[10] O. Mazumder, D. Roy, S. Bhattacharya, A. Sinha and A. Pal, "Synthetic PPG generation from haemodynamic model with baroreflex autoregulation: A Digital twin of cardiovascular system," in *41st Annual International Conference of the IEEE Engineering in Medicine and Biology Society (EMBC)*, pp. 5024–9, 2019. https://doi.org/10.1109/EMBC.2019.8856691

[11] E. Winokur, C. Sodini and D. He, "A continuous, wearable, and wireless heart monitor using head ballistocardiogram (BCG) and head electrocardiogram (ECG)," in *2011 Annual International Conference of the IEEE Engineering in Medicine and Biology Society*, pp. 4729–32, May 2011. https://doi.org/10.1109/IEMBS.2011.6091171

[12] N. Chakshu and I. Sazonov, "Towards enabling a cardiovascular digital twin for human systemic circulation using inverse analysis," *Biomechanics and Modeling in Mechanobiology*, pp. 449–65, 2021.

[13] C. N. Kavan, C. Jason, I. Sazonov and N. Perumal, "A semi-active human digital twin model for detecting severity of carotid stenoses from head vibration—a coupled computational mechanics and computer vision method: A semi-active human digital twin model for detecting carotid stenoses," *International Journal for Numerical Methods in Biomedical Engineering*, vol. 35, no. 5, p. e3180, Jan 2019.

[14] Y. Liu, L. Zhang, Y. Yang, L. Zhou, L. Ren, F. Wang and R. Liu, "A novel cloud-based framework for the elderly healthcare services using digital twin," *IEEE Access*, vol. 7, pp. 49088–101, 2019.

[15] M. Ianculescu, A. Alexandru, N.-D. Nicolau, G. Neagu and O. Bica, "IoHT and edge computing, warrants of optimal responsiveness of monitoring applications for seniors. A case study," in *22nd International Conference on Control Systems and Computer Science (CSCS)*, pp. 655–61, 2019. https://doi.org/10.1109/CSCS.2019.00118

[16] R. Rajavel, S. K. Ravichandran, K. Harimoorthy, P. Nagappan and K. R. Gobichettipalayam, "IoT-based smart healthcare video surveillance system using edge computing," *Journal of Ambient Intelligence and Humanized Computing*, vol. 13, pp. 3195–207, Mar 2021.

[17] A. Abir, K. T. Woo, L. Vincenzo and P. Jong, "Blockchain-based secure digital twin framework for smart healthy city," *Advanced Multimedia and Ubiquitous Engineering*, pp. 107–13, Dec 2020.

[18] A. Alrawais, A. Alhothaily, C. Hu and X. Cheng, "Fog computing for the internet of things: Security and privacy issues," *IEEE Internet Computing*, vol. 21, p. 2, 2017.

[19] K. Gai, M. Qiu, Z. Xiong and M. Liu, "Privacy-preserving multichannel communication in edge-of-things," *Future Generation Computer Systems*, vol. 85, pp. 190–200, 2018.

[20] P. P. Ray, D. Dash, K. Salah and N. Kumar, "Blockchain for IoT-based healthcare: Background, consensus, platforms, and use cases," *IEEE Systems Journal (Early Access)*, pp. 85–94, 2021.

[21] P. P. Ray, D. Dash, K. Salah and N. Kumar, "Blockchain for IoT-based healthcare: Background, consensus, platforms, and use cases," *IEEE Systems Journal (Early Access)*, pp. 85–94, 2021.

[22] N. Garg, M. Wazid, A. K. Das, D. P. Singh, J. J. P. C. Rodrigues and Y. Park, "BAKMP-IoMT: Design of blockchain enabled authenticated key management protocol for internet of medical things deployment," *IEEE Access*, vol. 8, pp. 95956–77, 2020.

[23] H.-N. Dai, M. Imran and N. Haider, "Blockchain-enabled internet of medical things to combat COVID-19," *IEEE Internet of Things Magazine*, vol. 3, no. 3, pp. 52–7, Sep 2020.

[24] W. Sihua and D. Jiang, "Electronic medical record security sharing model based on blockchain," in *Proceedings of the 3rd International Conference on Cryptography, Security and Privacy*, pp. 13–17, 2019. https://doi.org/10.1145/3309074.3309079

[25] H. L. W. Guo, N. Mark and S. Chien-Chung, "Access control for electronic health records with hybrid blockchain-edge architecture," *IEEE International Conference on Blockchain (Blockchain)*, 2019. https://doi.org/10.1109/Blockchain.2019.00015

[26] C. Community, *Principles of Chaos Engineering*, Mar 2019. [Online]. Available: http://principlesofchaos.org/?lang=ENcontent.

[27] S. Chandra, V. Paravastu, R. Jayarajasingam, R. Cottam, S. J. Palfreyman, J. A. Michaels and S. M. Thomas, "Endovascular repair of abdominal aortic aneurysm," *Cochrane Database of Systematic Reviews*, vol. 23, no. 1, p. CD004178, Jan 2014. https://doi.org/10.1002/14651858.CD004178.pub2

[28] M. E. Biancolini, K. Capellini, E. Costa, C. Groth and S. Celi, "Fast interactive CFD evaluation of hemodynamics assisted by RBF mesh morphing and reduced order models: The case of aTAA modelling," *International Journal on Interactive Design and Manufacturing (IJIDeM)*, pp. 1227–38, Sep 2020.

[29] N. K. Chakshu, I. Sazonov and P. Nithiarasu, "Towards enabling a cardiovascular digital twin for human systemic circulation using inverse analysis," *Biomechanics and Modeling in Mechanobiology*, vol. 20, pp. 449–65, Oct 2021.

[30] S. Weidmann, "Heart: Electrophysiology," *Annual Review of Physiology*, vol. 366, pp. 155–69, Mar 1974.

[31] T. Gerach, S. S. J. Fröhlich, L. Lindner, E. Kovacheva, R. Moss, E. M. Wülfers, G. Seemann, C. Wieners and A. Loewe, "Electro-mechanical whole-heart digital twins: A fully coupled multi-physics approach," *Development and Applications of Multi-Scale Mathematical Models in Cardiology*, vol. 9, no. 11, p. 1247, May 2021.

[32] E. Zeitler, W. Schoop, W. Zahnow, "The treatment of occlusive arterial disease by transluminal catheter angioplasty," *Diagnostic Radiology*, vol. 99, no. 1, Apr 1971.

[33] U. NHS, *Heart Attack: Overview*, NHS [Online]. Available: www.nhs.uk/conditions/heart-attack/.

[34] D. C. Hosting, *Distributed (Deep) Machine Learning Common*, DMLC Community Hosting, 2023 [Online]. Available: http://dmlc.io/.

[35] Fedesoriano, *Heart Failure Prediction Dataset*, Kaggle, September 2021 [Online]. Available: www.kaggle.com/datasets/fedesoriano/heart-failure-prediction.

[36] E. P. Networks, *Go Ethereum*, Dec 2019 [Online]. Available: https://geth.ethereum.org/docs/interface/private-network.

[37] S. Wu and J. Du, "Electronic medical record security sharing model based on blockchain," in *Proceedings of the 3rd International Conference on Cryptography, Security and Privacy*, pp. 13–17, 2019. https://doi.org/10.1145/3309074.3309079

[38] H. Guo, W. Li, M. Nejad and C.-C. Shen, "Access control for electronic health records with hybrid blockchain-edge architecture," in *IEEE International Conference on Blockchain (Blockchain)*, 2019. https://doi.org/10.1109/Blockchain.2019.00015

[39] M. E. Miller and E. Spatz, "A unified view of a human digital twin," *Human-Intelligent Systems Integration*, pp. 23–33, Jun 2022.

[40] A. Lombardo and C. Ricci, "Digital twins federation for remote medical care of de-hospitalized patients," in *EEE International Conference on Pervasive Computing and Communications Workshops and other Affiliated Events (PerCom Workshops)*, pp. 718–23, 2022. https://doi.org/10.1109/PerComWorkshops53856.2022.9767417

[41] A. E. Azzaoui, T. W. Kim, V. Loia and J. Park, "Blockchain-based secure digital twin framework for smart healthy city," *Advanced Multimedia and Ubiquitous Engineering*, pp. 107–13, Dec 2020.

[42] E. Winokur, C. Sodini and D. D. He, "A continuous, wearable, and wireless heart monitor using head ballistocardiogram (BCG) and head electrocardiogram (ECG)," in *2011 Annual International Conference of the IEEE Engineering in Medicine and Biology Society*, pp. 4729–32, May 2011. https://doi.org/10.1109/IEMBS.2011.6091171

Index

A

atomic swaps, 41
audit trail, 43

B

block, 167
blockchain, 1
Boston's MedRec system, 2

C

Cancer Gene Trust, 103, 235
cardiac arrhythmia, 294
chaos engineering, 292, 301
Cloud of Things, 177
cold chain, 5
consensus mechanisms, 39
consortium blockchains, 50, 226
contact tracing, 150
coral health, 232, 233
cross-chain bridges, 41
cryptographic keys, 125

D

DApp application, 80
data feeds, 295
decentralized applications (DApps), 41
DefectChecker, 111
distributed ledger technology, 225
distributed request system, 202
DNATIX, 231
double spending, 168

E

Echidna, 109, 121
e-Estonia, 234
electronic health records, 56, 100
electronic medical records (EMR), 81
EncrypGen, 11, 268, 277
Eth2Vec, 109, 121
Ethereum, 52, 107
Express.js, 53

F

FHIRChain, 19, 63
Forensics Toolkit, 172

G

Ganache, 53, 102, 107, 117, 296, 298, 299, 303
Gartner Hype Cycle, 253
GasChecker, 111, 122
Gasper, 111
Gastap, 110
Genecoin, 231, 243, 268, 271
General Data Protection Regulation, 213, 228, 267
genesis block, 54
Genesy, 269
Genesy model, 269, 270
Genomes.io, 235, 268, 269
Genomic Data Commons, 268
GEN token, 231
GeoAI, 141, 145, 146, 159
Geth, 108, 121

H

Hashlog, 143
HealthBank, 4
healthcare 4.0, 213
healthcare supply chain, 4
HoneyBadger, 111
hybrid blockchain, 50
hyperchain, 143
Hyperledger Caliper, 104, 148
Hyperledger Composer, 108
Hyperledger Fabric, 50, 81, 89, 99, 105, 108, 117, 154, 190, 191, 197, 202, 207, 210, 233, 247, 248
Hyperledger Sawtooth, 105, 121

I

immutability, 50
The Internet of Medical Things, 8
interoperability, 40
interoperability protocols, 41
InterPlanetary File System, 200

Iroha, 107, 121
IRYO, 232

L

LOCARD, 177
Luna DNA, 268

M

MadMax, 111, 122
Manticore, 112, 122
MATLAB, 108
MedBlock, 16, 24, 82, 92
MedHypChain, 7, 22
Medicalchain, 64, 233
Medichain, 15
MediLedger, 62
MedRec, 2, 58, 91, 231, 232, 243
mHealth system, 156
miners, 188
mining, 167
multi-party protected computing, 84
MyBitBlock, 268
Mythril, 111, 122

N

nebula genomics, 11, 229, 268, 277
nodes, 168
nonce, 168, 201

O

Open Zeppelin smart contract library, 137
OrganChain, 14
outbreak, 34
Oyente, 67, 111, 117, 158

P

patientory, 24, 233
peer-to-peer (P2P), 29
permissioned blockchain, 49
personal health records, 191
PGxChain, 103
PHBC, 143
Postman, 107
PoW, 144
private blockchain, 49, 226
ProCredEx, 62
proof-of-authority, 144, 298, 299
proof-of-work (PoW), 55
public blockchain, 49, 226

Q

QuorumChain, 103

R

real-time data analysis, 37
register contract, 3
Remix IDE, 110
remote health monitoring, 291
roles, 137

S

Satoshi Nakamoto's blockchain technology, 134
secure data sharing, 36
securify, 112, 117, 122
Shivom, 268, 271, 277
Slither, 109, 110, 122
SmartAnvil, 110
SmartBugs, 110, 122
SmartCheck, 110, 117, 122
SolCover, 67
SPSS, 109, 121
Spyder IDE, 105, 109
SynCare, 7, 22

T

telecare medicine infor- mation system, 100
telemedicine, 6
tokenization, 41
Truffle, 108, 117

U

un-permissioned blockchain, 49

V

Vandal, 112, 122
VANET, 278, 279, 280, 281, 282, 283, 285, 286, 287, 288, 289, 290
VeChain, 143

W

Wireshark, 105, 108

Z

Zenome, 230, 243, 268, 269, 271, 277
ZeppelinOS, 67
zero-knowledge protocol, 239
ZNA coin, 230